Disasters and Public Health: Planning and Response

Disasters and Public Health: Planning and Response

Editor: Lawanna Boone

AMERICAN
MEDICAL PUBLISHERS
www.americanmedicalpublishers.com

AMERICAN
MEDICAL PUBLISHERS
www.americanmedicalpublishers.com

Cataloging-in-Publication Data

Disasters and public health : planning and response / edited by Lawanna Boone.
p. cm.
Includes bibliographical references and index.
ISBN 979-8-88740-063-1
1. Disaster medicine. 2. Medical emergencies. 3. Public health. 4. Emergency medical services--Management.
5. Emergency management. I. Boone, Lawanna.
RA645.5 .D57 2023
362.18--dc23

American Medical Publishers,
41 Flatbush Avenue,
1st Floor, New York,
NY 11217, USA

ISBN 979-8-88740-063-1 (Hardback)

Contents

Preface

This book has been a concerted effort by a group of academicians, researchers and scientists, who have contributed their research works for the realization of the book. This book has materialized in the wake of emerging advancements and innovations in this field. Therefore, the need of the hour was to compile all the required researches and disseminate the knowledge to a broad spectrum of people comprising of students, researchers and specialists of the field.

Public health emergencies or disasters are events that negatively affect the public health system and its protective infrastructure. This includes water, sanitation, shelter, food, fuel and health, resulting in both direct and indirect consequences on the health of a population. These events result in a large number of deaths, a high number of serious or long-term disabled people, and a risk for future harm in the affected population. A public health emergency system should emphasize on the promotion of capabilities of health systems, communities and individuals to prevent, protect against, respond to, and recover from an event. Efficient planning is necessary for preparing, responding and recovering from a public health or disaster event afterwards. This book examines the critical intersection between disaster management and public health. The topics included herein provide a comprehensive knowledge of planning and response related to disasters. The book will serve as a valuable source of reference for students and professionals involved in this area at various levels.

At the end of the preface, I would like to thank the authors for their brilliant chapters and the publisher for guiding us all-through the making of the book till its final stage. Also, I would like to thank my family for providing the support and encouragement throughout my academic career and research projects.

Editor

1

Long-Term Impact of Disasters on the Public Health System

Nina Lorenzoni [1,*], Verena Stühlinger [1], Harald Stummer [1,2] and Margit Raich [1]

1 Department for Public Health, Health Services Research and Health Technology Assessment, UMIT TIROL—Private University for Health Sciences, Medical Informatics and Technology, 6060 Hall in Tirol, Austria; verena.stuehlinger@umit.at (V.S.); harald.stummer@umit.at (H.S.); margit.raich@umit.at (M.R.)

2 Department of Business, University Seeburg Castle, 5201 Seekirchen am Wallersee, Austria

* Correspondence: nina.lorenzoni@umit.at

Abstract: As past events have shown, disasters can have a tremendous impact on the affected population's health. However, research regarding the long-term impact on a systems level perspective is still scarce. In this multi-case study, we analyzed and compared the long-term impacts on the public health system of five disasters which took place in Europe: avalanche (Austria), terror attack (Spain), airplane crash (Luxembourg), cable-car tunnel fire (Austria), and a flood in Central Europe. We used a mixed-methods approach consisting of a document analysis and interviews with key stakeholders, to examine the various long-term impacts each of the disasters had on health-system performance, as well as on security and health protection. The results show manifold changes undertaken in the fields of psychosocial support, infrastructure, and contingency and preparedness planning. The holistic approach of this study shows the importance of analyzing long-term impacts from the perspective of the type (e.g., disasters associated with natural hazards) and characteristic (e.g., duration and extent) of a disaster, as well as the regional context where a disaster took place. However, the identified recurring themes demonstrate the opportunity of learning from case studies in order to customize the lessons and apply them to the own-disaster-management setting.

Keywords: long-term impact; disaster; public health; case study; disaster management; multi-case analysis; Europe

---

1. Introduction

The impact of disasters on the health of the people affected and on the public health system can be far-reaching and long lasting. However, studies examining these long-term influences months or even years (mid- to long-term periods) after the event are rare, although their importance is repeatedly underlined [1–3]. Nomura et al. (2016) emphasize the need for a better understanding of long-term health impacts of disasters, in order to be able to set measures and guide actions (before, during, and after the event) to reduce health risks [4]. Moreover, the Sendai Framework for Disaster Risk Reduction points out, in Priority 4 ("Enhancing disaster preparedness for effective response and to 'Build Back Better' in recovery, rehabilitation and reconstruction"), that the importance of post-disaster reviews as they offer a valuable source for learning lessons for the public health system and consequently raise disaster preparedness [5]. Such a systematic review of challenges, dysfunctions, and, consequently, changes, as well as impacts, would be essential to improve preparedness for future events [6]. A better understanding of the impacts of disasters on the public health system and which determinants influence these impacts would be an important contribution to reduce disaster risk. The Sendai Framework advocates for the collection and analysis of the impacts of disasters and consequently the dissemination of the resulting lessons learned across all relevant stakeholders. Researchers are asked for their contributions, sharing their evaluations with practitioners, government officials, and policy makers, to support decision-making and the implementation of good practices on local, regional, and national level [5]. Especially studies on mid- to long-term periods, i.e., months to years after the event, would be needed. A long-term study is difficult, since data are hardly available in a consistent form, and the quality of these data also varies greatly depending on jurisdiction and time frame [7]. Furthermore, the literature review provided no recommendations for the definition of "long-term". The studies differed in the use of time spans, but no discussion was found as to why the authors used specific time spans.

Investigations on the long-term impact of disasters on the health of people affected cover a wide field of research topics (e.g., disaster impacts such as economic losses of the affected population or effects on mental and/or physical health; or focus on specific target groups such as children or the elderly [8–13]). Research on economic and human loss or damage tends to focus on short-term effects, while longer-term effects are difficult to track, and public attention often shifts on the next disaster event [4,14]. Murthy et al. [15] analyzed the progress made in public health preparedness within the US after 9/11, until 2016, by using self-reports from "Centers for Disease Control and Prevention" and reports of congress funding. Fitter et al. [16] examined the recovery of the public health system of Haiti following the 2010 earthquake and cholera outbreak. By using a framework consisting of 10 essential public health services, their research demonstrated progress and improvement made regarding the public health system seven years after the disaster. Our literature review revealed that the research on long-term impact mainly focuses on individual or population health, but less on the systems perspective.

The purpose of this study was to investigate the various long-term impacts on the public health system of five different disasters occurring in Europe, from 1999 to 2013. The chosen holistic research approach allowed the representation of the complexity, specific circumstances, and undertaken measures for each disaster in detail. This process allowed us to identify undertaken adaptions and changes that result in longer-term impacts.

2. Materials and Methods

2.1. Design

We decided to use a case study approach, as it allowed for us to capture both the diversity in disaster management and the complexity of specific circumstances. An extensive collection of rich data makes an embedded multiple-case analysis and presentation possible. The selection of multiple cases resulted from replication logic [17]. We built upon contrasting cases [18], since a variety of contexts, circumstantial factors, and their impact on each case could offer a more complete picture of the longer-term impact of disasters on public health. Since the study was conducted within the EU project PsyCris (PSYchosocial support in CRISis Management), the selected case studies all took place in the European Union. The project consortium decided to use disasters, which are relevant for many EU countries. In addition to the high probability, further criteria for the decision of which cases to use were the scale of the disaster, complexity and number of institutions involved, long-term consequences, and data availability. Moreover, the analysis should include disasters caused by natural hazards, as well as human-caused disasters (e.g., technological or mass-violence).

We decided to use a mixed-method approach consisting of document analysis and expert interviews. As we could not identify a standardized assessment tool to investigate the long-term impact of disasters to the public health system in the literature, we decided to focus on impact models [19–22] that serve as a foundation for the development of the interview guide and the category grid used for the document analysis.

The main categories in the grid were as follows:

- Information about the chosen disaster (what happened, number of people affected, which organizations were involved in disaster management and response, and reaction of the healthcare system);
- General coping strategies and direct effects on health;
- Direct costs and follow-up costs;
- Long-term effects on the public healthcare system;
- Long-term effects on culture and the community.

For our analysis, we reviewed key documents relevant to the disaster-management process and the long-term impact of chosen disasters. The reviewed documents included governmental and organizational reports, legislative documents, journal articles, books, letters, TV documentaries, brochures, and newspaper articles.

As a reconstruction of the complex disaster management process is not possible with existing public documents only, we also conducted expert interviews.

The interview partners all played key roles in the management of the respective disaster. When selecting the interview partners, care was taken to obtain a picture as broad and holistic as possible of the most diverse organizations and units. The professional fields of the interview partners included fire department, emergency psychologists, politicians, armed forces, police, physicians, red cross, forensic, and priests. The average interview duration was 60 min. Table 1 shows the number of interviewees per case study.

Table 1. Overview of number of interviewees per case study.

Case Study	Number of Interviewees
Avalanche, 1999 (Austria)	7
Cable-Car Accident, 2000 (Austria)	7
Airplane Crash, 2002 (Luxembourg)	7
Terror Attack, 2004 (Spain)	7
Flood, 2013 (Austria/Germany)	8

The main themes of the interviews were as follows:

- Job description and responsibilities of the interviewed person;
- Description of the event and the disaster-management process;
- Organization and cooperation of rescue organizations and teams;
- Psychosocial support and challenges for the disaster managers;
- Community resilience;
- Security/protection of population.

For the interview analysis, we used GABEK® (Holistic Processing of Complexity) (Josef Zelger, Innsbruck, Austria), a qualitative method of knowledge organization developed by Josef Zelger, supporting analysis of unstructured texts on the basis of the theory of "linguistic gestalten". The method helps to handle individual thoughts and attitudes and present them in a structured and systematic way. GABEK allows for the transparent organization of knowledge and captures the holistic representation of complex social situations, like disasters, from the perspective of those affected [23]. The analysis was conducted with the corresponding software application GABEK–WinRelan, which combines qualitative content analysis (e.g., coding of keywords, evaluations, or causal relationships) and quantitative measures (e.g., frequencies of keywords and relations) and therefore offers a profound understanding of data, their interlinkages, and their weight [24].

2.2. *The Case Studies*

2.2.1. Avalanche, Austria, 1999

On 23 February 1999, shortly after 4:00 p.m., an avalanche buried around 100 people in the village of Galtuer (Austria). Ongoing snowfall in the previous days triggered high avalanche risk in the entire federal state of Tyrol. The Paznaun valley, in which Galtuer is located, was already cut off from the outside world before the avalanche, due to the snow conditions. The avalanche hit areas in the village center, which had previously been considered safe from avalanches. Due to the bad weather conditions, no rescue teams were able to reach Galtuer for assistance. The people affected were left to their own devices to rescue the buried victims. Only on the 24 February did the first helicopters could take off and bring the injured from the village to the surrounding hospitals. The Austrian government asked NATO (North Atlantic Treaty Organisation) and neighboring countries for support with additional helicopters. On 25 February, aerial evacuation of the whole valley began with 37 helicopters from Austria, Germany, Switzerland, France, and the US. Thirty-one people died in the avalanche, and 35 were injured (11 of them severely).

2.2.2. Cable-Car Accident, Austria, 2000

In Kaprun (Salzburg), on 11 November 2000, in the tunnel of the cable-car, a fire occurred in the ascending train. The glacier around the Kitzsteinhorn is a popular all-the-year skiing region. On 11 November, the train started at 8:57 in the morning, with 161 passengers aboard. At 9:02 a.m., the first smoke formed. At 9:05 a.m., the train stopped after 600 m in the tunnel; the total distance from the entrance to the exit was 3.8 km. Passengers broke the windows. Smoke rose from the train at the back. The operator saw the fire and gave alarm. Twelve passengers walked with their ski boots downstairs and survived. The other 149 passengers and the operator were in the tunnel. At 9:35 a.m., because of the danger of explosion, the outfall of electricity, and the formation of toxic smoke, the fire brigade had to stop the rescue mission. The mountain station had to be evacuated. At 10:16 a.m., a rescue team started to enter the tunnel. Three people died at the mountain station because of exhaust-gas poisoning. One person survived. At 12:00 p.m., a second team of the fire brigade entered the tunnel. In total, 155 passengers died on 11th of November.

2.2.3. Airplane Crash, Luxembourg, 2002

On Wednesday, 6 November 2002, an airplane of the national air company crashed during the approach to Luxembourg airport. At 10:05 a.m., the airplane reported difficulties during the landing procedure, and 42 s later, the plane disappeared from the radar. The reasons for the airplane crash are based on a mix of technical problems, human errors, and bad weather conditions. At 10:06 a.m., the plane ploughed into a field, and one side of the plane was ripped open. Six passengers were catapulted out. After the crash, the aviation fuel caught fire, and the plane began to burn. Both pilots were trapped in the wreckage. After fire brigades had extinguished the fire, the rescue of the trapped passengers began. The only survivors had been sitting in the front of the aircraft, which had been torn off during the crash, leaving the nose cone embedded in the ground. Twenty people died and two survived severely injured.

2.2.4. Terror Attack, Spain, 2004

On 11 March 2004, ten explosions occurred aboard four commuter trains in the city of Madrid. It was later reported that thirteen improvised explosive devices had been hidden on the trains. The explosions happened during rush hour, on a normal workday, between 7:37 a.m. and 7:39 a.m. At 7:37 a.m., three bombs exploded on train number 21,431, on track two, inside Atocha station, the main capital railway station. At 7:38 a.m., two bombs exploded in train number 21,435, at El Pozo del Tío Raimundo Station. One bomb exploded on train number 21,713, at Santa Eugenia Station, at 7:38 a.m. Then, at 7:39 a.m., four bombs exploded on train number 17,305, on Calle Téllez, approximately 500 m from Atocha station. The bombing was the deadliest terror attack in the history of Spain: 191 people died, and more than 2000 were injured.

2.2.5. Flood, Austria/Germany, 2013

Due to exceptionally heavy rainfalls in early June 2013, extreme flooding of the major river systems occurred throughout Central Europe (particularly Switzerland, Germany, Austria, Czech Republic, Slovakia Hungary, and Serbia). Thousands of people needed to be evacuated from their houses. Twice as much rainfall as average during the month in Austria resulted in the soil becoming saturated. Although forecasts predicted a high rise of water levels, the prognoses have been too low. The water level exceeded the levels seen during the disastrous "once in a century" Central European floods of 2002 in many areas. In Austria, six people died in the flood, and thousands of people had to be evacuated. The infrastructural damages were extensive; railway lines, roads, bridges, and houses were damaged severely.

3. Results

The following section describes the long-term effects of the disasters on the public health system. Figure 1 gives an overview of the framework of analysis. We decided to categorize the identified impact factors into the categories health system performance, and security and health protection. The increased demand during and after a disaster has a direct effect on the health system performance, i.e., the delivering of services, the creation of resources, the stewardship, and, finally, the related financing [25]. Security and health protection refers to post-disaster efforts aiming at optimizing leadership and governance, contingency and preparedness planning, infrastructure, and training, or may lead to an increase in security research funding activities, as well as information and communication activities. The information stated in this section was extracted from the stated sources, as well as from the expert interviews.

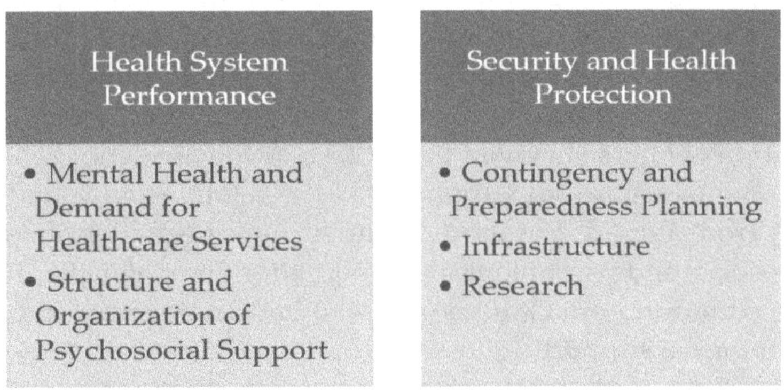

Figure 1. Overview of the aggregated long-term impacts of the analyzed disasters on the public health system (source: the authors).

3.1. Long-Term Impact on Health System Performance

3.1.1. Mental Health and Demand for Healthcare Services

For an adequate public health policy, different dimensions have to be taken into account to optimize the offer for healthcare services, including mental health. The identification and evaluation of how many people are affected by a disaster and develop adjustment disorders because of distress seems to be a challenge for health service providers. For the chosen disasters, statistics about the health status of people affected and derived demand for healthcare services are rare.

Distinction of Target Groups

For an analysis of the demand for healthcare services, a distinction of target groups has to be undertaken. Standardized programs for psychosocial and psychological support are not sufficient, as one crisis manager from Luxembourg stated. The demand for psychosocial and psychological support, but also for medical and physical treatments, mainly differs depending on who is affected. The target groups have to be defined carefully, to guarantee adequate support. A study conducted by the Complutense University of Madrid, with 526 victims of the bombings in Madrid, shows that, ten years later, almost 30% of them presented symptoms of anxiety, depression, and PTSD (posttraumatic stress disorder). Ten years later, nearly 200 victims still received psychological treatment [26]. Moreover, a care program has been launched for people with hearing disabilities after the terror attack in Madrid. The explosions and the effects of the blast caused hearing impairments resulting in total deafness in many victims of these attacks. The General Directorate of Support for Victims of Terrorism taught sign language to victims of these attacks and to their families to help them recover communication within their families [27].

Psychosocial Support for Specific Target Groups

An important lesson that has been identified in all cases is the demand for performance-linked psychosocial support. Target-oriented healthcare delivery has to consider the different needs of people affected (e.g., survivors, families, witnesses, and volunteers). Standardization in the provision of services is seen critically by most of the interview partners. One interview partner from Luxembourg explained: "The pilot survived, there was certainly a different need, with the family, than with those where people died; I also think that people had different approaches to dealing with the accident ... To accommodate these different "points of view", that's extremely difficult. It is often the case that you think you have a solution to a problem, but actually you have to realize in retrospect that you need many solutions for many types of people ... and you also have to give people the freedom to deal with the problem in their own way which is enormously difficult". Because of the fact that nearly all people in the airplane died, the psychosocial support for families played the most important role. The challenge for the disaster management team was the information management to the relatives of the victims, the organization of their arrivals and accommodation, and how to offer psychosocial support.

Compared to our analyzed disasters associated with natural hazards (avalanche and flood), only a small number of passengers survived in the case of the airplane crash or cable-car accident. The main target group for psychosocial support was the relatives who had to arrive from longer distance or respectively from abroad. Locals and tourists have been identified as important relevant target groups for psychosocial and psychological support after the avalanche. Results have shown that the cohesiveness of the community in Galtuer (=locals) had an essential impact on the demand for psychosocial and psychological support.

The terror attack in Spain, with its destructive power for humans and infrastructure, caused a large number of deaths and people injured. Because of the characteristic of the disaster that occurred in this urban area, more walk-in volunteers entered the scene during the acute phase of the disaster, for help. This has an effect on the demand of psychosocial and psychological support in order to consider a large number of walk-in volunteers.

People Affected Who Originate from Abroad

Additionally, in some of the analyzed disasters, no information about psychosocial and psychological support, as well as medical or physical treatment of people who originate from other countries, was given. Especially in the case of the airplane crash, the avalanche and the cable-car accident many victims came from abroad. They were tourists or traveling persons. Survivors and relatives stayed for a certain period time in the country of the event. This leads to the inability to diagnose disorders and reactions, especially of those who were not directly affected by the disaster since some diagnoses cannot be identified immediately after the event, but occur later on (e.g., flashbacks and posttraumatic stress reaction). About 100 of the evacuated tourists in Galtuer were traumatized seriously, and some eventually were confronted with posttraumatic stress disorders later on [28,29].

Refusal of Psychosocial or Psychological Support

Individuals or a community may refuse psychosocial or psychological support. An interview partner involved in psychosocial support after the terror attack in Spain explained the following: "I've learned not to take it personally but as a normal reaction to emotional trauma. Sometimes we had to work with volunteers who were affected by the comments of relatives, like "if you're not going to return my son to me I don't know what you're doing here ... Emotional trauma can cause aggressive reactions and that's normal". Some families who lost relatives during the airplane crash in Luxembourg refused psychosocial support. One survivor of the avalanche was buried for several hours. He preferred to talk with his family to cope with the disaster. It was reported that only one woman with adjustment disorders consulted a psychologist after the avalanche disaster in Galtuer [30].

A community may also refuse psycho0social and psychological support. In Galtuer, locals dealt intensively with the event and experienced common grief. In the first year, they talked among themselves about the disaster and about their experiences, until they felt some relief from their burden. From the cultural point of view, the locals preferred to talk with family, relatives, or friends, but not with outsiders. Locals also had negative associations with psychologists because of two reasons. First, they experienced an insufficient management of psychosocial support directly after the event. Second, a big distance from and distrust of mental healthcare services were observed. The trust into the community was more helpful for the locals to recreate a meaningful life, as compared to professional organized support.

Risk Perceptions

Results gave interesting insights in the awareness of possible causes of risks. People living in endangered zones may perceive possible causes of risks induced by predictable disasters (e.g., risk of a flood or avalanche) as neutral compared to events that arise abruptly without any advanced warning (e.g., airplane crash or terror attack). The resistance of people living in an endangered zone can be influenced of their motivation and individual risk perception living in such an area. This conscious decision has an impact on the mental and physical health in the context of a disaster. The persons may dispose of a higher acceptance of the forces of nature, given the fact that the inhabitants of Galtuer do not evaluate the avalanches negatively [30]. Moreover, in the investigated flood case, in an area that is prone to flood, people are used to dealing with the flood. One interview partner explained the following: "The people down there, they can handle the water... they have their own strategies, they can handle it. And the humility and the acceptance with which they take the flood there, that's fascinating for me. I couldn't imagine that every 10 years I clean out my house, clear out the silt, pump out the water. For them, it's just the water, it's as simple as that". Moreover, most people had family or friends close by with whom they could stay during evacuation, when needed. These two factors are assumed to be a huge reduction of stress for the effected people.

Legal Proceedings

A relevant aspect in dealing with disasters is the way of legal response, especially in the case of organizational failures. One important impact on health was identified in the context of legal proceedings after the cable-car accident. Many family members of the victims complained about the lack of empathy during the legal proceedings. The trial was experienced as unfair by many families, leading to a lot of anger and disappointment. The need for clarity and mental processing was not fulfilled [31,32]. During the trial, a self-help initiative was founded which fought for years for resumption of the legal process [33]. Moreover, after the airplane crash, the legal proceedings lasted over years. One interview partner said the following: "[These] court proceedings have simply taken far too long, and that is disastrous for the people who are affected, who simply want decisions and that they can finish their mourning at some point. It has simply taken far too long".

3.1.2. Structure and Organization of Psychosocial Support

Different longer-term impacts in the structure and organization of psychosocial support have been identified. In one case, the formation of a new organization was induced; in other cases, major or smaller organizational improvements were undertaken. After the avalanche, the disorganization of psychosocial support caused enormous costs for the life assurances, public authorities, and governments. Good management of psychosocial and psychological support, distinct functional attributions, structures, and responsibilities lead to the reduction of conflicts between organizations and institutions involved in the management of a disaster. After the disaster, a discussion was started with regard to financial responsibilities of long-term mental treatments. In the context of psychosocial support, the responsibilities and financing structures for further events were revised.

Formation of New Organizations and Units

A completely new organization for psychosocial support was formed after the Galtuer avalanche. The management of psychosocial support was not organized by one central responsible body. Competition between psychologists and psychotherapists was the source of many conflicts. Additionally, journalists disguised themselves as psychologists and psychotherapists to access the disaster scene. In the years following the disaster, the Austrian Red Cross established the crisis intervention team (KIT—Kriseninterventionsteam). Moreover, it was decided to provide uniforms for the emergency psychologists as they were not associated as professionals by the surviving dependents. An interview partner who was in Galtuer after the avalanche explained the following: "Today it is taken for granted that already the emergency doctor asks if you want a crisis intervention team. But it was different in the past. We didn't wear a uniform, that was a big problem. And nobody knew the service. The care of uninjured survivors simply didn't exist". Although Kaprun, where the cable-car accident happened, is located in Salzburg, in the neighboring province of Tyrol, no structure for psychosocial support existed there at the time of the disaster. However, the tunnel fire was seen as trigger event to also establish a crisis intervention team in Salzburg. In the context of psychosocial support, the extent of the event has led to the formation of a special psychological care unit which takes over the organization and management of psychosocial support. Because of the huge dimension of the terror attack, a systemized supply of psychosocial support for rescue workers in their organizations was established. The awareness for the necessity of psychosocial support for people affected (victims, relatives, and also rescue teams) has grown after all of the analyzed disasters.

3.2. Long-Term Impact on Security and Health Protection

3.2.1. Contingency and Preparedness Planning

Plans and Checklists

An important long-term impact that was identified in all analyzed disasters is the update of existing emergency, civil protection, and national rescue plans and the development or adaption of checklists. Protocols for different contexts have been developed (e.g., intervention protocols for psychological intervention), as well protocols for recruiting people to participate in emergency volunteer management and psychological interventions. The emergency plans and the interfaces between the participating organizations were modified to improve the cooperation and coordination between security teams, armed forces, medical teams (doctors and nurses) in hospitals, social workers, and psychologists. After the airplane crash, psychosocial support was officially integrated as a necessary component into the national rescue plan of Luxembourg.

Establishment of Working Groups and New Units

As a central long-term impact, many different units and working groups were created after the disasters. The established working groups with experts and persons concerned analyzed past events, with the objective of developing recommendations for further improvements. The National Counter-Terrorism Coordination Centre has also been created, aiming to improve coordination between the National Police and the Guardia Civil, and terrorism experts have been sent from the Ministry of Interior to key embassies, to improve exchanges of information. After the airplane crash, an airline emergency committee was rebuilt, and a crisis-support center for Luxair accidents abroad was established. After the avalanche, the local government established a center to link research institutions, non-profit organizations, and businesses in the field of environmental hazards, to improve security measures, create databases, and develop efficient and up-to-date scenario plans.

Legal Changes

Several changes in laws (fire safety regulations and railway act, which also includes funiculars) have occurred after the Kaprun tunnel fire [34]. As a response to the disaster in Galtuer, the federal minister decided to update the guidelines of the danger areas. Basics of the administration procedures are the danger-zone plans, state-specific land-use planning laws, and the forest law of 1975. As a consequence of the flood, the land registry plans have been re-evaluated, and danger zones have been updated. However, various interview partners pointed out the difficulty of keeping danger zones up in the long-term: "The danger is simply that the pressure on the administrative employees comes when nothing has happened for a long time, that one says the yellow zone is no longer necessary. Or people demand the red zone to become a yellow zone in which building, under certain conditions, is possible. The pressure is certainly there, because we are in need of soil that can be built on". Moreover, concepts for resettlement from the endangered areas have been developed. However, it is unclear if and how many people have agreed to resettlement. A decision of the airline management after the crash in Luxembourg led to the implementation of all recommendations from aircraft designers concerning technical details in a compulsory way.

3.2.2. Infrastructure

For all investigated disasters, measures concerning infrastructure were initiated. These measures are referred to as items that improve security, in general, or specific measures to optimize processes, to be better prepared for future disasters. The costs of these infrastructure measures differ substantially.

Large-Scale Investments

After the avalanche, the avalanche barriers around Galtuer were improved and extended. In order to protect the houses of Galtuer in the future, an avalanche barrier was built in the middle of the village center. This special construction, called "Alpinarium", combines avalanche protection and an integrated museum, which deals with the history of Galtuer and the avalanche risk in the area. Further infrastructural measures were the improvement of the meteorological station, a reforestation project, and the extension of the security tunnels at the access road to Galtuer.

High investments were also undertaken in the case of the Austrian flood. Improvements and extended flood protection measures with 34 new building projects were realized. The building process had to be sped up after the flood because 17 projects had not been realized until then. Compared to the building projects, public authorities weighed the importance of the security of the public and decided not to invest in a dam, because of the complex construction project, the enormous monetary investment, and low benefit [35]. For affected public buildings like kindergartens and community buildings, the high possibility of future floods was considered, and a flood-proof way of construction and the addition of flood-resistant materials were implemented. For better forecasts and accurate prognosis, automated water-level measurement stations have been installed. However, improved technical equipment does not automatically lead to better flood protection, as one interview partner explains: "The most difficult thing is the final interpretation of the measured values. A river is a living organism, constantly changing". The damage of the transport medium—as what took place in Kaprun—catalyzed the building of a new ropeway instead of a new funicular due to security reasons. Due to the legal adaptions, many existing funiculars in Austria had to be adapted to guarantee a high level of security for the passengers. Finally, new helicopters with a higher load capacity were purchased for the Austrian Armed Forces, to ensure access to the valleys in the event of natural hazards restricting access to the population.

Small- and Medium-Scale Investments

Small- and medium-sized investments were undertaken in the case of Luxembourg, to improve transport by using more containers for meeting places or restrooms for rescue teams for future operations. These decisions were based on low costs and high flexibility. Additionally, a new operation control car was acquired. In Spain, public infrastructures were controlled more intensively after the terror attack, and constructional adaptions were undertaken. Security measures, like video surveillance, emergency exits, controls of specific infrastructure, and future usage of flak vests, were implemented.

3.2.3. Research

After the Galtuer avalanche, the local government invested in research projects which should reduce future disaster risks. One project was the "Alpine Safety and Information Centre (ASI)". The mission of this non-profit organization was to promote safety mountain environment and to act as a communication bridge between all participating institutions and local organizations. One product of these research investments that is now being used in practice is the "ESIS Tirol" mission information system, an internet platform that facilitates communication and coordination in the event of a disaster. Moreover, new calculations for avalanche simulation models have been developed.

3.3. Others

Because there were some problems in the flow of information between the response organizations, the communication processes have been updated in all investigated disasters. Moreover, technological improvements like the implementation of a uniform radio system in Tyrol and special software have been undertaken. The high media interest after the avalanche and the tunnel fire had a negative impact on the well-being and health of people affected. Therefore, improvements in media management were undertaken. Changes regarding the trainings and exercises (e.g., special topics such as media or psychosocial support, more joint trainings, and cross-border cooperation) could also be observed in all cases. Measures for improvements in the coordination of processes between the organizations and of the handling of professionals and volunteers have been initialized in all cases. Formal and informal networking was identified as a valuable basis for future cooperation. An interview partner pointed out the following: "I would add that in order to improve our response in emergencies, all the teams intervening in an emergency should have more meetings and we should learn to coordinate ourselves better, defining new plans on coordination, structure and control to make sure we all know who's in charge, where we have to go and what we have to do".

Tables 2 and 3 summarize the various impacts each disaster had on the public health system.

Table 2. Overview of long-term impacts on health-system performance.

	Avalanche	Cable Car Accident	Airplane Crash	Terror Attack	Flood
Mental health and demand for health care services	• Significance of different needs of target groups • Refusal of external psychosocial support	• Influence of legal proceedings on mental health and coping	• Significance of different needs of target groups	• Special long-term care for people with hearing impairment due to explosions needed • Sign language courses for families	
Structure and organisation of psychosocial support	• Establishment of KIT by Austrian Red Cross • Financing structure for psychological treatment • Uniforms for emergency psychologists	• Establishment of KIT by Austrian Red Cross		• Formation of special psychological care units	

Table 3. Overview of long-term impacts on security and health protection.

	Avalanche	Cable Car Accident	Airplane Crash	Terror Attack	Flood
Contingency and Preparedness Planning	• Adaption of danger areas • Creation of new working groups and units • Update emergency plans	• Update emergency plans • Changes in fire safety regulations and railway act	• Psychosocial support officially integrated in national rescue plan • Creation of new working groups and units • Update emergency plans	• Creation of new working groups and units • Update emergency plans • Creation of new psychological protocols and plans	• Re-evaluation of land registry pans
Infrastructure	• Avalanche barriers • Reforestation> • Extension security tunnel • Higher load capacity helicopters	• Ropeway instead of funicular	• Extended use of containers • Acquisition of operation control car	• More video surveillance • Adaptions of emergency exits • Flak vests	• Flood protection building measures • Flood-proof way of construction for public buildings • Automated water level measurement
Research	• ASI Centre • ESIS mission information system • Avalanche simulation models		-	-	-

Many of the identified impacts overlap with the recommendations in the Sendai Framework [5]: update of preparedness and contingency plans (Paragraph 33a), forecasting and early warning system (Paragraph 33b), trainings and exercises (Paragraphs 33f, 33h, 34f, and 34h), land-use planning (Paragraph 33j), provision of psychosocial support (Paragraph 33o), and revision of laws (Paragraph 33p). It can be concluded from this that the opportunity to "Build Back Better" and consequently enhance disaster preparedness has been taken.

4. Discussion

Based on the results of the literature review, we identified highly fragmented studies without any standardized approach to investigating the long-term impacts of disasters on public healthcare. We did not find any standard definition of long-term impact on the healthcare system. In the context of long-term impacts, the literature mainly focuses on long-term psychological impact effects on affected populations. A broader approach is missing. The studies have also chosen different time frames that do not allow any comparative conclusions.

The investigation of the case studies has shown that each disaster causes aftermaths in various fields. Learning circles [36] play a substantial role in the context of disaster management, as many of the identified long-term impacts on the public health system are the result of a learning process because of inadequate outputs in the past.

The changes observed all seem to have been sustained over the years. One exception is the ASI center, which, according to one interviewee, was closed for political reasons. The necessity of the acquired helicopters is regularly discussed in politics and media. However, landslides and roadblocks due to avalanche risk repeatedly demonstrate their importance for the protection of the affected population.

The study showed us that federalism and organizational boundaries can be a hindrance to improvements: After the 1999 avalanche in Galtuer, the Red Cross created a crisis intervention team in the province of Tyrol. In the neighboring province of Salzburg, however, there was no such infrastructure for psychosocial support yet established when the tunnel fire happened in November 2000. Christensen, Lægreid, and Rykkja (2013) describe something similar in their study: A major obstacle after the terrorist attack in Oslo was the fragmentation of responsibility within government departments. This might have hindered information-sharing and, consequently, taking measures which could have reduced the impact of the Oslo terror attack in 2011, as plans for improving the security of the building had already been established prior the attacks, but not implemented yet [37].

There is the need to analyze the individual and social circumstances of people affected. Results show the importance of analyzing long-term impacts from the perspective of the type (e.g., disaster associated with natural hazards or human-made disaster) and characteristic (e.g., duration and extent) of a disaster, as well as the regional context where a disaster took place. The effectiveness of disaster management procedures is dependent on a number of contingencies (e.g., not only how accurately one system is implemented, but also how well aligned a system is with cultural subsystems) [5,38,39]. As became apparent in Galtuer, the inhabitants applied coping strategies that are rooted in local traditions (e.g., importance of spiritual support). Nevertheless, the consequences of the avalanche led the local population to increasingly open up and cope with this specifically challenging situation by augmented communication. The ex post facto identification of local practices could be highly valuable as basis for discussion within a broader audience of special interest groups (e.g., experts for avalanche risk areas in Austria, Italy, and France).

The chosen cases include disasters caused by natural hazards, as well as human-made disasters. Both types of disasters have been demonstrated to have a potentially high impact on the public health system. However, they might have different consequences concerning preparedness planning. As avalanches and floods are often foreseeable, proactive actions like early warning and evacuation are possible in many cases. On the other hand, avalanches and floods result in relatively large impact areas, which makes response more difficult and requires thorough preparedness regarding mobilization and equipment. Differences between disasters caused by natural hazards and human-caused disasters are also observed with regards to mental health.

Dynes and Quarantelli [40] describe disasters caused by natural hazards as "consensus crises", leading to an increase of community cohesiveness and moral, whereas human-made disasters are characterized by human blame [41]. This has consequences for the coping process and the need for psychological support. Although the disasters analyzed in the case studies may have different characteristics, they share many similarities in their impact. Recurring themes in all the case studies were infrastructural measures, update of emergency plans, changes in communication procedures, and a raised awareness for the importance of mental health and providing psychosocial support. It might prove difficult to compare different individual disaster-management cases in order to elect one best practice example. However, the use of historical lessons can be a valuable source for improvements regarding disaster preparedness [38]. Gaining insights from out-of-sector lessons is often overlooked or considered as not relevant [42]. The recurring themes we identified across the various disasters analyzed in this study, however, demonstrate the learning opportunities from other fields or kinds of disasters. Crichton et al. [42] recommend broadening the perspective and trying to apply lessons beneficially to the own environment. Therefore, the learnings from these European cases can also be of use for countries with other structures and regulations regarding their public health system and disaster management structure. Even though political, socioeconomic, cultural, environmental, and hazard circumstances vary in every state, good practices might be transferable. This learning can be achieved when using a customized approach by "making use of others' experience, for instance by reviewing the contexts of particular measures and the nature of good practices and lessons learned, and then tailoring these to implement policies and activities that are appropriate for the local contexts" [43] (p. 5). Moreover, the Sendai Framework [5] points out the need for adaptions to the respective jurisdictions, capacities, and capabilities of each country.

Although each disaster is unique in its progress and coping, we ask for the design of a standardized assessment system for long-term disaster impacts. This would help to increase comparability of disasters. We share the recommendation expressed in the WHO Health-EDRM framework [1] regarding future research needs: a holistic all-hazard perspective across all disaster-management phases which includes physical, mental, and psychosocial needs. In order to achieve this, multidisciplinary and multi-sectoral collaboration between science, policy makers and practitioners is needed [39,44,45]. Such an exchange and dialogue between stakeholders is important in order to identify knowledge gaps, jointly develop knowledge, and, finally, to put scientific findings into practice [5].

5. Limitations

The chosen case-study methodology can be criticized because of its limited generalizability. The results of our case studies are a preliminary investigation with the intention of generating a first understanding of long-term impact and its underlying determinants. Although it is hardly possible to derive a holistic model covering all cumulative effects of disasters, such case studies can serve as a guide for researchers, policy makers, and disaster managers [3].

The case studies refer to disasters that have occurred in the European Union. Analyzing cases from other countries, which have different disaster management structures and health system regulations, might be an interesting task for future research offering further insights.

6. Conclusions

In this study, we investigated the long-term impacts of disasters on the public health system. We used a mixed-method approach consisting of document analysis and expert interviews. For our analysis, we chose the following cases: an avalanche, a cable-car accident, an airplane crash, a terror attack, and a flood. The analysis of the case studies revealed the variety of direct and indirect impacts on population health and health systems major incidents can have. We grouped the identified impacts into the categories of health-system performance, and security and health protection. Subcategories in health-system performance were mental health and demand for healthcare services, as well as structure and organization of psychosocial support. The subcategories for security and health protection were contingency and preparedness planning, infrastructure, and research. Although we chose contrasting cases, we identified recurring themes in all the cases investigated. A change in communication processes, updates of emergency plans, infrastructural measures, and a higher awareness for psychosocial support was observed in each case study. Our chosen holistic strategy gave us deep insights into each case study and helped us to better understand the undertaken or missing reactions concerning public health. By analyzing past events and their consequences on the public health system, one can develop strategies for better dealing with similar events in the future.

Author Contributions: Conceptualization, M.R., V.S., N.L., and H.S.; methodology, M.R. and V.S.; formal analysis, M.R. and N.L.; investigation, M.R., N.L., and V.S.; writing—original draft preparation, N.L.; writing—review and editing, N.L., M.R., V.S., and H.S.; supervision, M.R. and H.S.; project administration, M.R., N.L., and H.S.; funding acquisition, M.R. All authors have read and agreed to the published version of the manuscript.

Acknowledgments: We thank all disaster managers and other stakeholders who shared their experiences with us, gave us feedback during these initial steps, and helped us develop the current concept. We would also like to thank all our project partners for their tireless support during the past months, to finally reach this point, where we can start to discuss our current research.

References

1. WHO. *Health Emergency and Disaster Risk Management Framework*; World Health Organization: Geneva, Switzerland, 2019; Available online: https://www.who.int/hac/techguidance/preparedness/health-emergency-and-disaster-risk-management-framework-eng.pdf?ua=1 (accessed on 30 July 2020).
2. Lucchini, R.G.; Hashim, D.; Acquilla, S.; Basanets, A.; Bertazzi, P.A.; Bushmanov, A.; Crane, M.; Harrison, D.J.; Holden, W.; Landrigan, P.J. A comparative assessment of major international disasters: The need for exposure assessment, systematic emergency preparedness, and lifetime health care. *BMC Public Health* **2017**, *17*, 46. [CrossRef] [PubMed]
3. Oloruntoba, R.; Sridharan, R.; Davison, G. A proposed framework of key activities and processes in the preparedness and recovery phases of disaster management. *Disasters* **2018**, *42*, 541–570. [CrossRef] [PubMed]
4. Nomura, S.; Parsons, A.J.; Hirabayashi, M.; Kinoshita, R.; Liao, Y.; Hodgson, S. Social determinants of mid- to long-term disaster impacts on health: A systematic review. *Int. J. Disaster Risk Reduct.* **2016**, *16*, 53–67. [CrossRef]
5. UNISDR. *Sendai Framework for Disaster Risk Reduction 2015–2030*; UNISDR: Geneva, Switzerland, 2015.
6. Sundnes, K.O. 18. Preparedness process. *Scand. J. Public Health* **2014**, *42*, 151–172. [CrossRef]
7. Hettige, S.; Haigh, R. An integrated social response to disasters: The case of the Indian Ocean tsunami in Sri Lanka. *Disaster Prev. Manag.* **2016**, *25*, 595–610. [CrossRef]
8. Dell'Osso, L.; Carmassi, C.; Massimetti, G.; Daneluzzo, E.; Di Tommaso, S.; Rossi, R. Full and partial PTSD among young adult survivors 10months after the L'Aquila 2009 earthquake: Gender differences. *J. Affect. Disord.* **2011**, *131*, 79–83. [CrossRef]
9. Hussain, Y.; Bagguley, P. Funny Looks: British Pakistanis' experiences after 7 July 2005. *Ethn. Racial Stud.* **2013**, *36*, 28–46. [CrossRef]
10. Dorn, T.; Yzermans, J.C.; Spreeuwenberg, P.M.M.; Schilder, A.; Van Der Zee, J. A cohort study of the long-term impact of a fire disaster on the physical and mental health of adolescents. *J. Trauma. Stress* **2008**, *21*, 239–242. [CrossRef]
11. Rafiey, H.; Momtaz, Y.A.; Alipour, F.; Khankeh, H.; Ahmadi, S.; Khoshnami, M.S.; Haron, S.A. Are older people more vulnerable to long-term impacts of disasters? *Clin. Interv. Aging* **2016**, *11*, 1791–1795. [CrossRef]
12. Goenjian, A.K.; Roussos, A.; Steinberg, A.M.; Sotiropoulou, C.; Walling, D.; Kakaki, M.; Karagianni, S. Longitudinal study of PTSD, depression, and quality of life among adolescents after the Parnitha earthquake. *J. Affect. Disord.* **2011**, *133*, 509–515. [CrossRef]
13. Annang, L.; Wilson, S.; Tinago, C.; Sanders, L.W.; Bevington, T.; Carlos, B.; Cornelius, E.; Svendsen, E. Photovoice: Assessing the Long-Term Impact of a Disaster on a Communitys Quality of Life. *Qual. Health Res.* **2016**, *26*, 241–251. [CrossRef] [PubMed]

14. Coffman, M.; Noy, I. Hurricane Iniki: Measuring the long-term economic impact of a natural disaster using synthetic control. *Environ. Dev. Econ.* **2011**, *17*, 187–205. [CrossRef]
15. Murthy, B.P.; Molinari, N.-A.M.; Leblanc, T.T.; Vagi, S.J.; Avchen, R.N. Progress in Public Health Emergency Preparedness-United States, 20012016–. *Am. J. Public Health* **2017**, *107*, S180–S185. [CrossRef] [PubMed]
16. Fitter, D.L.; Delson, D.B.; Guillaume, F.D.; Schaad, A.W.; Moffett, D.B.; Poncelet, J.-L.; Lowrance, D.; Gelting, R.J. Applying a New Framework for Public Health Systems Recovery following Emergencies and Disasters: The Example of Haiti following a Major Earthquake and Cholera Outbreak. *Am. J. Trop. Med. Hyg.* **2017**, *97*, 4–11. [CrossRef] [PubMed]
17. Yin, R.K. *Case Study Research Design*; SAGE Publications: Thousand Oaks, CA, USA, 2009.
18. Mabry, L. Case study in social research. In *The Sage Handbook of Social Research Methods*; SAGE Publications Inc.: London, UK, 2008.
19. Shoaf, K.I.; Rottman, S.J. The role of public health in disaster preparedness, mitigation, response, and recovery. *Prehosp. Disaster Med.* **2000**, *15*, 18–20. [CrossRef]
20. A Scoping Study of Emergency Planning and Management in Health Care: What Further Research is Needed? Available online: http://www.netscc.ac.uk/netscc/hsdr/files/project/SDO_FR_09-1005-01_V01.pdf (accessed on 17 July 2020).
21. Lindell, M.K.; Prater, C.; Perry, R.W. *Introduction to Emergency Management*; John Wiley & Sons: Hoboken, NJ, USA, 2006.
22. Lindell, M.K. Disaster studies. *Curr. Sociol.* **2013**, *61*, 797–825. [CrossRef]
23. Zelger, J. Twelve Steps of GABEKWinRelan A Procedure for Qualitative Opinion Research, Knowledge Organization and Systems Development. In *GABEK II. Zur Qualitativen Forschung. On Qualitative Research*; Buber, R., Zelger, J., Eds.; Studienverlag: Innsbruck, Austria, 2000; pp. 205–220.
24. Raich, M.; Mueller, J.; Abfalter, D. Hybrid analysis of textual data. *Manag. Decis.* **2014**, *52*, 737–754. [CrossRef]
25. Evans, D.B.; Murray, C.; WHO. *Health Systems Performance Assessment: Debates, Methods and Empiricism*; World Health Organization: Geneva, Switzerland, 2003.
26. Seguimiento y Tratamiento Psicológico de las Víctimas de los Atentados. Available online: https://www.youtube.com/watch?v=_AdXnr_oWEA (accessed on 17 July 2020).
27. Ministerio de Interior Gobierno de España. *El Ministerio del Interior ha Indemnizado y Ayudado a las Víctimas de los Atentados del 11-M con 318,2 Millones de Euros en Diez Años*; Ministerio de Interior Gobierno de España: Madrid, Spain, 2014.
28. Brauchle, G.; Juen, B.; Hötzendorfer, C.; Bänninger-Huber, E. Notfallpsycho logie oder Psychotherapie. Aufgaben und Einsatzkriterien psychologischen Handelns in Großschadensereignissen. *Psychol. Österreich* **2000**, *20*, 260–264.
29. Brauchle, G.; Juen, B.; Hötzendorfer, C.; Bänninger-Huber, E. *Die "Entdeckung" der Katastrophe als Betätigungsfeld—Kritische Betrachtungen über Helfer als "Helden" am Beispiel der Lawinenkatastrophe von Galtür Brauchle Gernot, Juen Barbara, Hötzendorfer Christian, Bänninger-Huber Eva*; Texte der Fachhochschule Villingen-Schwenningen, Hochschule für Polizei: Villingen-Schwenningen, Germany, 2000; pp. 1–14.
30. Rieken, B. *Schatten über Galtür? Gespräche mit Einheimischen über die Lawine von 1999*; Waxmann: Münster, Germany, 2010.
31. Kaprun: Zurück ins Leben. Available online: https://tvthek.orf.at/history/Die-Katastrophe-von-Kaprun/9840723/Kaprun-Zurueck-ins-Leben/9485772 (accessed on 30 July 2020).
32. Kaprun Disaster Protokoll einer Katastrophe Teil 4. 2014. Available online: https://www.youtube.com/watch?v=s5jSnY4vKRE (accessed on 30 July 2020).
33. Godeysen, H. *Gerechtigkeit für Kaprun*; Die Zeit: Hamburg, Germany, 2009.
34. Meyer, H.J. The Kaprun cable car fire disaster—Aspects of forensic organisation following a mass fatality with 155 victims. *Forensic Sci. Int.* **2003**, *138*, 1–7. [CrossRef]
35. *Bures will Hochwasserschutz beschleunigen*; Die Presse: Vienna, Austria, 2013.
36. Hedberg, B. How organizations learn and unlearn. In *Handbook of Organziational Design*; Nyström, P.C., Starbuck, W.H., Eds.; Oxford University Press: New York, NY, USA, 1981; pp. 3–26.
37. Christensen, T.; Lægreid, P.; Rykkja, L.H. After a terrorist attack: Challenges for political and administrative leadership in Norway. *J. Contingencies Cris. Manag.* **2013**, *21*, 167–177. [CrossRef]

38. Roth, F.; Prior, T. Learning from Disaster Events and Exercises in Civil Protection Organizations. *Risk Resil. Rep.* **2016**, *5*, 1–27.
39. Généreux, M.; Lafontaine, M.; Eykelbosh, A. From science to policy and practice: A critical assessment of knowledge management before, during, and after environmental public health disasters. *Int. J. Environ. Res. Public Health* **2019**, *16*, 587. [CrossRef] [PubMed]
40. Dynes, R.R.; Quarantelli, E.L. *Organization Communications and Decision Making in Crises*; Disaster Research Center: Columbus, OH, USA, 1976.
41. Tierney, K.; Lindell, M.; Perry, R.W. *Facing the Unexpected: Disaster Preparedness and Response in the United States*; Natural Hazards and Disasters; Joseph Henry Press: Washington, DC, USA, 2001; Volume 2001, p. 281.
42. Crichton, M.T.; Ramsay, C.G.; Kelly, T. Enhancing Organizational Resilience Through Emergency Planning: Learnings from Cross-Sectoral Lessons. *J. Contingencies Cris. Manag.* **2009**, *17*, 24–37. [CrossRef]
43. UNISDR & UNOCHA. *Disaster Preparedness for Effective Response Guidance and Indicator Package for Implementing Priority Five of the Hyogo Framework, Hyogo Framework for Action: 2005–2015 Building the Resilience of Nations and Communities to Disasters*; United Nations: New York, NY, USA, 2008; p. 60.
44. Lo, S.T.T.; Chan, E.Y.Y.; Chan, G.K.W.; Murray, V.; Abrahams, J.; Ardalan, A.; Kayano, R.; Yau, J.C.W. Health Emergency and Disaster Risk Management (Health-EDRM): Developing the Research Field within the Sendai Framework Paradigm. *Int. J. Disaster Risk Sci.* **2017**, *8*, 145–149. [CrossRef]
45. Kayano, R.; Chan, E.Y.Y.; Murray, V.; Abrahams, J.; Barber, S.L. WHO thematic platform for health emergency and disaster risk management research network (TPRN): Report of the kobe expert meeting. *Int. J. Environ. Res. Public Health* **2019**, *16*, 1232. [CrossRef] [PubMed]

2

Personal Cold Protection Behaviour and its Associated Factors in 2016/17 Cold Days in Hong Kong: A Two-Year Cohort Telephone Survey Study

Holly Ching Yu Lam [1,2,3], Zhe Huang [2,3], Sida Liu [2,3], Chunlan Guo [2,3], William Bernard Goggins [3] and Emily Ying Yang Chan [2,3,4,*]

1 National Heart and Lung Institute, Imperial College London, Emmanuel Kaye Building, London SW3 6LR, UK; ching.lam@imperial.ac.uk

2 Collaborating Centre for Oxford University and CUHK for Disaster and Medical Humanitarian Response (CCOUC), Faculty of Medicine, The Chinese University of Hong Kong, Shatin, Hong Kong SAR, China; huangzhe@cuhk.edu.hk (Z.H.); kevin.liu@cuhk.edu.hk (S.L.); theresachunlanguo@gmail.com (C.G.)

3 Jockey Club School of Public Health and Primary Care, Chinese University of Hong Kong, New Territories, Hong Kong, China; wgoggins@cuhk.edu.hk

4 Nuffield Department of Medicine, University of Oxford, Oxford OX3 7LF, UK

* Correspondence: emily.chan@cuhk.edu.hk

Abstract: *Background:* Despite larger health burdens attributed to cold than heat, few studies have examined personal cold protection behaviours (PCPB). This study examined PCPB during cold waves and identified the associated factors in a subtropical city for those without central heating system. *Methods*: A cohort telephone survey was conducted in Hong Kong during a colder cold wave (2016) and a warmer cold wave (2017) among adults (≥15). Socio-demographic information, risk perception, self-reported adverse health effects and patterns of PCPB during cold waves were collected. Associated factors of PCPB in 2017 were identified using multiple logistic regression. *Results:* The cohort included 429 subjects. PCPB uptake rates were higher during the colder cold wave ($p < 0.0005$) except for ensuring indoor ventilation. Of the vulnerable groups, 63.7% had low self-perceived health risks. High risk perception, experience of adverse health effects during the 2016 cold wave, females and older groups were positive associated factors of PCPB in 2017 ($p < 0.05$). *Conclusions:* PCPB changed with self-risk perception. However vulnerable groups commonly underestimated their own risk. Indoor ventilation may be a concern during cold days in settings that are less prepared for cold weather. Targeted awareness-raising promotion for vulnerable groups and practical strategies for ensuring indoor ventilation are needed.

Keywords: cold; personal health protective behaviour; associated factors; risk perception; subtropical city

---

1. Introduction

Low ambient temperatures are associated with adverse health effects such as hypothermia and higher risk of cardiovascular diseases, respiratory diseases and infectious diseases globally [1–5]. The elderly, people with illnesses and outdoor workers are more vulnerable during conditions of extreme temperatures [3]. In warmer regions, although winters may be considered milder than in colder regions, due to the less appropriate housing design for low temperatures and acclimatization [4], effects of unusual low temperature might increase mortality and morbidity. Previous studies have shown that populations residing in lower latitudes were more vulnerable to cold temperature [5] and had higher threshold temperatures at which cold effects began to be observed [1]. Adverse health effects related to low temperatures and cold waves have been reported in subtropical regions including Hong Kong, Guangzhou, China, Taiwan and Brisbane, Australia [4,6–13].

As highlighted in the Sendai Framework [14], understanding risks and enhancing preparedness are priorities to support bottom up risk reduction and resilience in communities. Despite the scientific evidence showing the adverse health effects of extreme low temperatures [1,15,16], studies examining personal cold protection behaviours (PCPB) are rare [17]. Several studies focusing on heat protective measures and associated factors have been published, probably due to raising concerns about increasing global temperature [18–22]. Studies from temperate regions have shown socio-demographic factors such as sex and economic status were associated with the uptake of personal protection measures against extreme temperatures [17,18]. In the United Kingdom (UK), females and people with higher income were more likely to apply personal heat protection measures during heat waves [18]. A European study also found females were more likely to wear more outdoor clothes on cold days but the insulation of clothes was poorer than those of males [17].

Risk perception is another important determinant of health behaviours [23,24] Studies from the UK [19], China [20] and Pakistan [21] have reported positive associations between risk perception and protective behaviour against high temperatures. Vulnerable groups, however, had been reported more likely to underestimate their health risks during extreme high temperatures [25]. A focus group study from New York City, United States, found that seniors and people with fair or poor health conditions were not aware of their own risk during hot days [22].

Despite the expected increase in number of hot days and average temperature [26], cold effects on human health are, however, still more severe than the effects of heat and should not be neglected [1,4]. Individual cold protection behaviour, risk perception and other potential associated factors, such as experience of adverse health effects in previous cold waves and socio-demographic factors, are mostly unknown and make the formulation of evidence-based cold-related health protection policy and promotion challenging.

This two-year telephone survey cohort study, conducted immediately after an extreme cold wave in 2016 and a regular cold wave in 2017: (1) explored the perceived health risks and risk perception accuracy at low temperatures; (2) examined the pattern of PCPB; and (3) identified the associated characteristics of PCPB in a subtropical city. The results of this study will support the facilitation of drafting health protection strategy to reduce avoidable health risk during cold waves in warmer regions.

2. Materials and Methods

2.1. Study Period

In Hong Kong, there is no clear definition of a cold wave. The Hong Kong Observatory takes into consideration multiple meteorological parameters and issues a cold weather warning signal when cold weather may incur harm to the public. In this study, cold waves are defined as periods when cold weather warning signals were issued by the Hong Kong Observatory.

This is a two-year telephone survey-based cohort study. Two telephone surveys were conducted, during February of 2016 and March of 2017, one week after the cold weather warning signals were issued by the Hong Kong Observatory on 21–27 January 2016 and 23–27 February 2017, respectively. The surveys were conducted shortly after the cold waves to reduce recall bias. The 2016 survey was completed in eight days while the 2017 survey was finished in eleven days. The cold wave in 2016 was severe and 24 January 2016 was the coldest day in Hong Kong since 1957. The average daily mean temperature during the 2016 cold wave was 10.6 °C (average daily mean temperature in January in 1981, 2010: 16.3 °C). The 2017 cold wave was relatively milder in intensity. The average daily mean temperature within the study cold wave period was 14.8 °C (average daily mean temperature in February in 1981, 2010: 16.8 °C).

Sampling and Subject Recruitment

A random digit dialling approach was used to select households from a full list of landline telephone numbers in Hong Kong and the last birthday method, inviting the household member with birthday closest to the interview date, was used to select Cantonese speaking subjects ≥ 15 years old for the baseline survey in 2016. Quota sampling was adopted to match the population characteristics in terms of age-group, gender and residential districts in the Hong Kong SAR Census in 2011 (2016 Census information was not available at the time of the baseline study). The baseline sample size of 1000 was based on being able to estimate the percentage of people applying a particular cold protection measure with maximum margin of error of 3.5% at a 95% confidence level. Phone calls were made in the evening on weekdays and throughout the day on weekends to minimize bias based on employment status. Oral consent had been sought from each participant at the beginning of the surveys. The study was conducted in accordance with the Declaration of Helsinki and the protocol was approved by the Survey and Behavioural Research Ethics Board, The Chinese University of Hong Kong.

2.2. *Variables*

Socio-demographic characteristics, self-report history of chronic diseases (conditions that require medical treatment for more than six months), health risk perceptions of cold weather, self-reported health outcomes and protection behaviour patterns within the study period were collected in the survey. Based on the health guidelines provided by the Hong Kong Observatory [27], four personal cold protection measures, which included 'putting on more clothes', 'avoid staying in windy areas', 'use of heating equipment' and 'ensuring adequate indoor ventilation', were studied. The possible biological associations between the four behaviours and human health are shown in Table 1. Details of questionnaire design and phone call algorithm for the 2016 data have been published elsewhere [28]. Follow-up surveys were conducted with the same cohort and using same questions after the 2017 cold wave.

Table 1. Biological association between personal cold protective behaviours and health outcomes.

Protective Measure	Linkage with Human Health	Related Health Benefits from Literature	Personal Characteristics Associated with the Behaviour from Literature
Wearing More clothes	Prevent heat loss through insulation and resistance to evaporation, wind and water. Inner layer to control body temperature and humidity, middle layer for insulation and outer layer to protect against the outer environment [29].	Control heat loss, insulate current temperature and reduce discomfort due to cold injury and hypothermia. Increase manual working performance. High moisture absorbing material can keep the skin dry even when sweating. Ventilating garments prevent post-chilling effect when the wet garment is drying [29].	Elderly people in the UK with problems such as thyroid, poor circulation, anaemia and heart irregularities wore more clothes. To supplement appliance to keep warm [30], Japanese female cooperative workers were more likely to wear one or more items of clothing [31].
Avoid Windy Areas	Protect wind chills from reducing skin temperature through rapid evaporation, especially when weather is overcast. [32]	Reduce the risk of hip fractures, incidence of asthma, sickle cell disease and acute pain. [33]	Hong Kong Observatory released advice to "avoid prolonged exposure to wintry winds." [34] No literature was found to evaluate the local population's wind-related behaviour.

Table 1. *Cont.*

Protective Measure	Linkage with Human Health	Related Health Benefits from Literature	Personal Characteristics Associated with the Behaviour from Literature
Use of Heaters	Maintaining adequate indoor temperature. [35]	Increase resistance to respiratory and vascular complications, such as myocardial infractions. Improvement in symptoms of asthma in children and reduced time off school. [8,36]. Ensure thermoregulatory function in elderly people, as the minimum indoor temperature for them should be a few degrees higher than average. [35]	Availability of heating system(s) such as heaters, fireplace, central heating, etc. [30]
Ensure Indoor Ventilation	Intended to remove pollutants emitted from indoor sources, e.g., building materials, furnishings, unvented combustions, etc.	Associated with reduced prevalence of sick building syndrome and allergic manifestation in children. Literature suggests low ventilation rates are associated with inflammation and respiratory infections [37].	A few elders in the UK opened windows for air circulation, mostly for a short while. Most considered it potentially wasteful of heat. [30] Some elders opened windows at night to sleep and turned off the heater [35].

Remark: Protective measures included were references from the Hong Kong Observatory.

Measurement of Risk Perception Accuracy

To assess the risk perception accuracy of subjects, the objective risk of subjects was compared with their self-risk perception. Subjects fulfilling at least one of these four factors in 2017, old age (≥60 years), history of chronic diseases, living alone and receiving comprehensive social security assistance (CSSA), were considered to be at high health risk during low temperatures. This assumes that old age and a history of chronic diseases increase vulnerability physiologically, while living alone and receiving CSSA are related to less resources and support. Underestimation of risk was defined as subjects who fulfilled one or more of these risk factors (the high-risk group) but did not consider themselves high risk. Considering that there might be other risk factors of cold related health problems not included in this study, people who appeared to be overestimating their risk (reported themselves as high risk but fulfilled none of the four pre-set criteria) were grouped as "potentially overestimated". Subjects from the high-risk group who considered themselves high risk, and those who did not have any of the pre-set criteria and considered themselves low risk were defined as having correct perception.

2.3. Statistical Method

Chi-square test was used to compare the uptake rate of the PCPB between the two cold waves. Associated factors for the uptake of protective behaviours in 2017 cold wave were identified using multiple logistic regression models. A two-stage model selection approach, univariate analyses (chi-square test) followed by multiple logistic regression, was adopted. Factors with $p < 0.2$ in univariate analyses were entered a logistic regression for examining the independent associations in the second stage. Chi-square test was performed to examine the characteristics of the lost-to-follow-up group. All analyses were performed using IBM SPSS 21(IBM, Armonk, NY, USA).

2.4. Model Selections in Identifying Associated Factors of PCPB

Socio-demographic factors such as age, sex and income have been reported to be associated factors of heat protective behaviours [17,18]. Age-group, gender, household income and residential district were therefore included in all regression models as the core model. Other independent variables considered in the model selection process included education level, CSSA status, occupation, marital status, history of chronic diseases, risk perception, risk perception accuracy, feeling cold at home during the 2017 cold period and experience of adverse health effect during the 2016 cold waves that needed medical treatment or medicine. Dependent variables, the uptake of the four PCPBs during the 2017 cold wave (Yes/ No), were examined separately.

3. Results

3.1. Descriptive Results

A total of 1017 subjects were recruited for the 2016 baseline survey and 429 of these subjects have completed the follow-up survey in 2017 (follow-up rate 42.2 %). A diagram demonstrating the subject recruitment process is shown in Supplementary Figure S1.

Descriptive statistics of the personal characteristics of the 2016–2017 cohort are shown in Table 2 with the comparison to the characteristics of the Census. Although the baseline sample was comparable to the 2011 census characteristics, it should be noted that the proportion of the elderly ≥65 years old in the follow-up sample in 2017 was higher than that in the baseline, due to the lower follow-up rate among the working population (25–44 years) (lost-to-follow-up analysis available in Supplementary Table S2).

Table 2. Descriptive statistics of socio-demographic variables, history of chronic diseases and health perception of subjects in 2017 follow-up survey, with comparison to the major socio-demographic characteristics in Hong Kong Census 2016 and 2016 baseline sample.

Demographics	HK 2016 Population By-Census Data (n = 6,506,130)		Sampled Participants in 2016 (n = 1017)		Follow-Up Participants in 2017 (n = 429)		2017 Sample vs. Census
	n	%	n	%	n	%	p-Value [a]
Gender							1 [b]
Male	2,947,073	45.3%	437	43.0%	194	45.20%	
Female	3,559,057	54.7%	580	57.0%	235	54.80%	
Age							<0.001
15–24	785,981	12.1%	126	12.4%	49	11.40%	
25–44	2,228,566	34.3%	315	31.0%	109	25.40%	
45–64	2,328,430	35.8%	384	37.8%	165	38.50%	
≥65	1,163,153	17.9%	192	18.9%	106	24.70%	
Geographical distribution *							0.43
Hong Kong Island	1,120,143	17.2%	182	17.9%	83	19.30%	
Kowloon	1,987,380	30.6%	315	31.0%	133	31.00%	
New Territories	3,397,499	52.2%	518	51.0%	213	49.70%	
Education attainment							<0.01
Primary and below	1,673,431	25.7%	137	13.5%	59	13.80%	
Secondary	2,841,510	43.7%	501	49.4%	215	50.10%	
Post-secondary	1,991,189	30.6%	377	37.1%	154	35.90%	
Marital status							0.34 [b]
Single	2,708,709	41.6%	410	40.5%	188	43.80%	
Married	3,797,421	58.4%	602	59.5%	239	55.70%	
Monthly household income (HKD)							
<10,000					67	15.60%	
10,000–19,999					72	16.80%	
20,000–29,999					72	16.80%	
30,000–39,999					60	14.00%	
40,000 or above					128	29.80%	

Table 2. *Cont.*

Demographics	HK 2016 Population By-Census Data (*n* = 6,506,130)		Sampled Participants in 2016 (*n* = 1017)		Follow-Up Participants in 2017 (*n* = 429)		2017 Sample vs. Census *p*-Value [a]
	n	%	*n*	%	*n*	%	
Comprehensive social security assistant (CSSA)							
Yes					17	4.00%	
No					412	96.00%	
Occupation							
Clerical					66	15.40%	
Non clerical					108	25.20%	
Housewife					88	20.50%	
Student					37	8.60%	
Retired/ unemployed					123	28.70%	
History of chronic diseases							
Yes					113	26.30%	
No					316	73.70%	
Living alone							
Yes					38	8.90%	
No					388	91.40%	
Own heating equipment at home							
Yes					252	58.70%	
No					175	40.80%	
Felt cold at home during the study cold period in 2017							
Very cold					24	5.60%	
Cold					253	59.00%	
Not cold					149	34.70%	
Reporting any adverse health effects during the 2016 cold waves (needed medical treatment or medicine)							
Yes					49	11.40%	
No					380	88.60%	
Self- risk perception in low temperature							
High					100	23.30%	
Low					324	75.50%	
Risk at low temperature based on pre-defined factors							
High					193	45.00%	
Low					234	54.50%	
Health perception accuracy [c]							
Correct					267	62.2%	
Underestimated					123	28.7%	
Potentially overestimated					32	7.5%	

[a] $\chi 2$ test was used to measure the overall difference in proportions between this survey and the 2016 Hong Kong Population Census data. p-value < 0.05 indicates significant difference. [b] $\chi 2$ test with continuity correction was used. [c] Underestimated: People fulfilled at least one of the four preset criteria (old age, history of chronic diseases, living alone and receiving CSSA) but did not consider themselves high risk. Correct: People fulfilled at least one of the four preset criteria and considered themselves high risk AND People did not have any of the preset criteria and considered themselves low risk. Overestimated: People did not have any of the preset criteria but considered themselves high risk. * Marine population are excluded. Remarks: Percentage may not add up to 100% due to missing data.

3.1.1. Risk Perception and Risk Perception Accuracy

In the 2017 survey, 45.0% of the subjects fulfilled at least one of the pre-defined risk factors and were considered as high risk in low temperatures. Overall, 23.3% of subjects considered themselves having higher health risk during low temperature (Table 2). Regarding risk perception accuracy,

62.2% had correct risk perception, 28.7% had underestimated their risk and 7.5% had potentially overestimated the risk. Among the high-risk group, 63.7% (123/193) had underestimated their risk.

3.1.2. PCPB Patterns

In general, warm-keeping PCPB uptake rate was statistically significantly higher during the colder cold wave in 2016 ($p < 0.0005$ in chi-square test) (Figure 1). During the colder cold wave in 2016, 95.3% had reported putting on more clothes, 83.4% had avoid staying in windy area and 55.0% has used heating equipment during the cold wave (80.2 % among those owning heating equipment). In the milder cold wave in 2017, 81.4% had reported putting on more clothes, 59.2% had avoided staying in windy area and 28.7% had used heating equipment (41.0 % among those owning heating equipment). In contrast, the proportion of subjects that had ensured indoor ventilation increased from 79.0% in 2016 to 89.5% in 2017.

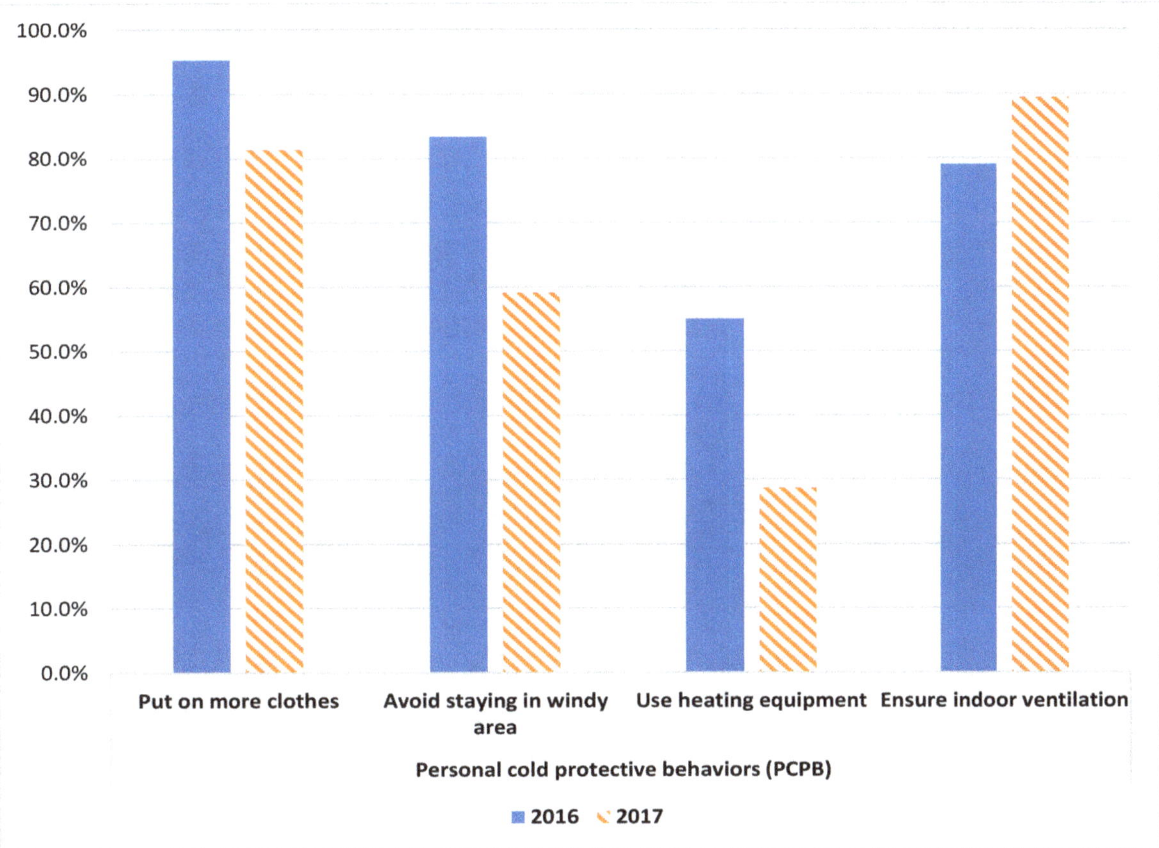

Figure 1. Uptake rate of personal cold protection behaviour among the same group of subjects in 2016 and 2017 cold wave ($n = 429$). Remarks: p-values of Chi-square test comparing the four personal cold protective behaviours between 2016 (the colder cold wave) and 2017 (a warmer cold wave) are all <0.0005.

3.2. *Associated Factors of PCPB*

The selected distribution of PCPB across levels of covariates and the respective chi-square test results are presented in Table 3. A full table of results of all variables considered can be found in Supplementary Table S1. Subjects with previous experience of adverse health effect in the 2016 cold wave were more likely to consider themselves as high risk at low temperature (p-value for chi-square test = 0.003). To avoid multicollinearity, self-risk perception was excluded from multiple logistic regression models whenever previous experience of adverse health effect was included in the model, and vice versa.

Table 3. Association between personal characteristics and uptake of personal cold protection behaviour in 2017 cold wave using Chi-square test.

Personal Characteristics	Put on More Cloths			Avoid Staying at Windy Area			Use Heating Equipment			Keep Indoor Ventilation		
	No	Yes	* p-Value	No	Yes	* p-Value	No	Yes	* p-Value	No	Yes	* p-Value
Gender												
Male	39	155	0.37	89	104	0.03	155	39	<0.0005	21	173	0.84
	50.0%	44.4%		51.4%	40.9%		50.7%	31.7%		46.7%	45.1%	
Female	39	194		84	150		151	84		24	211	
	50.0%	55.6%		48.6%	59.1%		49.3%	68.3%		53.3%	54.9%	
Age												
15–24	10	39	0.64	21	28	0.09	42	7	0.08	13	36	<0.0005
	12.8%	11.2%		12.1%	11.0%		13.7%	5.7%		28.9%	9.4%	
24–39	18	65		36	47		58	25		11	72	
	23.1%	18.6%		20.8%	18.5%		19.0%	20.3%		24.4%	18.8%	
40–59	22	117		45	94		98	41		18	121	
	28.2%	33.5%		26.0%	37.0%		32.0%	33.3%		40.0%	31.5%	
60–69	18	68		35	52		64	23		2	85	
	23.1%	19.5%		20.2%	20.5%		20.9%	18.7%		4.4%	22.1%	
≥70	10	60		36	33		44	27		1	70	
	12.8%	17.2%		20.8%	13.0%		14.4%	22.0%		2.2%	18.2%	
Education												
Primary or below	8	51	0.46	28	30	0.29	41	18	0.78	3	56	0.06
	10.3%	14.6%		16.2%	11.9%		13.4%	14.8%		6.7%	14.6%	
Secondary	38	176		80	134		157	58		19	196	
	48.7%	50.4%		46.2%	53.0%		51.3%	47.5%		42.2%	51.2%	
Post-secondary or above	32	122		65	89		108	46		23	131	
	41.0%	35.0%		37.6%	35.2%		35.3%	37.7%		51.1%	34.2%	

Table 3. *Cont.*

Personal Characteristics	Put on More Cloths			Avoid Staying at Windy Area			Use Heating Equipment			Keep Indoor Ventilation		
	No	Yes	* *p*-Value	No	Yes	* *p*-Value	No	Yes	* *p*-Value	No	Yes	* *p*-Value
Residential districts												
Hong Kong Island	17	65	0.05	48	35	0.001	64	19	0.15	12	71	0.41
	21.8%	18.6%		27.7%	13.8%		20.9%	15.4%		26.7%	18.5%	
Kowloon	15	117		53	80		87	46		12	121	
	19.2%	33.5%		30.6%	31.5%		28.4%	37.4%		26.7%	31.5%	
New Territories	46	167		72	139		155	58		21	192	
	59.0%	47.9%		41.6%	54.7%		50.7%	47.2%		46.7%	50.0%	
Self-risk perception at low temperature												
Low risk	64	259	0.03	137	185	0.18	249	75	<0.0005	34	290	0.89
	86.5%	74.4%		79.7%	74.0%		81.9%	65.5%		75.6%	76.5%	
High risk	10	89		35	65		55	45		11	89	
	13.5%	25.6%		20.3%	26.0%		18.1%	37.5%		24.4%	23.5%	
Risk-perception accuracy												
Correct	50	207	0.12	102	156	0.34	188	70	0.26	28	230	0.05
	68.5%	59.7%		59.6%	62.7%		62.0%	58.8%		63.6%	60.8%	
Under-estimate	22	115		61	75		100	38		10	128	
	30.1%	33.1%		35.7%	30.1%		33.0%	31.9%		22.7%	33.9%	
Potentially over-estimate	1	25		8	18		15	11		6	20	
	1.4%	7.2%		4.7%	7.2%		5.0%	9.2%		13.6%	5.3%	
Experience of adverse health effect in 2016 cold wave and needed medical consultation/ any form of treatment												
No	75	303	0.02	157	221	0.23	278	102	0.02	37	343	0.16
	96.2%	86.8%		90.8%	87.0%		90.8%	82.9%		82.2%	89.3%	
Yes	3	46		16	33		28	21		8	41	
	3.8%	13.2%		9.2%	13.0%		9.2%	17.1%		17.8%	10.7%	

*p-value for Chi-square test.

Table 4. Adjusted Odds-ratio (OR) of associated factors of personal cold protective behaviours in 2017 cold wave using multiple logistic regression.

Associated Factor	Personal Cold Protective Measures											
	Put on More Cloths (n = 398)			Avoid Staying at Windy Area (n = 398)			Use Heating Equipment (n = 399)			Keep Indoor Ventilation (n = 398)		
	OR	95%CI		OR	95%CI		OR	95%CI		OR	95%CI	
		Lower	Upper		Lower	Upper		Lower	Upper		Lower	Upper
^ Gender												
Male	1.00	-	-	1.00	-	-	1.00	-	-	1.00	-	-
Female	1.08	0.62	1.85	1.34	0.88	2.04	**1.85**	**1.14**	**3.00**	0.92	0.46	1.85
^Age												
15–24	1.00	-	-	1.00	-	-	1.00	-	-	1.00	-	-
25–39	0.86	0.33	2.23	1.22	0.57	2.62	**3.31**	**1.12**	**9.77**	1.74	0.64	4.73
40–59	1.70	0.66	4.35	**2.15**	**1.03**	**4.50**	**3.34**	**1.18**	**9.50**	1.12	0.38	3.36
60–69	0.74	0.27	2.06	1.52	0.68	3.41	2.52	0.82	7.74	**7.22**	**1.13**	**46.02**
≥70	1.02	0.32	3.26	0.95	0.39	2.30	**4.00**	**1.210**	**13.19**	**14.57**	**1.33**	**159.55**
^ Residential districts												
Hong Kong Island	1.00	-	-	1.00	-	-	1.00	-	-	1.00	-	-
Kowloon	**2.64**	**1.15**	**6.04**	**2.18**	**1.20**	**3.97**	1.94	0.97	3.91	**3.07**	**1.16**	**8.16**
New Territories	1.15	0.57	2.29	**2.65**	**1.50**	**4.67**	1.44	0.73	2.84	2.10	0.88	5.02
^ Income												
<10000	1.00	-	-	1.00	-	-	1.00	-	-	1.00	-	-
10000–19999	0.70	0.24	2.03	1.50	0.69	3.26	0.51	0.221	1.18	2.02	0.36	11.34
20000–29999	0.66	0.22	1.99	1.14	0.53	2.45	0.73	0.32	1.68	0.77	0.15	3.85
30000–39999	0.42	0.14	1.29	1.20	0.52	2.74	0.63	0.25	1.56	1.22	0.22	6.73
≥40000	0.42	0.15	1.18	1.00	0.47	2.11	0.70	0.31	1.56	1.49	0.29	7.74
^ Marital status												
Currently not married	-	-	-	-	-	-	-	-	-	1.00	-	-
Currently married	-	-	-	-	-	-	-	-	-	**3.33**	**1.34**	**8.28**
^ Felt cold at home during the cold period in 2017												
No	-	-	-	-	-	-	1.00	-	-	-	-	-
Cold	-	-	-	-	-	-	1.24	0.77	2.08	-	-	-
Very cold	-	-	-	-	-	-	**3.72**	**1.29**	**10.72**	-	-	-

Table 4. *Cont.*

Associated Factor	Personal Cold Protective Measures											
	Put on More Cloths (n = 398)			**Avoid Staying at Windy Area (n = 398)**			**Use Heating Equipment (n = 399)**			**Keep Indoor Ventilation (n = 398)**		
	OR	**95%CI**		**OR**	**95%CI**		**OR**	**95%CI**		**OR**	**95%CI**	
		Lower	**Upper**		**Lower**	**Upper**		**Lower**	**Upper**		**Lower**	**Upper**
^ Experience of adverse health effect in 2016 cold wave and needed medical consultation/ any form of treatment												
No	1.00	-	-	-	-	-	1.00	-	-	-	-	-
Yes	**5.48**	**1.26**	**23.83**	-	-	-	1.89	0.97	3.71	-	-	-
# Health risk perception at low temperatures												
Low	**1.00**	-	-	-	-	-	1.00	-	-	-	-	-
High	**2.30**	**1.03**	**5.16**	-	-	-	**2.57**	**1.48**	**4.44**	-	-	-

ORs were estimated from Logistic Regression models. **Bold**: p-value < 0.05 in Logistic Regression. ^ Not adjusted for "Health risk perception at low temperatures". # Not adjusted for "Experience of adverse health effect in 2016 cold wave and needed medical consultation/any form of treatment".

3.2.1. Put on More Clothes

Those who lived in Kowloon (compared to those who lived on Hong Kong Island) (Odds Ratios (OR) (95% confidence interval) 2.64 (1.15 to 6.04)), those who had experienced adverse health effects during the 2016 cold wave (5.48 (1.26 to 23.83)) and those who perceived high health risk at low temperatures (2.30 (1.03 to 5.16)) were more likely to put on more clothes (Table 4).

3.2.2. Avoid Staying in Windy Area

Compared to residents from the Hong Kong Island, those living in Kowloon (2.18 (1.20 to 3.97)) and the New Territories (2.65 (1.50 to 4.67)) were more likely to avoid staying in a windy area. Age group 40-59 (2.15 (1.03 to 4.50)) were also more likely to stay away from the wind compared to the youngest age-group 15–24.

3.2.3. Use Heating Equipment

Females (1.85 (1.14 to 3.00)), those who felt very cold at home (3.72 (1.29 to 10.72)), the older age-groups (vs. 15–24) and those who had high health risk perception (2.57 (1.48 to 4.44)) were more likely to use heating equipment during the cold wave. The ORs of using heating equipment for the older age-groups (vs. 15–24) ranged from 3.31 to 4.00 (Table 4). In subgroup analysis among those who owned any heating equipment at home by age, feeling cold at home remained statistically significant.

3.2.4. Ensure Indoor Ventilation

The elderly aged above 60 years (ORs range from 7.22 to 14.57), those who lived in Kowloon (3.07 (1.16 to 8.16)) and were married (3.33 (1.34 to 8.28)) were more likely to ensure indoor ventilation.

4. Discussion

In summary, 45.0% of the subjects were considered under high health risk during cold weather but more than 60% (28.7% of all subjects) of this vulnerable group had underestimated their health risk. The uptake rates of cold protective measures were generally higher in a stronger cold wave except for ensuring indoor ventilation. Regarding associated factors of PCPB, those who had experienced adverse health effects during the 2016 cold wave, who perceived high health risk in low temperatures, females and the older groups (≥60) were more likely to apply PCPB in the cold waves studie.

Risk perception was associated with warm-keeping, cold protective behaviours in this study (wearing more clothes and using heating equipment). This was consistent with the results from previous hot effect studies from the UK [19], China [20] and Pakistan [21]. However, a significant proportion of subjects did not consider themselves more vulnerable in extremely low temperatures regardless of their age and history of chronic diseases and similar results have been reported in UK [38] and North American based cities (proportions not reported) [39]. The findings did highlight the gap in health literacy and self-risk perception and reconfirmed the need for targeted health education and services for the vulnerable groups, such as people with chronic disease and the elderly, to reduce exposures, and also highlighted the corresponding health outcomes and the related health burden. The two-year survey-based study has also suggested the adaptation ability of the population to low temperature by implementing personal protective measures based on personal experiences.

Our study found that females were more likely to uptake cold protective behaviours which agreed with the findings from previous studies [17,18]. Previous studies suggested this may be associated with less willingness to seek care or help among men than women, as reported previously [40]. Targeted health promotion can be considered for the male group. Older age was another demographic factor associated with higher adoption of PCPB, which was contradictory to the previous hot effect studies in the UK [18] and New York City [22]. Although the effect of age on uptake of health protection behaviours is unclear, the differences in physiological conditions that affect homeostatic process between age groups may explain our result. Older people generally have lower metabolic rate and compromised thermoregulation [41,42], which may make the elderly more sensitive to cold than heat [43]. Income or CSSA status, which was associated with hot protective behaviour in the UK [18], and education level, which was associated with cold protective behaviour in Europe, were not found to be associated in this study. One possibility is that most of the PCPBs in this study are straight forward, well-promoted by the Hong Kong Observatory and financially affordable (e.g., avoid staying in windy area), which made them less likely to affected by income and education level.

Special attention should be paid to results for ensuring indoor ventilation. While the population were more likely to adopt warm-keeping measures in the colder winter (2016), they were less likely to manage indoor ventilation. Hong Kong is a subtropical city in which central heating and housing design for cold insulation are not common. On cold days, people tend to shut doors and windows to reduce the drop in indoor temperature. Unlike regions with colder climates, facilities enhancing ventilation, such as trickle vent on window frames, are rarely found in Hong Kong. Shutting doors and windows leads to poor indoor ventilation. Poor ventilation is associated with higher risk of infectious diseases [4]. Indoor air quality and heating have been raised as an important element in building a sustainable living environment [44]. More investigation is needed to seek practical solutions in balancing indoor warming and ventilation during cold days in different settings to reduce relevant health risks.

To the authors' knowledge, this is the first study examining personal cold protective behaviours in a setting without central heating systems and cold-insulation housing design. This study covered PCPB on the coldest day in the region in the past six decades which allowed us to capture PCPB in response to an unusual cold wave and compare it to a that in a normal cold wave. The sample was representative in terms of gender and residential districts. The immediate outreach to subjects after the cold waves also helped reduce recall bias. This study has several limitations. Although the land-based telephone list covered 94% of fix line telephones in Hong Kong, the households that were not in the list of land-based telephone service were not included [28]. The follow-up rate was low due to the length of the survey (about 30 minutes). Thus, the age distribution of the 2017 follow-up sample might not be comparable to that of the general population. We adjusted age-group in statistical models for identifying associated factors of PCPB to reduce the bias. Due to the relatively small sample size, all chronic diseases were grouped and assessed as a single variable which might also introduce bias as behaviour may vary by disease. Effects of microclimate that might affect personal protective behaviours were not included in this study. The prompt interviews conducted, starting one week after the cold waves, might not be able to capture all adverse health effects, as cold-related health effects tended to have long lags [45–47]. The proportion of reporting unwell might be underestimated.

5. Conclusions

Our results showed that PCPB changed according to the intensity of cold waves, age, gender, past experiences and risk perception. Study findings agree with previous studies that vulnerable groups commonly underestimated their health-risk which might deter PCPB and increase risk of adverse health effects. Targeted health promotion should be provided to vulnerable groups, such as those with chronic diseases, old aged and living alone, to increase risk perception, and to males to raise their awareness of health protection against cold to reduce avoidable cold-related health risks. This study also raised the concern in balancing indoor warming and ventilation in warmer regions that are less prepared for low temperature. Studies investigating warm-keeping solutions without compromising ventilation should inform cold-related health protection strategies.

Supplementary Materials:
Table S1: Association between personal characteristics and uptake of personal cold protection behaviour in 2017 cold wave using Chi-square test; Table S2: Table showing age distribution in participants in the lost-to-follow-up group and 2016-17 cohort group; Figure S1: Diagram showing subject recruitment process.

Author Contributions: Conceptualization, E.Y.Y.C.; methodology, E.Y.Y.C., Z.H., S.L. and C.G.; data curation, Z.H., S.L., and C.G.; formal analysis, Z.H. and H.C.Y.L.; investigation, Z.H. and H.C.Y.L.; writing—original draft:

H.C.Y.L.; writing—review & editing and approval of the final version, E.Y.Y.C., Z.H., S.L., C.G., W.B.G., Z.H. and H.C.Y.L. All authors have read and agreed to the published version of the manuscript.

Acknowledgments: The authors would like to thank Hong Kong Observatory and all the participants for their support.

References

1. Gasparrini, A.; Guo, Y.; Hashizume, M.; Lavigne, E.; Zanobetti, A.; Schwartz, J.; Tobias, A.; Tong, S.; Rocklöv, J.; Forsberg, B.; et al. Mortality risk attributable to high and low ambient temperature: A multicountry observational study. *Lancet* **2015**, *386*, 369–375. [CrossRef]
2. Bunker, A.; Wildenhain, J.; Vandenbergh, A.; Henschke, N.; Rocklöv, J.; Hajat, S.; Sauerborn, R. Effects of air temperature on climate-sensitive mortality and morbidity outcomes in the elderly; A systematic review and meta-analysis of epidemiological evidence. *EBioMedicine* **2016**, *6*, 258–268. [CrossRef] [PubMed]
3. Handmer, J.; Honda, Y.; Arnell, N.; Benito, G.; Hatfield, J.; Fadl Mohamed, I.; Peduzzi, P.; Wu, S.; Sherstyukov, B.; Takahashi, K.; et al. Changes in impacts of climate extremes: Human systems and ecosystems. In *Managing the Risks of Extreme Events and Disasters to Advance Climate Change Adaptation*; Field, C.B., Barros, V., Stocker, T.F., Eds.; Cambridge University Press: Cambridge, UK; New York, NY, USA, 2012; pp. 231–290.
4. Seltenrich, N. Between extremes: Health effects of heat and cold. *Environ. Health Perspect.* **2015**, *123*, A275–A280. [CrossRef] [PubMed]
5. Curriero, F.C.; Heiner, K.S.; Samet, J.M.; Zeger, S.L.; Strug, L.; Patz, J.A. Temperature and mortality in 11 cities of the Eastern United States. *Am. J. Epidemiol.* **2002**, *155*, 80–87. [CrossRef] [PubMed]
6. Xu, Z.; Huang, C.; Hu, W.; Turner, L.R.; Su, H.; Tong, S. Extreme temperatures and emergency department admissions for childhood asthma in Brisbane, Australia. *Occup. Environ. Med.* **2013**, *70*, 730–735. [CrossRef]
7. Yu, W.; Guo, Y.; Ye, X.; Wang, X.; Huang, C.; Pan, X.; Tong, S. Science of the total environment the effect of various temperature indicators on different mortality categories in a subtropical city of Brisbane, Australia. *Sci. Total Environ.* **2011**, *409*, 3431–3437. [CrossRef]
8. Lin, Y.; Wang, Y.; Lin, P.; Li, M.; Ho, T. Science of the total environment relationships between cold-temperature indices and all causes and cardiopulmonary morbidity and mortality in a subtropical island. *Sci. Total Environ.* **2013**, *461–462*, 627–635. [CrossRef]
9. Chan, E.Y.Y.; Goggins, W.B.; Kim, J.J.; Griffiths, S.M. A study of intracity variation of temperature-related mortality and socioeconomic status among the Chinese population in Hong Kong. *J. Epidemiol. Community Health* **2012**, *66*, 322–327. [CrossRef]
10. Zhou, M.G.; Wang, L.J.; Liu, T.; Zhang, Y.H.; Lin, H.L.; Luo, Y.; Xiao, J.P.; Zeng, W.L.; Zhang, Y.W.; Wang, X.F.; et al. Health impact of the 2008 cold spell on mortality in subtropical China: The climate and health impact national assessment study (CHINAs). *Environ. Health* **2014**, *13*, 60. [CrossRef]
11. Goggins, W.B.; Chan, E.Y.Y.; Yang, C.; Chong, M. Associations between mortality and meteorological and pollutant variables during the cool season in two Asian cities with sub-tropical climates: Hong Kong and Taipei. *Environ. Health* **2013**, *12*, 59. [CrossRef]
12. Chau, P.H.; Wong, M.; Woo, J. Ischemic heart disease hospitalization among older people in a subtropical city — Hong Kong: Does winter have a greater impact than summer? *Int. J. Environ. Res. Public Health* **2014**, *11*, 3845–3858. [CrossRef] [PubMed]
13. Qiu, H.; Sun, S.; Tang, R.; Chan, K.-P.; Tian, L. Pneumonia hospitalization risk in the elderly attributable to cold and hot temperatures in Hong Kong, China. *Am. J. Epidemiol.* **2016**, *184*, 555–569. [CrossRef] [PubMed]
14. *United Nations Sendai Framework for Disaster Risk Reduction 2015–2030*; UNISDR: Geneva, Switzerland, 2015.
15. Ryti, N.R.I.; Guo, Y.; Jaakkola, J.J.K. Global association of cold spells and adverse health effects: A systematic review and meta-analysis. *Environ. Health Perspect.* **2016**, *124*, 12–22. [CrossRef] [PubMed]
16. Turner, L.R.; Barnett, A.G.; Connell, D.; Tong, S. Ambient temperature and cardiorespiratory morbidity: A systematic review and meta-analysis. *Epidemiology* **2012**, *23*, 594–606. [CrossRef]
17. Donaldson, G.; Rintamäki, H.; Näyhä, S. Outdoor clothing: Its relationship to geography, climate, behaviour and cold-related mortality in Europe. *Int. J. Biometeorol.* **2001**, *45*, 45–51. [CrossRef]
18. Khare, S.; Hajat, S.; Kovats, S.; Lefevre, C.E.; De Bruin, W.B.; Dessai, S.; Bone, A. Heat protection behaviour in the UK: Results of an online survey after the 2013 heatwave. *BMC Public Health* **2015**, *15*, 1–12. [CrossRef]

19. Lefevre, C.E.; Bruine de Bruin, W.; Taylor, A.L.; Dessai, S.; Kovats, S.; Fischhoff, B. Heat protection behaviors and positive affect about heat during the 2013 heat wave in the United Kingdom. *Soc. Sci. Med.* **2015**, *128*, 282–289. [CrossRef]
20. Ban, J.; Shi, W.; Cui, L.; Liu, X.; Jiang, C.; Han, L.; Wang, R.; Li, T. Health-risk perception and its mediating effect on protective behavioral adaptation to heat waves. *Environ. Res.* **2019**, *172*, 27–33. [CrossRef]
21. Rauf, S.; Bakhsh, K.; Abbas, A.; Hassan, S.; Ali, A.; Kächele, H. How hard they hit? Perception, adaptation and public health implications of heat waves in urban and peri-urban Pakistan. *Environ. Sci. Pollut. Res.* **2017**, *24*, 10630–10639. [CrossRef]
22. Lane, K.; Wheeler, K.; Charles-Guzman, K.; Ahmed, M.; Blum, M.; Gregory, K.; Graber, N.; Clark, N.; Matte, T. Extreme heat awareness and protective behaviors in New York City. *J. Urban Health* **2014**, *91*, 403–414. [CrossRef]
23. Burns, W.J.; Slovic, P. Risk perception and behaviors: Anticipating and responding to crises. *Risk Anal.* **2012**, *32*, 579–582. [CrossRef]
24. Ferrer, R.; Klein, W.M. Risk perceptions and health behavior. *Curr. Opin. Psychol.* **2015**, *5*, 85–89. [CrossRef] [PubMed]
25. Sund, B.; Svensson, M.; Andersson, H. Demographic determinants of incident experience and risk perception: Do high-risk groups accurately perceive themselves as high-risk? 2017, 20, 99–117. *J. Risk Res.* **2017**, *20*, 99–117. [CrossRef]
26. IPCC Summary for policymakers. In *Climate Change 2014: Impacts, Adaptation, and Vulnerability. Part A: Global and Sectoral Aspects. Contribution of Working Group II to the Fifth Assessment Report of the Intergovernmental Panel on Climate Change*; Field, C.B.; Barros, V.R.; Dokken, D.J. (Eds.) Cambridge University Press: Cambridge, UK; New York, NY, USA, 2014; pp. 1–32.
27. Hong Kong Observatory Cold and Very Hot Weather Warnings. Available online: http://www.hko.gov.hk/wservice/warning/coldhot.htm. (accessed on 2 March 2020).
28. Ying, E.; Chan, Y.; Huang, Z.; Ka, C.; Mark, M. Weather information acquisition and health significance during extreme cold weather in a subtropical city: A cross-sectional survey in Hong Kong. *Int. J. Disaster Risk Sci.* **2017**, *8*, 134–144.
29. Færevik, H. Clothing and protection in arctic environments. *J. Amb. Intel. Smart En.* **2015**, *14*, 7–9.
30. Day, R.; Hitchings, R. *Older People and Their Winter Warmth Behaviours: Understanding the Contextual Dynamics*; University of Birmingham: Birmingham, UK, 2009.
31. Tanner, L.M.; Moffatt, S.; Milne, E.M.G.; Mills, S.D.H.; White, M. Socioeconomic and behavioural risk factors for adverse winter health and social outcomes in economically developed countries: A systematic review of quantitative observational studies. *J. Epidemiol. Community Health* **2013**, *67*, 1061–1067. [CrossRef]
32. Budd, G.M. Ergonomic aspects of cold stress and cold adaptation. *Scand. J. Work Environ. Health* **2017**, *1*, 15–26.
33. Jones, S.; Duncan, E.R.; Thomas, N.; Walters, J.; Dick, M.C.; Height, S.E.; Stephens, A.D.; Thein, S.L.; Rees, D.C. Windy weather and low humidity are associated with an increased number of hospital admissions for acute pain and sickle cell disease in an urban environment with a maritime temperate climate. *Br. J. Haematol.* **2005**, *131*, 530–533. [CrossRef]
34. Li, P.; Chan, S. Application of a weather stress index for alerting the public to stressful weather in Hong Kong. *Meteorol. Appl.* **2000**, *7*, 369–375. [CrossRef]
35. McKee, C.M. Deaths in winter: Can Britain learn from Europe? *Eur. J. Epidemiol.* **1989**, *5*, 178–182. [CrossRef]
36. Olsen, N.D. Prescribing warmer, healthier homes. *Br. Med. J.* **2001**, *322*, 748–749. [CrossRef]
37. Sundell, J.; Levin, H.; Nazaroff, W.W.; Cain, W.S.; Fisk, W.J.; Grimsrud, D.T.; Gyntelberg, F.; Li, Y.; Persily, A.K.; Pickering, A.C.; et al. Ventilation rates and health: Multidisciplinary review of the scientific literature. *Indoor Air* **2011**, *21*, 191–204. [CrossRef]
38. Abrahamson, V.; Wolf, J.; Lorenzoni, I.; Fenn, B.; Kovats, S.; Wilkinson, P.; Adger, W.N.; Raine, R. Perceptions of heatwave risks to health: Interview-based study of older people in London and Norwich, UK. *J. Public Health (Bangkok)* **2008**, *31*, 119–126. [CrossRef]
39. Sheridan, S.C. A survey of public perception and response to heat warnings across four North American cities: An evaluation of municipal effectiveness. *Int. J. Biometeorol.* **2007**, *52*, 3–15. [CrossRef]
40. Doward, J. Men Risk Health by Failing to Seek NHS Help, Survey Finds. Available online: https://www.theguardian.com/society/2012/nov/04/men-failing-seek-nhs-help (accessed on 11 August 2017).

41. Frisard, M.I.; Broussard, A.; Davies, S.S.; Roberts, L.J.; Rood, J.; Jonge, L.D.; Fang, X.; Jazwinski, S.M.; Deutsch, W.A.; Ravussin, E. Aging, resting metabolic rate, and oxidative damage results from the Louisiana healthy aging study. *J. Gerontol. A Biol. Sci. Med. Sci.* **2007**, *62*, 752–759. [CrossRef]
42. Barzilai, N.; Huffman, D.M.; Muzumdar, R.H.; Bartke, A. The critical role of metabolic pathways in aging. *Diabetes* **2012**, *61*, 1315–1322. [CrossRef]
43. Guergova, S.; Dufour, A. Thermal sensitivity in the elderly: A review. *Ageing Res. Rev.* **2011**, *10*, 80–92. [CrossRef]
44. Sharpe, R.A.; Machray, K.E.; Fleming, L.E.; Taylor, T.; Henley, W.; Chenore, T.; Hutchcroft, I.; Taylor, J.; Heaviside, C.; Wheeler, B.W. Household energy efficiency and health: Area-level analysis of hospital admissions in England. *Environ. Int.* **2019**, *133*. [CrossRef]
45. Liu, J.; Ma, Y.; Wang, Y.; Li, S.; Liu, S.; He, X.; Li, L.; Guo, L.; Niu, J.; Luo, B.; et al. The impact of cold and heat on years of life lost in a Northwestern Chinese city with temperate continental climate. *Int. J. Environ. Res. Public Health* **2019**, *16*, 3529. [CrossRef]
46. Chai, G.; He, H.; Su, Y.; Sha, Y.; Zong, S. Lag effect of air temperature on the incidence of respiratory diseases in Lanzhou, China. *Int. J. Biometeorol.* **2020**, *64*, 83–93. [CrossRef]
47. Yi, W.; Chan, A.P.C. Effects of temperature on mortality in Hong Kong: A time series analysis. *Int. J. Biometeorol.* **2015**, *59*, 927–936. [CrossRef]

3

The Asia Pacific Disaster Mental Health Network: Setting a Mental Health Agenda for the Region

Elizabeth A. Newnham [1,2,*], Peta L. Dzidic [1], Enrique L.P. Mergelsberg [1], Bhushan Guragain [3], Emily Ying Yang Chan [2,4,5], Yoshiharu Kim [6], Jennifer Leaning [2], Ryoma Kayano [7], Michael Wright [8], Lalindra Kaththiriarachchi [9], Hiroshi Kato [10], Tomoko Osawa [10] and Lisa Gibbs [11]

1 School of Psychology, Curtin University, Perth 6845, Australia; peta.dzidic@curtin.edu.au (P.L.D.); enrique.mergelsberg1@curtin.edu.au (E.L.P.M.)
2 François-Xavier Bagnoud Center for Health & Human Rights, Harvard University, Boston, MA 02115, USA; emily.chan@cuhk.edu.hk (E.Y.Y.C.); jleaning@hsph.harvard.edu (J.L.)
3 Centre for Victims of Torture, Kathmandu 44600, Nepal; bhushan@cvict.org.np
4 Division of Global Health and Humanitarian Medicine, CUHK, Hong Kong 999077, China
5 Nuffield Department of Medicine, University of Oxford, Oxford OX3-7LF, UK
6 National Institute of Mental Health, Tokyo 187-0031, Japan; joice21@yc4.so-net.ne.jp
7 World Health Organization Kobe Centre, Kobe 651-0073, Japan; kayanor@who.int
8 School of Occupational Therapy, Social Work and Speech Pathology, Curtin University, Perth 6845, Australia; m.wright@curtin.edu.au
9 Department of Physiology, Faculty of Medicine, General Sir John Kotelawala Defense University, Rathmalana 10390, Sri Lanka; lasakamd@ymail.com
10 Hyogo Institute for Traumatic Stress, Kobe 651-0073, Japan; kato@j-hits.org (H.K.); osawa@j-hits.org (T.O.)
11 Child and Community Wellbeing Unit, Melbourne School of Population and Global Health, University of Melbourne, Melbourne 3010, Australia; lgibbs@unimelb.edu.au
* Correspondence: Elizabeth.Newnham@curtin.edu.au

Abstract: Addressing the psychological mechanisms and structural inequalities that underpin mental health issues is critical to recovery following disasters and pandemics. The Asia Pacific Disaster Mental Health Network was established in June 2020 in response to the current disaster climate and to foster advancements in disaster-oriented mental health research, practice and policy across the region. Supported by the World Health Organization (WHO) Thematic Platform for Health Emergency and Disaster Risk Management (Health EDRM), the network brings together leading disaster psychiatry, psychology and public health experts. Our aim is to advance policy, research and targeted translation of the evidence so that communities are better informed in preparation and response to disasters, pandemics and mass trauma. The first meetings of the network resulted in the development of a regional disaster mental health agenda focused on the current context, with five priority areas: (1) Strengthening community engagement and the integration of diverse perspectives in planning, implementing and evaluating mental health and psychosocial response in disasters; (2) Supporting and assessing the capacity of mental health systems to respond to disasters; (3) Optimising emerging technologies in mental healthcare; (4) Understanding and responding appropriately to addressing the mental health impacts of climate change; (5) Prioritising mental health and psychosocial support for high-risk groups. Consideration of these priority areas in future research, practice and policy will support nuanced and effective psychosocial initiatives for disaster-affected populations within the Asia Pacific region.

Keywords: disaster; mental health; psychosocial; Asia Pacific; COVID-19; Health EDRM

1. Introduction

Disasters create an environment of disruption, trauma and grief, with potential for sustained mental health impacts. Heightened stress during pandemics and disasters can impair individual wellbeing (with effects on psychological health and sleep), cognitive function (memory, concentration and executive function), high-risk behaviours (alcohol and substance use, increased rates of domestic violence) and behavioural outcomes (such as compliance or disregard for public health orders) [1,2]. The mental health effects of disasters result not only from trauma exposure but may also arise from the implementation of public health response strategies such as quarantine, physical and social distancing or evacuation [3,4]. Economic insecurity, unemployment or underemployment, school closures and the shutdown of regional infrastructure can have devastating effects for population mental health. In addition, concerns regarding safety measures and sufficient supply of personal protective equipment can contribute to psychological distress [4,5]. Moreover, while many people demonstrate tremendous resilience during emergencies and in the immediate aftermath [6], the long-term psychological effects of disasters and pandemics are often debilitating [7,8].

The Asia Pacific region records the highest frequency of hazards and greatest number of people affected by disasters annually [9,10]. The immense psychological consequences are particularly concerning in nations with developing mental health systems and services [11]. A significant proportion of mental health need is unmet, and this has substantial effects on the social ecology and economic stability of affected communities. As climate change, growing urbanization, population density and animal–human viral transmission generate increasingly severe impacts of hazards and health emergencies, attention to mental health will be critical.

In response, the Asia Pacific Disaster Mental Health Network was established in June 2020 to create a collaborative platform for rigorous research, evidence-based practice and tailored policy designed to support improvements in mental health among disaster-affected communities. The network is supported by the World Health Organization (WHO) Thematic Platform for Health Emergency and Disaster Risk Management (Health EDRM) and its research network [12]. At its formation, the network represented seven Asian-Pacific nations, and it is growing. The network's membership represents practitioners and scholars with broad interdisciplinary expertise in the fields of humanitarian response, psychiatry, psychology, public health, disaster risk reduction, human rights and security, indigenous mental health, emergency and mental health services and climate change action. In its first meetings, the network sought to determine an agenda for the advancement of disaster mental health evidence and practice within the region that would inform the design of future collaborative research, policy development and delivery of services.

2. Materials and Methods

The Asia Pacific Disaster Mental Health Network comprises fifteen representatives (57% female), selected for their expertise in responding to health emergencies and natural disasters, and work with trauma-affected communities within the region. The network is open to all Asia Pacific nations and currently includes representatives from Australia, Japan, China, Nepal, Sri Lanka, India and the USA. The purpose of the network's early meetings was to establish a collaborative platform for future research and policy development and set overarching priorities in line with the goals of the WHO Thematic Platform for Health EDRM and its research network. Monthly meetings are conducted via videoconference. The selection of research priorities was conducted through open consultation within the network. An iterative-generative reflective method was adopted, whereby experiential knowledge of network members gleaned through their immersion with affected communities allowed for iterative debate [13]. As reflective-generative practitioners, each network member provided community-relevant insights as to potential priority areas. An iterative and deliberative discussion occurred across two meetings, held in June and July 2020. A list of key priorities identified by the group as central to mental health practice, research and policy within the region was generated. Thirteen representatives attended the first meeting and ten representatives attended the second. Impromptu responses on the priority list were systematically collated; the list was adapted following a second round of discussion and then circulated among the representatives for feedback. An additional round of input from representatives on the priorities and supporting evidence was incorporated into the write-up. All network members contributed to and provided feedback on the final priority list.

3. Results

3.1. *Key Priorities for Disaster Mental Health*

Large-scale climate disasters, severe wildfires and the COVID-19 pandemic have drawn renewed global attention to disaster response this year. The COVID-19 pandemic has amplified the structural injustices of race, faith, gender, age, migration and economic inequality within and across societies, with significant implications for mental health (e.g., [14–18]). Addressing structural disadvantage and inequality is vital, and without attention to these issues, many mental health difficulties during and after disasters may not be amenable to psychological treatment. Mental health practitioners and researchers play a vital role in highlighting injustice, community needs and the role of economic empowerment in supporting mental health. It is critical that psychological first aid and evidence-based interventions suitable for response to mass trauma events are implemented to support individual, family and community level improvements in mental health, recognizing that psychological distress occurs on a continuum and multi-level strategies are required [19,20]. First, broad public health strategies such as psychological first aid, mental health education, family reunification and child-friendly spaces, should be implemented at the community level to address general distress following an event; second, delivery of low-intensity programs to assist those dealing with sustained distress and psychological difficulties; third, clinical treatment provided for those with diagnosable conditions [19,21,22]. However, the effectiveness of treatments will vary due to the sociocultural context in which they are delivered [23]. A nuanced, solution-based approach will support significant advancements in this field. In line with this point, we identified the following priorities for a regional disaster mental health agenda.

3.2. *Strengthening Community Engagement and the Integration of Diverse Perspectives in Planning, Implementing and Evaluating Mental Health Response*

Reinforcing local social networks, social solidarity and engagement with community groups in responding to disasters and other mass trauma events will enhance psychosocial outcomes [24–26]. Community-driven responses are led by the community and may invite external agency partnership, whereas community-supported responses are facilitated by an external agency with the endorsement of the community [27]. Central to both approaches is that the community be recognised as valued authorities on their own lived experience. Listening to and incorporating diverse knowledges and multiple perspectives are essential to ensure that mental health services and psychosocial initiatives designed for any community are accessible, acceptable, culturally secure and developmentally appropriate [28] and that intervention models, disaster risk reduction strategies and mental health policy are designed and delivered in ways that are meaningful and relevant [29]. Furthermore, emerging evidence suggests that mutual reinforcement of public health messages and actions among community members has positive implications for health-related behaviors and compliance with public health directives during pandemics [30]. Restoring connections to the natural environment will have additional mental health benefits [31]. Working within existing community social structures and across a broad cross section of the community—with Elders, youth, local faith leaders and community groups—helps to establish respectful and collaborative relationships. Measures to access broad input and community guidance will result in treatment models, services and strategies that meet the diversity of mental health needs [32–34].

3.3. *Supporting the Capacity of Mental Health Systems to Respond to Disasters*

Disasters create multiple waves of healthcare need. Early response requires a focus on physical injuries, bereavement and re-establishing critical infrastructure for survival [35]. Establishing conditions for safe recovery will lessen distress for a vast majority of the population [19,36]. Mental illness tends to emerge in a second surge of health need, often months and years following the initial emergency [37]. However, the COVID-19 pandemic highlighted mental health needs that required immediate support during this crisis [2,5]. Health systems need to be prepared to address the short- and long-term mental health needs that arise within disaster-affected settings. Disaster response must begin with a diverse and well-supported workforce and include ensuring that workers are trained and supported with ongoing supervision and further training in psychological care for traumatized people—including how to cope with the added overlay of mass trauma impacts. Where disasters are more likely to affect remote areas, infrastructure to support regional health workers and digital health platforms will be important [38]. Lessons learned from the COVID-19 pandemic have already sparked significant expansion of mental health systems in many nations, including in China, where an increased workforce was engaged in order to address the psychological distress and grief arising from the pandemic in Wuhan [39,40]. Similar initiatives have been developed in other parts of the Asia Pacific region, including increased mental health budget funding in Australia [41], improved and expanded mental health helpline services in Nepal [42] and increased in-person and remote counselling services in Japan [43]. The challenge will be an ongoing commitment to the long-term sustainability of services to address the growing incidence of disaster-related trauma and grief within our region and ensuring that first responders, medical, nursing and allied health staff are well supported [44,45]. Mental health services research is both urgent and critical to evaluate the efficacy of models for rapid upskilling and ongoing support of the healthcare workforce, and to design and implement the appropriate expansion of access; acceptability and cultural security of services; effectiveness of trauma-informed treatments in low resource settings and community-based strategies to prevent the escalation of psychological distress.

3.4. *Optimising the Integration of Digital Platforms in Mental Healthcare to Support Access and Acceptability of Care*

The COVID-19 pandemic has fast-tracked the development and widespread adoption of technology in mental healthcare in many settings. Digital mental health services include treatment sessions conducted via video call, telephone helplines, clinical text messaging services, digital health applications and platforms, online streaming and therapy services and mass dissemination of mental health resources on social media [39,46]. Enabling the safe continuation of mental health services during lockdown or physical distancing, tele-mental health services have been widely implemented in many nations including China, Japan, Australia and New Zealand and have received additional funding for development and dissemination globally [39,47,48]. New and adapted technologies have the potential to transform the delivery of mental healthcare, as care can be tailored on a personal level, provided anywhere, be perceived as less stigmatizing and can empower people to take a more active role in their own healthcare decisions [49–51]. Although many settings within the Asia Pacific region still lack reliable access to electricity, internet and phone coverage, all limiting the use of digital mental healthcare [52]; the growing ubiquity of smartphone use has enabled rapid communication of disaster and mental health messaging, reaching populations less likely to be engaged with mainstream health services, such as international migrant workers [53]. Technology may also enable people to maintain the social connections that are critical to mental health and wellbeing outcomes. However, the digitalization of mental healthcare has possible negative implications. Reliance on technology can lead to social disengagement, and there are increasing concerns about the potential for misinformation with unregulated online information, as well as technical issues, unreliable internet access, low digital competences of health providers and clients, safety of data handling and perceived loss of therapeutic relationships [49,54]. It is thus essential to now identify which services and strategies have proven to be protective and efficient in improving mental health outcomes in the context of COVID-19 so as to design approaches that will have relevance beyond this pandemic.

3.5. *Addressing the Mental Health Impacts of Climate Change*

Climate change has increased the frequency and severity of natural disasters in the Asia Pacific region, with resulting risks for mental health problems [55–57]. The relationship between climate change and mental health impacts can be direct, by experiencing trauma caused by climate hazards, or indirect, through resulting physical health consequences, increased economic vulnerability and detrimental effects on community cohesion [55,56]. Further indirect effects from climate change may arise through a reduced sense of hope and self- and community-efficacy, identified as essential elements in recovery from mass trauma events such as natural disasters [58]. Within the Asia Pacific region, Indigenous communities and those dependent on agricultural production or coastal fishing experience disproportionate adverse impacts of climate change [55,56,59]. However, the effects are broadening—the Australian 2020 wildfires demonstrated widespread ecological and economic damage—with substantial psychological effects [38,60]. Similarly, climate change has had significant effects on mental health in the Pacific Island of Tuvalu [59], where the changing climate threatens irreversible changes to the way of life [61]. Climate-related hazards (i.e., tropical cyclones and increasing ocean temperatures) combined with urbanization, land shortages, overcrowding, limitations in infrastructure, services and poor governance have resulted in high levels of stress, anxiety and depressive symptoms among the Tuvaluan population [59]. Similar issues accompanied the impact of 2013 super typhoon Haiyan in the Philippines [62]. Direct and indirect mental health consequences from climate change are current and understudied [57]. This gap in our knowledge requires our immediate and collective attention in order to bring about an efficient, effective and holistic approach to mitigating the inequity of climate change impacts on mental health, led by local experts. This effort must become a central focus of disaster risk reduction in the coming decades.

3.6. *Prioritising Mental Health and Psychosocial Support for High-Risk Groups*

High-risk groups, including those disadvantaged or discriminated against due to the characteristics and intersection of age, gender, sexuality, ethnicity, faith, ability, migration and economic status, may be at greater risk of mental health difficulties during and after disasters [63,64]. In addition, those affected by domestic violence, chronic mental illness, forced displacement, job loss or homelessness will require tailored solutions [65]. The damage to the natural environment from climatic hazards may also generate an additional level of pain and loss for First Nations people with historical and cultural connections to the land [66], as well as for many others who find solace and peace in the persistence of nature. Failure to recognize historical circumstances and cultural values can result in interventions reinforcing existing patterns of disadvantage and prejudice [67]. Risk factors are dynamic, and an individual's level of vulnerability during disasters is dependent on a range of contextual factors, resulting in resilience at times and vulnerability at others [63]. For example, there is a complex relationship between disaster exposure and suicide risk, with increased risk associated with large-scale disaster impacts and length of time following exposure [68]. Specific groups, such as working-age men and older women, and factors including limited social connections, economic insecurity, living in temporary housing and pre-existing or new mental health conditions may increase suicide risk following disasters [68,69]. COVID-19 has demonstrated the potential for mental health risks to emerge as a result of both disaster-related trauma and the public health safety measures implemented to reduce transmission. This has been highlighted in Nepal, where widespread job loss and economic insecurity arising from government lockdown measures during the pandemic has resulted in a tragic spike in suicides, with 1200 deaths reported due to suicide during the 74 day lockdown [70,71]. Established mental health services in Nepal are working to provide helpline services through telephone and social media and further improve the capacity of community psychosocial workers to respond to individuals experiencing psychological distress [42]. Thus, effective services working within high-risk communities must be supported to continue and, where needed, expand their services during and after disasters. As we see an increasingly sophisticated global response to disaster risk reduction, inclusion and support for high-risk groups will be vital for effective mental healthcare.

4. Conclusions

The Asia Pacific Disaster Mental Health Network was established to foster advancements and coordination of psychosocial supports and mental health service delivery, policy development and collaborative research in the region. In line with the priorities of the WHO Thematic Platform for Health EDRM and its research network [12,72], the Asia Pacific Network aims to contribute to improvements in mental healthcare and psychosocial support through rigorous research and policy. Within the context of the COVID-19 pandemic and recent climatic hazards, the network set an agenda that prioritises strengthened community engagement, improved capacity for mental health and community services to respond to the needs of disaster-affected populations, integrating emerging technologies, addressing the impacts of climate change and supporting high-risk groups. Through multidisciplinary regional partnerships, the network will contribute to effective and culturally secure intervention design and delivery, translation of evidence to support community preparedness and response, and the collection of high-quality data to inform knowledge, policy and practice specific to the Asia Pacific region and relevant across the globe.

Author Contributions: Conceptualization, E.A.N., E.Y.Y.C., P.L.D., L.G.; B.G., Y.K., J.L., L.K., H.K., writing—original draft preparation, E.A.N., E.L.P.M., P.L.D.; writing—review and editing, E.A.N., P.L.D., E.L.P.M., B.G., E.Y.Y.C., Y.K., J.L., R.K., M.W., L.K., H.K., T.O., L.G., funding acquisition, E.A.N., Y.K., H.K., L.G., P.L.D., J.L. All authors have read and agreed to the published version of the manuscript.

References

1. Holmes, E.A.; O'Connor, R.C.; Perry, V.H.; Tracey, I.; Wessely, S.; Arseneault, L.; Ballard, C.; Christensen, H.; Silver, R.C.; Everall, I. Multidisciplinary research priorities for the COVID-19 pandemic: A call for action for mental health science. *Lancet Psychiatry* **2020**, *7*, 547–560. [CrossRef]
2. Pfefferbaum, B.; North, C.S. Mental health and the Covid-19 pandemic. *N. Engl. J. Med.* **2020**, *383*, 510–512. [CrossRef] [PubMed]
3. Brooks, S.K.; Webster, R.K.; Smith, L.E.; Woodland, L.; Wessely, S.; Greenberg, N.; Rubin, G.J. The psychological impact of quarantine and how to reduce it: Rapid review of the evidence. *Lancet* **2020**, *395*, 912–920. [CrossRef]
4. Li, H.Y.; Cao, H.; Leung, D.Y.; Mak, Y.W. The psychological impacts of a COVID-19 outbreak on college students in China: A longitudinal study. *Int. J. Environ. Res. Public Health* **2020**, *17*, 3933. [CrossRef] [PubMed]
5. Choi, E.P.H.; Hui, B.P.H.; Wan, E.Y.F. Depression and anxiety in Hong Kong during COVID-19. *Int. J. Environ. Res. Public Health* **2020**, *17*, 3740. [CrossRef] [PubMed]
6. Bonanno, G.A.; Brewin, C.R.; Kaniasty, K.; Greca, A.M.L. Weighing the costs of disaster: Consequences, risks, and resilience in individuals, families, and communities. *Psychol. Sci. Public Interest* **2010**, *11*, 1–49. [CrossRef] [PubMed]
7. Beaglehole, B.; Mulder, R.T.; Frampton, C.M.; Boden, J.M.; Newton-Howes, G.; Bell, C.J. Psychological distress and psychiatric disorder after natural disasters: Systematic review and meta-analysis. *Br. J. Psychiatry* **2018**, *213*, 716–722. [CrossRef] [PubMed]
8. Bryant, R.A.; Gibbs, L.; Gallagher, H.C.; Pattison, P.; Lusher, D.; MacDougall, C.; Harms, L.; Block, K.; Sinnott, V.; Ireton, G. Longitudinal study of changing psychological outcomes following the Victorian black Saturday bushfires. *Aust. N. Z. J. Psychiatry* **2018**, *52*, 542–551. [CrossRef] [PubMed]
9. CRED; UNISDR. *2018 Review of Disaster Events*; Centre for Research on the Epidemiology of Disasters: Brussels, Belgium, 2019.
10. Below, R.; Wallemacq, P. *Annual Disaster Statistical Review 2017*; Centre for Research on the Epidemiology of Disasters: Brussels, Belgium, 2018.

11. Henderson, L.J. Emergency and disaster: Pervasive risk and public bureaucracy in developing nations. *Public Organ. Rev.* **2004**, *4*, 103–119. [CrossRef]
12. Kayano, R.; Chan, E.Y.; Murray, V.; Abrahams, J.; Barber, S.L. WHO Thematic Platform for Health Emergency and Disaster Risk Management Research Network (TPRN): Report of the Kobe Expert Meeting. *Int. J. Environ. Res. Public Health* **2019**, *16*, 1232. [CrossRef]
13. Dokecki, P.R. On knowing the community of caring persons: A methodological basis for the reflective-generative practice of community psychology. *J. Community Psychol.* **1992**, *20*, 26–35. [CrossRef]
14. Matache, M.; Bhabha, J. Anti-Roma Racism is Spiraling during COVID-19 Pandemic. *Health Hum. Rights* **2020**, *22*, 379. [PubMed]
15. Tai, D.B.G.; Shah, A.; Doubeni, C.A.; Sia, I.G.; Wieland, M.L. The Disproportionate Impact of COVID-19 on Racial and Ethnic Minorities in the United States. *Clin. Infect. Dis.* **2020**. [CrossRef] [PubMed]
16. Kihato, C.W.; Landau, L.B. Coercion or the social contract? COVID 19 and spatial (in) justice in African cities. *City Soc.* **2020**, *32*. [CrossRef] [PubMed]
17. Xafis, V. 'What is Inconvenient for You is Life-saving for Me': How Health Inequities are playing out during the COVID-19 Pandemic. *Asian Bioeth. Rev.* **2020**, 1. [CrossRef] [PubMed]
18. Pirtle, W.N.L. Racial capitalism: A fundamental cause of novel coronavirus (COVID-19) pandemic inequities in the United States. *Health Educ. Behav.* **2020**. [CrossRef]
19. Tol, W.A.; Barbui, C.; Galappatti, A.; Silove, D.; Betancourt, T.S.; Souza, R.; Golaz, A.; Van Ommeren, M. Mental health and psychosocial support in humanitarian settings: Linking practice and research. *Lancet* **2011**, *378*, 1581–1591. [CrossRef]
20. Zhang, Y.; Ma, Z.F. Impact of the COVID-19 pandemic on mental health and quality of life among local residents in Liaoning Province, China: A cross-sectional study. *Int. J. Environ. Res. Public Health* **2020**, *17*, 2381. [CrossRef]
21. Forbes, D.; O'Donnell, M.; Bryant, R. Psychosocial recovery following community disasters: An international collaboration. *Aust. N. Z. J. Psychiatry* **2017**, *51*, 660–662. [CrossRef]
22. Kim, Y.; Akiyama, T. Post-disaster mental health care in Japan. *Lancet* **2011**, *378*, 317–318. [CrossRef]
23. Newnham, E.A.; McBain, R.K.; Hann, K.; Akinsulure-Smith, A.M.; Weisz, J.; Lilienthal, G.M.; Hansen, N.; Betancourt, T.S. The Youth Readiness Intervention for war-affected youth. *J. Adolesc. Health* **2015**, *56*, 606–611. [CrossRef] [PubMed]
24. Bryant, R.; Gallagher, H.; Waters, E.; Gibbs, L.; Pattison, P.; MacDougall, C.; Harms, L.; Block, K.; Baker, E.; Sinnott, V. Mental health and social networks after disaster. *Am. J. Psychiatry* **2017**, *173*, 277–285. [CrossRef] [PubMed]
25. Gallagher, H.C.; Block, K.; Gibbs, L.; Forbes, D.; Lusher, D.; Molyneaux, R.; Richardson, J.; Pattison, P.; MacDougall, C.; Bryant, R.A. The effect of group involvement on post-disaster mental health: A longitudinal multilevel analysis. *Soc. Sci. Med.* **2019**, *220*, 167–175. [CrossRef] [PubMed]
26. Hawdon, J.; Räsänen, P.; Oksanen, A.; Ryan, J. Social solidarity and wellbing after critical incidents: Three cases of mass shootings. *J. Crit. Incid. Anal.* **2012**, *3*, 2–25.
27. Rodriguez-García, R.; Bonnel, R.; N'Jie, N.D.; Olivier, J.; Pascual, F.B.; Wodon, Q. *Analyzing Community Responses to HIV and AIDS: Operational Framework and Typology*; The World Bank: Washington, DC, USA, 2011.
28. Wright, M.; Lin, A.; O'Connell, M. Humility, inquisitiveness, and openness: Key attributes for meaningful engagement with Nyoongar people. *Adv. Ment. Health* **2016**, *14*, 82–95. [CrossRef]
29. Tol, W.A.; Song, S.; Jordans, M.J. Annual research review: Resilience and mental health in children and adolescents living in areas of armed conflict–a systematic review of findings in low-and middle-income countries. *J. Child Psychol. Psychiatry* **2013**, *54*, 445–460. [CrossRef]
30. Lim, S.; Nakazato, H. The emergence of risk communication networks and the development of citizen health-related behaviors during the COVID-19 pandemic: Social selection and contagion processes. *Int. J. Environ. Res. Public Health* **2020**, *17*, 4148. [CrossRef]
31. Block, K.; Molyneaux, R.; Gibbs, L.; Alkemade, N.; Baker, E.; MacDougall, C.; Ireton, G.; Forbes, D. The role of the natural environment in disaster recovery: "We live here because we love the bush". *Health Place* **2019**, *57*, 61–69. [CrossRef]
32. Harr, C.R.; Yancey, G.I. Social work collaboration with faith leaders and faith groups serving families in rural areas. *J. Relig. Spiritual. Soc. Work Soc. Thought* **2014**, *33*, 148–162. [CrossRef]

33. Israel, B.A.; Schulz, A.J.; Parker, E.A.; Becker, A.B. Review of community-based research: Assessing partnership approaches to improve public health. *Annu. Rev. Public Health* **1998**, *19*, 173–202. [CrossRef]
34. Wright, M.; Crisp, N.; Newnham, E.A.; Flavell, H.; Lin, A. Addressing mental health in Aboriginal young people in Australia. *Lancet Psychiatry* **2020**. [CrossRef]
35. Bar-On, E.; Abargel, A.; Peleg, K.; Kreiss, Y. Coping with the challenges of early disaster response: 24 years of field hospital experience after earthquakes. *Disaster Med. Public Health Prep.* **2013**, *7*, 491–498. [CrossRef] [PubMed]
36. North, C.S.; Pfefferbaum, B. Mental health response to community disasters: A systematic review. *JAMA* **2013**, *310*, 507–518. [CrossRef] [PubMed]
37. Gibbs, L.; Waters, E.; Bryant, R.A.; Pattison, P.; Lusher, D.; Harms, L.; Richardson, J.; MacDougall, C.; Block, K.; Snowdon, E. Beyond Bushfires: Community, Resilience and Recovery-a longitudinal mixed method study of the medium to long term impacts of bushfires on mental health and social connectedness. *BMC Public Health* **2013**, *13*, 1036. [CrossRef]
38. Newnham, E.A.; Titov, N.; McEvoy, P. Preparing mental health systems for climate crisis. *Lancet Planet. Health* **2020**, *4*, e89–e90. [CrossRef]
39. Liu, S.; Yang, L.; Zhang, C.; Xiang, Y.T.; Liu, Z.; Hu, S.; Zhang, B. Online mental health services in China during the COVID-19 outbreak. *Lancet Psychiatry* **2020**, *7*, e17–e18. [CrossRef]
40. Li, W.; Yang, Y.; Liu, Z.H.; Zhao, Y.J.; Zhang, Q.; Zhang, L.; Cheung, T.; Xiang, Y.T. Progression of mental health services during the COVID-19 outbreak in China. *Int. J. Biol. Sci.* **2020**, *16*, 1732. [CrossRef]
41. Australian Government, Department of Health. *Supporting the Mental Health of Australians through the Coronavirus Pandemic*; Australian Government: Canberra, Australia, 2020.
42. MHIN. A global Community of Mental Health Innovators, and Department of Mental Health and Substance Use WHO. Resources for Mental Health and Psychosocial Support during the COVID-19 Pandemic. Available online: https://www.mhinnovation.net/collaborations/resources-mental-health-and-psychosocial-support-during-covid-19-pandemic (accessed on 23 July 2020).
43. Health, Centre for Japanese Mental. In-Person and Remote Counseling. Available online: https://cjmh.org/counseling/ (accessed on 23 July 2020).
44. Matsuishi, K.; Kawazoe, A.; Imai, H.; Ito, A.; Mouri, K.; Kitamura, N.; Miyake, K.; Mino, K.; Isobe, M.; Takamiya, S. Psychological impact of the pandemic (H1N1) 2009 on general hospital workers in Kobe. *Psychiatry Clin. Neurosci.* **2012**, *66*, 353–360. [CrossRef]
45. Krystal, J.H.; McNeil, R.L. Responding to the hidden pandemic for healthcare workers: Stress. *Nat. Med.* **2020**, *26*, 639. [CrossRef]
46. Ben-Zeev, D. The digital mental health genie is out of the bottle. *Psychiatr. Serv.* **2020**. [CrossRef]
47. Zhou, X.; Snoswell, C.L.; Harding, L.E.; Bambling, M.; Edirippulige, S.; Bai, X.; Smith, A.C. The role of telehealth in reducing the mental health burden from COVID-19. *Telemed. E-Health* **2020**, *26*, 377–379. [CrossRef] [PubMed]
48. Marshall, J.M.; Dunstan, D.A.; Bartik, W. The role of digital mental health resources to treat trauma symptoms in australia during COVID-19. *Psychol. Trauma Theory Res. Pract. Policy* **2020**, *12*, S269–S271. [CrossRef] [PubMed]
49. Bucci, S.; Schwannauer, M.; Berry, N. The digital revolution and its impact on mental health care. *Psychol. Psychother. Theory Res. Pract.* **2019**, *92*, 277–297. [CrossRef] [PubMed]
50. Hollis, C.; Sampson, S.; Simons, L.; Davies, E.B.; Churchill, R.; Betton, V.; Butler, D.; Chapman, K.; Easton, K.; Gronlund, T.A. Identifying research priorities for digital technology in mental health care: Results of the James Lind Alliance Priority Setting Partnership. *Lancet Psychiatry* **2018**, *5*, 845–854. [CrossRef]
51. World Economic Forum. *Empowering 8 Billion Minds: Enabling Better Mental Health for All Via the Ethical Adoption of Technologies*; World Economic Forum: Geneva, Switzerland, 2019.
52. Statica. Internet Penetration Rate in Asia Compared to the Global Penetration Rate from 2009 to 2020. Available online: https://www.statista.com/statistics/265156/internet-penetration-rate-in-asia/ (accessed on 23 July 2020).
53. Liem, A.; Wang, C.; Wariyanti, Y.; Latkin, C.A.; Hall, B.J. The neglected health of international migrant workers in the COVID-19 epidemic. *Lancet Psychiatry* **2020**, *7*, e20. [CrossRef]

54. Christensen, H.; Griffiths, K.M.; Farrer, L. Adherence in internet interventions for anxiety and depression: Systematic review. *J. Med. Internet Res.* **2009**, *11*, e13. [CrossRef]
55. Berry, H.L.; Bowen, K.; Kjellstrom, T. Climate change and mental health: A causal pathways framework. *Int. J. Public Health* **2010**, *55*, 123–132. [CrossRef]
56. Fritze, J.G.; Blashki, G.A.; Burke, S.; Wiseman, J. Hope, despair and transformation: Climate change and the promotion of mental health and wellbeing. *Int. J. Ment. Health Syst.* **2008**, *2*, 13. [CrossRef]
57. Hayes, K.; Blashki, G.; Wiseman, J.; Burke, S.; Reifels, L. Climate change and mental health: Risks, impacts and priority actions. *Int. J. Ment. Health Syst.* **2018**, *12*, 28. [CrossRef]
58. Hobfoll, S.E.; Watson, P.; Bell, C.C.; Bryant, R.A.; Brymer, M.J.; Friedman, M.J.; Friedman, M.; Gersons, B.P.; De Jong, J.T.; Layne, C.M. Five essential elements of immediate and mid–term mass trauma intervention: Empirical evidence. *Psychiatrynterpers. Biol. Process.* **2007**, *70*, 283–315. [CrossRef]
59. Gibson, K.; Haslam, N.; Kaplan, I. Distressing encounters in the context of climate change: Idioms of distress, determinants, and responses to distress in Tuvalu. *Transcult. Psychiatry* **2019**, *56*, 667–696. [CrossRef] [PubMed]
60. Miller, V.M.; Davies, M.J.; Etherton-Beer, C.; McGough, S.; Schofield, D.; Jensen, J.F.; Watson, N. Increasing patient activation through diabetes self-management education: Outcomes of DESMOND in regional Western Australia. *Patient Educ. Couns.* **2020**, *103*, 848–853. [CrossRef]
61. Nunn, P.D. The end of the P acific? Effects of sea level rise on P acific I sland livelihoods. *Singap. J. Trop. Geogr.* **2013**, *34*, 143–171. [CrossRef]
62. Chan, C.; Tang, K.; Hall, B.; Yip, S.; Maggay, M. Psychological sequelae of the 2013 Super Typhoon Haiyan among survivor-responders. *Psychiatry Interpers. Biol. Process.* **2016**, *79*, 282–296. [CrossRef]
63. Newnham, E.A.; Ho, J.Y.; Chan, E.Y.Y. Identifying and engaging high-risk groups in disaster research. In *World Health Organization Guidance on Research Methods for Health Emergency and Disaster Risk Management*; Clarke, M., Murray, V., Chan, E.Y.Y., Kayano, R., Abrahams, J., O'Sullivan, T., Eds.; World Health Organization: Geneva, Switzerland, 2020, in press.
64. Collins, P.H.; Bilge, S. *Intersectionality*; Polity Press: Cambridge, UK, 2016.
65. Chan, E.Y.Y.; Gobat, N.; Kim, J.H.; Newnham, E.A.; Huang, Z.; Hung, H.; Dubois, C.; Hung, K.K.C.; Wong, E.L.Y.; Wong, S.Y.S. Informal home care providers: The forgotten health-care workers during the COVID-19 pandemic. *Lancet* **2020**, *395*, 1957–1959. [CrossRef]
66. Williamson, B.; Markham, F.; Weir, J. *Aboriginal Peoples and the Response to the 2019–2020 Bushfires*; Centre for Aboriginal Economic Policy Research, Australian National University: Canberra, Australia, 2020.
67. Hsu, M.; Howitt, R.; Miller, F. Procedural Vulnerability and Institutional Capacity Deficits in Post-Disaster Recovery and Reconstruction: Insights from Wutai Rukai Experiences of Typhoon Morakot. *Hum. Organ.* **2015**, *74*, 308–318. [CrossRef]
68. Matsubayashi, T.; Sawada, Y.; Ueda, M. Natural disasters and suicide: Evidence from Japan. *Soc. Sci. Med.* **2013**, *82*, 126–133. [CrossRef]
69. Safarpour, H.; Sohrabizadeh, S.; Malekyan, L.; Safi-Keykaleh, M.; Pirani, D.; Daliri, S.; Bazyar, J. Suicide death rate after disasters: A meta-analysis study. *Arch. Suicide Res.* **2020**. [CrossRef]
70. Singh, R.; Baral, K.P.; Mahato, S. An urgent call for measures to fight against increasing suicides during COVID-19 pandemic in Nepal. *Asian J. Psychiatry* **2020**, *54*, 102259. [CrossRef]
71. Poudel, A. Over 1,200 people killed themselves during 74 days of lockdown in Nepal. *The Kathmandu Post*, 21 August 2020.
72. Newnham, E.A.; Reifels, L.; Gibbs, L. Disaster mental health research. In *World Health Organization Guidance on Research Methods for Health Emergency and Disaster Risk Management*; larke, M., Murray, V., Chan, E.Y.Y., Kayano, R., Abrahams, J., O' Sullivan, T., Eds.; World Health Organization: Geneva, Switzerland, 2020, in press.

4

Batten Down the Hatches—Assessing the Status of Emergency Preparedness Planning in the German Water Supply Sector with Statistical and Expert-Based Weighting

Lisa Bross [1,*], Ina Wienand [2] and Steffen Krause [1]

1 Research Center RISK, Bundeswehr University Munich, Werner-Heisenberg-Weg 39, 85577 Neubiberg, Germany; steffen.krause@unibw.de
2 Federal Office of Civil Protection and Disaster Assistance, Provinzialstrasse 93, 53127 Bonn, Germany; ina.wienand@bbk.bund.de
* Correspondence: lisa.bross@unibw.de

Abstract: Emergency preparedness planning in the water supply sector includes preventive measures to minimize risks as well as aspects of crisis management. Various scenarios such as floods, power failures or even a pandemic should be considered. This article presents a newly developed composite indicator system to assess the status of emergency preparedness planning in the German water supply. Two weighting methods of the indicators are compared: the indicator system was applied to a case study and a Germany-representative data set. The results show that there is a need for action in emergency preparedness planning in the German water supply. This is in particular due to a lack of risk analyses and insufficient crisis management. Numerous water supply companies and municipalities are already well-prepared, however, there is a need for action at several levels, especially in the area of risk analysis and evaluation of measures. In Germany, responsibility for this lies primarily with the municipalities.

Keywords: crisis; critical infrastructure; disaster; drinking water; risk management; risk reduction

1. Introduction

The corona pandemic in 2020 affects society, as well as essential services such as the water utilities, in a new and profound way [1]. Critical infrastructures like water utilities and the provision of their vital services in such a scenario have an outstanding importance to a nation's society. Their failure or degradation could result in sustained supply shortages, which affect public health, economy and national security. Quarantined personnel, working from home to distance employees and unpredictable supply chains for consumables are new and unfamiliar conditions that make the operation of water supply companies more difficult and potentially endangers overall water supply [2].

A resilient drinking water supply is consequently one of the basic requirements for a stable social and economic system. However, impairments cannot be completely avoided, so that water supply companies have to deviate from normal operation, e.g., in the event of pipe bursts. Such minor disturbances occur comparatively frequently and have only minor effects [3]. They can usually be quickly identified and repaired. As a consequence they usually remain unnoticed to the consumers [4]. On the contrary, failures or more extensive impairments of the water supply systems can have serious impacts on the affected population and the economy [3,5–7]. Causes can be serious natural events, man-made accidents or intentional attacks [8,9], whose probability of occurrence is constantly increasing [10].

The corona pandemic puts the importance of critical infrastructures, and the need for proactive emergency preparedness planning to increase their resilience, at the forefront of civil protection and disaster management [1]. The understanding, analysis and quantification of resilience by water utilities, authorities, decision-makers and other stakeholders is a prerequisite for this.

The resilience of water supply systems can be increased by appropriate emergency preparedness planning instead of ad hoc coping responses. This includes the conceptual, organisational and technical preconditions for risk reduction and prepares structures for response in the event of a crisis [11]. Emergency preparedness planning in the water supply sector thus comprises, in addition to measures to avoid damaging events, especially preventive, safeguarding, reactive and restorative aspects of risk and crisis management.

Effective emergency preparedness planning is characterised, among other things, by the fact that the planning is carried out as preventive measures and the measures can be implemented in emergency situations. Beyond preventive measures to minimise risks, emergency preparedness planning in the water supply sector includes in particular aspects of crisis management [12]. Such emergency preparedness planning takes into account different scenarios and their possible effects on the water supply. In addition to preventive measures, the numerous aspects of crisis management also lead to risk minimization by limiting the extent of damage. Figure 1 shows the five steps of risk and crisis management according to the German Federal Ministry of the Interior [13] and the Federal Office of Civil Protection and Disaster Assistance [12,14].

Thorough preliminary planning forms as the first process step the basis for the successful establishment of risk and crisis management [13]. Basic specifications should be made in advance of the establishment or expansion of a risk and crisis management system. These include the promotion of risk awareness and the definition of key players as well as responsibilities in the course of the emergency preparedness planning process [14].

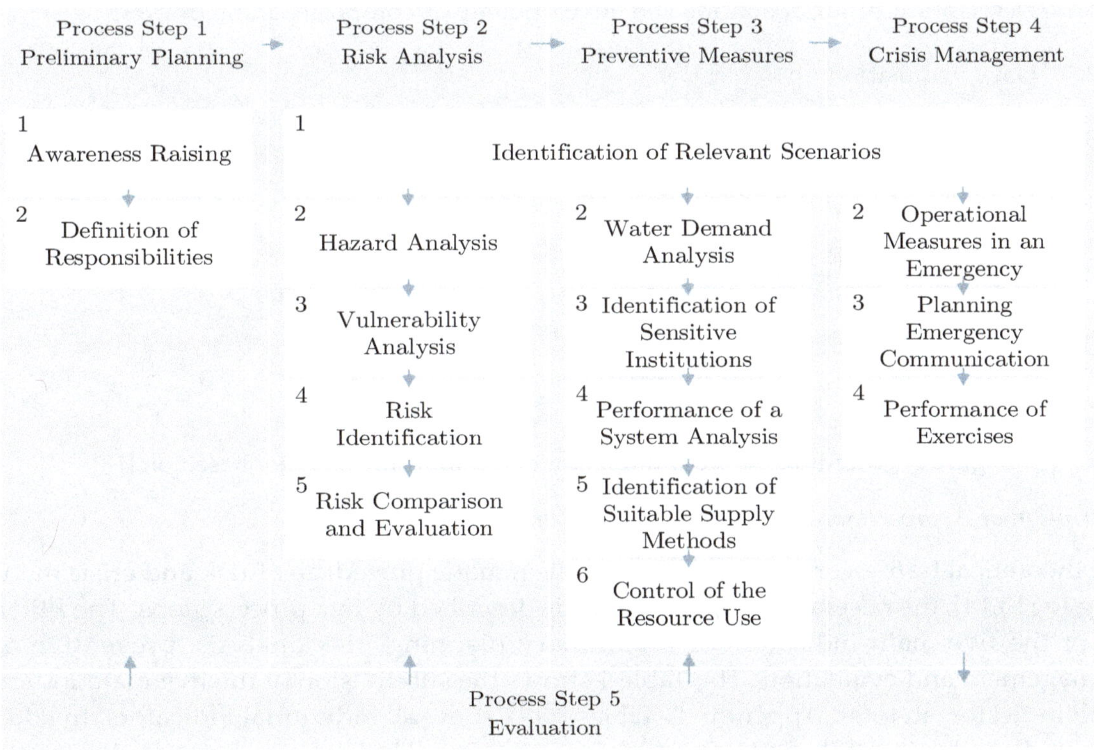

Figure 1. Structuring of the procedure for emergency preparedness planning in water supply based on [12,13,15].

A risk analysis structures and objectifies the collection of information on existing and potential risks to the water supply [14]. The analysis considers the reasons and causes of risks, examines the possible effects and determines the framework within which these consequences can occur [16]. In addition, risk analysis provides the basis for effective and efficient use of limited resources by comparing the various identified risks of processes and components of water supply.

Preventive measures contribute to the reduction of risks for critical processes. They also contribute to achieve operational protection goals and thus raise the barrier for events with crisis potential in the facility [12]. In this way, the number of crisis-prone events can be minimized or the intensity of the events can be reduced.

The processes of crisis management help to protect facilities and thus critical infrastructures and the population. Interactions exist with risk management, since not all risks can be reduced by risk-minimizing measures and a residual risk always remains [12]. Crisis management therefore offers a structure for coping with crises that cannot be prevented [13,17].

The evaluation refers to all phases, i.e., both the examination of points defined in the preliminary planning, the examination of the topicality of the information on existing risks, the examination of the effectiveness of the implemented preventive measures and the examination of the crisis management [14]. It should be repeated regularly.

2. Materials and Methods

The emergency preparedness planning indicator (EPP) developed in this study is based on a number of main, partial and individual indicators. These indicators cover organisational as well as technical aspects of emergency preparedness planning. The contents of the indicator correspond to the processes and components of effective emergency preparedness planning in water supply. For the development and calculation of the EPP, a multi-stage and iterative process according to [18] was carried out (Figure 2).

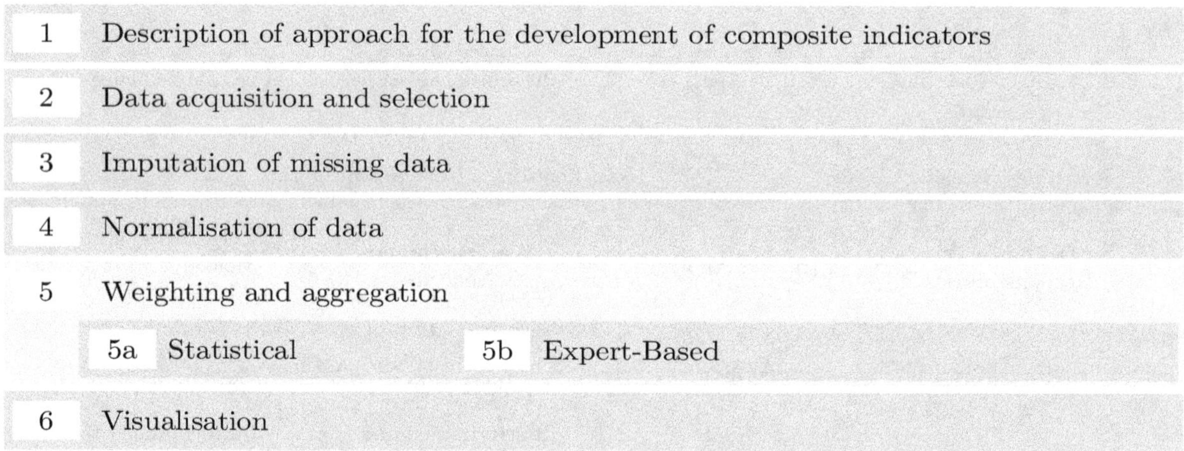

Figure 2. Procedure for the compilation of a composite indicator based on [18].

2.1. Description of Approach for the Development of Composite Indicators

The theoretical framework of the EPP is the systematic procedure of risk and crisis management according to [13,14], the necessary scope of which is described by five process steps. The EPP therefore consists of the five main indicators of preliminary planning, risk analysis, preventive measures, crisis management and evaluation. The Table 1 shows the subdivision of the five main indicators and the 19 sub-indicators in total. Appendix A Tables A1–7 show all individual indicators. In addition to a literature study and existing theoretical models, the individual indicators representative for emergency preparedness planning were developed on the basis of expert and stakeholder knowledge in different workshops, thus applying a stakeholder-oriented methodology. This methodology is usually used in the development of composite indicators (e.g., [19,20]), if, as in the present case, their use is intended as a self-assessment tool for municipalities or authorities.

Table 1. Composition and hierarchy of the emergency preparedness planning indicator through five main indicators as well as their sub and individual indicators.

	Main Indicator		Sub Indicator	Individual Indicator	Source	In NoWa I Dataset
PP	Preliminary Planning	PP_1	awareness raising	$PP_{1,1}$ to $PP_{1,9}$	[12,14,21,22]	Yes
		PP_2	definition of responsibilities	$PP_{2,1}$ to $PP_{2,3}$	[14,21,23]	No
RA	Risk Analysis	RA_1	hazard analysis	$RA_{1,1}$ to $RA_{1,8}$	[14,17,24]	Yes
		RA_2	vulnerability analysis	$RA_{2,1}$ to $RA_{2,8}$	[14,17]	No
		RA_3	risk identification	$RA_{3,1}$ to $RA_{3,7}$	[14,16,17,25]	Yes
		RA_4	risk comparison and assessment	$RA_{4,1}$ to $RA_{4,2}$	[14]	No
PM	Preventive Measures	PM_1	structural redundancies	$PM_{1,1}$ to $PM_{1,2}$	[14,17]	Yes
		PM_2	interrelation of supply	$PM_{2,1}$	[14,17,26]	Yes
		PM_3	grid construction	$PM_{3,1}$ to $PM_{3,2}$	[17,27,28]	No
		PM_4	remote monitoring, control systems	$PM_{4,1}$ to $PM_{4,2}$	[14,17,29,30]	No
		PM_5	general measures	$PM_{5,1}$ to $PM_{5,3}$	[17,31,32]	Yes
CM	Crisis Management	CM_1	organisation and coordination	$CM_{1,1}$ to $CM_{1,7}$	[12,14,17,23,33–35]	Yes
		CM_2	provision of resources	$CM_{2,1}$ to $CM_{2,2}$	[12,14]	Yes
		CM_3	exercises	$CM_{3,1}$ to $CM_{3,2}$	[12,14,17,23]	Yes
		CM_4	communication	$CM_{4,1}$	[14,17,36,37]	Yes
E	Evaluation	E_1	evaluation preliminary planning	$E_{1,1}$ to $E_{1,2}$	[14,17]	No
		E_2	evaluation risk analysis	$E_{2,1}$ to $E_{2,4}$	[14,17,38]	Yes
		E_3	evaluation preventive measures	$E_{3,1}$ to $E_{3,5}$	[14]	No
		E_4	evaluation crisis management	$E_{4,1}$ to $E_{4,4}$	[14,17,23,36]	Yes

2.2. *Data Acquisition and Selection*

The indicators shown in Table 1 are necessary for the quantitative assessment of the status of implementation of emergency preparedness planning. Thus, data are required that allow both a review of the applicability and significance of the EPP and the determination of the status quo in Germany. However, the required information cannot be determined from publicly available data, as this is utility-specific and relevant to the security of the water utility and its services. A targeted assessment is therefore necessary.

2.2.1. Case Study for Verification of Indicator

To check the applicability and significance of the EPP, all indicators were collected on the basis of a questionnaire for a water supply company as a case study. The case study shows a real water supply utility which supplies a total of 230,000 inhabitants in 120 municipalities and districts. In total, the water supply company delivers about 10 million cubic meters of water annually.

2.2.2. Germany-Representative Dataset

In order to assess the status quo of emergency preparedness planning in Germany, an existing dataset of a nationwide survey on emergency preparedness planning in water supply was analysed. The data set was collected in 2015 by means of a partially standardised questionnaire within the framework of the NoWa I research project with the assistance of the federal level in order to obtain a general, supra-regional overview of the current status of emergency planning in the districts and municipalities. As the responsible bodies, the districts and municipalities had to ask for input from the water supply companies to fill out the data collection form, if the information was not already available. In total, a completed survey questionnaire was returned by 194 districts and 166 municipalities. The data thus consists of 360 individual data sets, which contain data from nationwide distributed municipalities and districts with a population of around 39 million inhabitants.

Each dataset contains information on 37 questions concerning different aspects of emergency preparedness planning and existing water supply systems. To determine the status quo, 21 relevant individual indicators from the data entry form with 37 questions were identified and considered in the EPP. In total, the data sets are assigned to twelve of the 19 sub-indicators (Table 1).

A subsequent data collection or data supplement could not be implemented, since the data collection within the framework of the NoWa I project and an additional collection of a representative data set could not be repeated. Thus, the determination of the status quo does not include all identified indicators.

2.3. *Imputation of Missing Data*

Missing data impairs the development and evaluation of composite indicators and can lead to a distortion of the results [18]. In the present study, a case-by-case elimination of data sets is only applied if the data that are absolutely necessary for the situation analysis (e.g., allocation of the data set to the municipality) are not available.

The analysed data of the NoWa I project were collected before the methodology of the emergency preparedness planning indicator was developed. They do not include all indicators relevant to the EPP. Since it was not possible to collect such a data set subsequently, the NoWa I data sets were used to determine the indicator, although they did not include complete indicator data sets (as shown in Table 1). The missing individual indicators are therefore not included in the evaluation.

2.4. *Normalisation of Data*

In order to be able to compare the indicators of different municipalities or the individual sub-indicators with each other, a normalisation process is necessary. This is especially true if the data sets differ in their units of measurement [18].

The questions with "yes-no" or "yes-partial-no" possible answers are converted into a [0,1] scale. Likert scales with a given answer scale were also transformed into a [0,1] scale. The answer option "not known" was equated to the answer option "no", since this is equivalent in terms of content for the evaluation of the indicator. This was necessary because the originally planned survey in the NoWa I project had a different assignment of the questions.

2.5. Weigthing and Aggregation

The individual indicators are integrated into the composite indicator with different weightings (see Equation (1)). This is because the composite indicator is calculated by the weighted sum of its main indicators (see Equation (2)). For the contingency planning indicator, the weighted sum of the five main indicators is determined. As described in [39], there are several ways to determine the weighting of composite indicators.

$$CI = \sum_{j=1}^{m} x_j X_j \tag{1}$$

$$EPP = x_{PP} \cdot \mathrm{PP} + x_{RA} \cdot \mathrm{RA} + x_{PM} \cdot \mathrm{PM} + x_{CM} \cdot \mathrm{CM} + x_E \cdot \mathrm{E} \tag{2}$$

CI Composite indicator
m Number of main indicators
x_j weight of main indicator j
X_j normalized value of the main indicator (PP, RA, PM, CM and E)

For the EPP this paper compares the results of a statistical and an expert-based weighting approach. The main difference between the two approaches is how the indicator weights are derived. Since the weighting of the main and sub-indicators significantly influences the result of the EPP, the composite indicator is determined with identical main and sub-indicators for both weighting approaches.

If the main indicators are equally weighted, they are equally included in the composite indicator. Due to the different weighting of the individual summands (main indicators or sub-indicators), they are assigned a differentiated significance for the composite indicator.

To determine the expert-based weighting, the weights were derived from expert opinions. Using a budget allocation approach, fourteen experts with different specialist backgrounds were asked to assess the main and sub-indicators in a questionnaire using a Likert scale according to their relevance for target-oriented emergency preparedness planning. The weightings of the main indicators derived from the equal distribution and from the expert opinions are presented in Section 3.1.

2.6. Visualisation

The results of the composite and main indicators are visualized in an anonymized representation using treemap diagrams. This type of presentation was chosen because the data set depicts a large number of municipalities and water supply utilities, but the number of inhabitants varies greatly. The hierarchical structure of the treemap diagrams makes the proportions of the municipalities and water supply companies under consideration clear. At the same time all results are visible. Rectangles of different sizes are used to display the number of inhabitants of the district or the district-free city or municipalities (E_i) in relation to the inhabitants of the entire data set (E_{ges}) (see Figure 3). Thus, each rectangle corresponds to a municipality, which is always at the same position in the respective diagrams. The color of the rectangles represents the value of the indicator. The evaluation of the data sets is carried out anonymously. In addition, the possibilities of drawing conclusions about individual municipalities are minimized by the following selected representation.

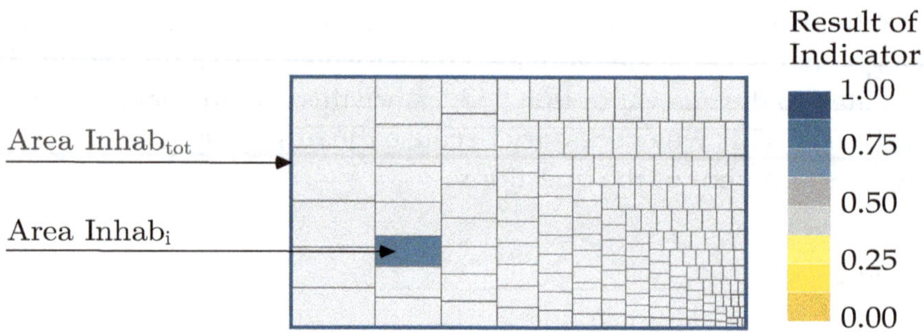

Figure 3. Explanation of the visualization of the analysis of the status of emergency preparedness planning through treemap diagrams.

3. Results

3.1. Determination of the Weighting of the Indicators

Emergency preparedness planning comprises the five process steps preliminary planning (1), risk analysis (2), preventive measures (3), crisis management (4) and evaluation (5). In case of equal distribution, the weighting of the five process steps corresponds to 20% or $x_j = 0,2$ each. The expert-based weights are between 17 and 22% (Figure 4). The mean value of the expert-based weight of the process step Preliminary Planning (1) is 0.22, the highest value, and the mean value of the expert-based weight of the process step Evaluation (5) is 0.17, the lowest value of the five weight. The expert opinion regarding the weight of the process step Evaluation (5) varies the strongest. The difference in the mean values of the expert-based weightings is statistically significant ($p < 0.05$).

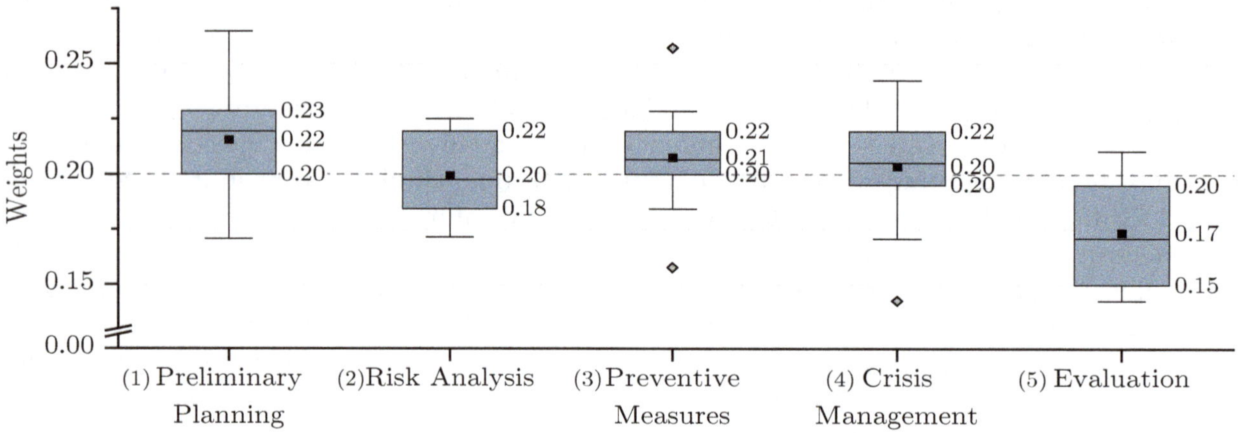

Figure 4. Expert-based weighting of the five process steps of emergency preparedness planning ($n = 14$).

3.2. Assessment of the Applicability and Significance of the Emergency Preparedness Planning Indicator Based on the Case Study

In order to determine the status quo of emergency preparedness planning, a data collection form was compiled from the indicators listed. This was answered by the water supply company and the responsible disaster control authority from the case study and the data was evaluated.

For the case study, this results in an EPP_S of 0.66 and an EPP_E of 0.67 (Figure 5). The main indicator PP with a value of 0.96 corresponds to the highest result of the five main indicators. The lowest value is obtained for the main indicator CM with 0.43 and 0.44. This means that in the area of preliminary planning almost all aspects have been implemented in the company and district, but in the area of preventive crisis management aspects are not yet sufficiently practiced.

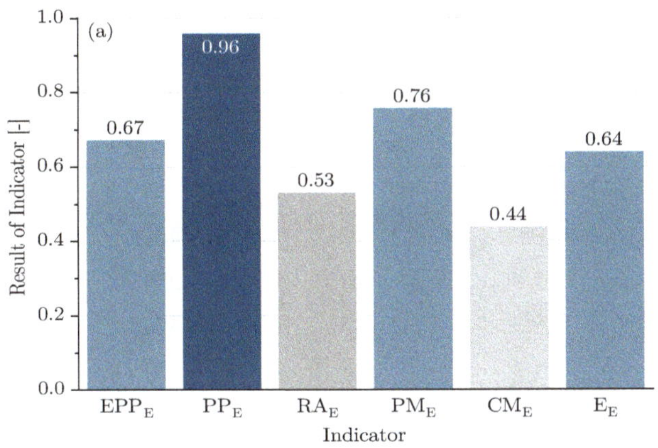

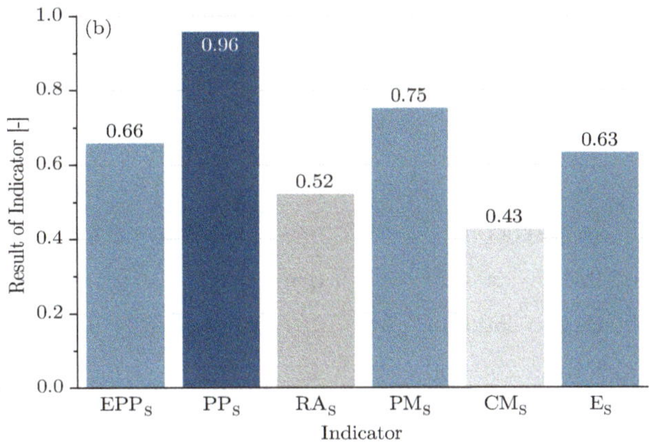

Figure 5. Results of the EPP and the main indicators for the case study based on the different weightings (**a**) Expert-based Weights (**b**) Equal Weights.

The methodology developed in this study to assess the status of emergency preparedness planning is applicable in practice. The applied questionnaire captures the relevant aspects for assessing the status quo and deriving the need for action. The quantitative results also enable a comparison between municipalities and the prioritisation of planned measures to address the need for action.

3.3. Status of Emergency Preparedness Planning in Germany

3.3.1. Data Basis for the Analysis of the Status Quo of Emergency Preparedness Planning

In order to determine the status of emergency preparedness planning in the water supply sector, a total of 360 data sets were analysed and evaluated. These comprise 194 data sets from districts and 166 data sets at the municipal level. Due to the different responsibilities in Germany, the data sets of the districts and municipalities are evaluated separately from the data sets at the municipal level (Table 2). The data sets are each divided into four groups of approximately equal size according to the number of inhabitants covered. In addition, a distinction was made between the areas of responsibility of the senders of the data collection forms. It is therefore necessary to examine, whether differences can be identified with regard to the level of preparation of the different senders and the size of the municipality.

Table 2. Size of the municipalities and districts as well as the field of activity of the senders of the survey forms.

Inhabitants	Proportion of Survey Forms					
	Water Utility	Administration	Civil Protection	Health Department	Multiple Senders	Line Sum
			Municipalities (n = 166)			
to 3.000	7%	20%	0%	0%	0%	27%
3.001 to 5.000	4%	16%	0%	0%	0%	20%
5.001 to 10.000	11%	14%	0%	0%	0%	25%
more than 10.000	19%	3%	0%	3%	3%	28%
Column Sum	41%	53%	3%	0%	3%	100%

Table 2. *Cont.*

Inhabitants	Proportion of Survey Forms					
	Water Utility	**Administration**	**Civil Protection**	**Health Department**	**Multiple Senders**	**Line Sum**
			Districts (n = 194)			
to 100.000	0%	6%	10%	3%	4%	23%
100.001 to 150.000	0%	7%	12%	4%	2%	25%
150.001 to 250.000	2%	5%	18%	1%	4%	30%
more than 250.000	2%	1%	11%	6%	2%	22%
Column Sum	4%	19%	51%	14%	12%	100%

3.4. Assessment of the Status of Emergency Preparedness Planning in Germany

In order to assess the status of the emergency preparedness planning of the districts as well as the municipalities, the composite indicator EPP and the main indicators PP, RA, PM, CM and E were determined on the basis of the data sets presented. For this purpose, the results of the emergency preparedness planning indicators with weighting according to expert opinion (EPP_E) and with equally distributed weighting (EPP_S) are presented below.

The results of the EPP_E and EPP_S vary for the districts in a few cases (Figure 6) The mean value of the EPP_E as well as the EPP_S is equal to 0.42 (Table 3). The small differences in the weighting show only a little effect in the result. Moreover, these differences are not statistically significant ($p > 0.05$).

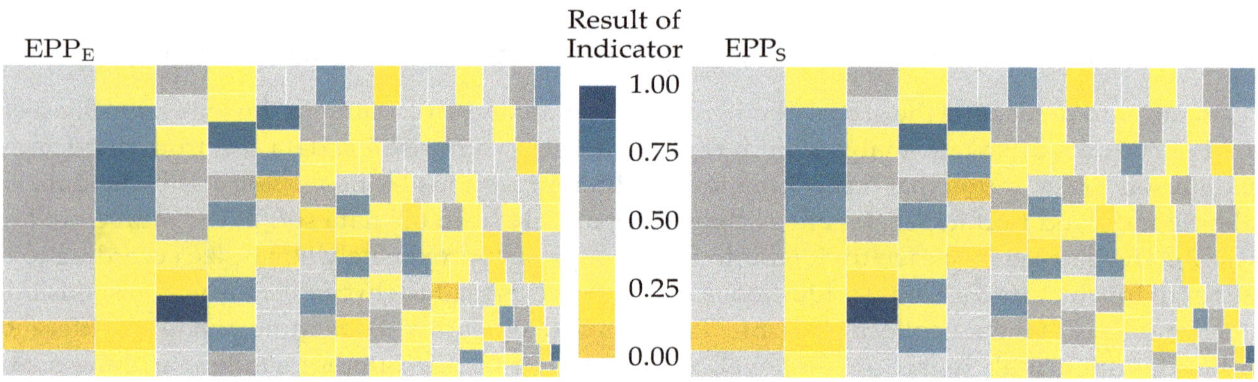

(**a**) Expert-based Weights (**b**) Equal Weights

Figure 6. Emergency preparedness planning indicator according to the size of the districts.

Table 3. Results of the emergency preparedness planning indicator with expert based and equally distributed weighting and the main indicators.

	Indicator	Mean Value of Indicator (Standard Derivation)	
		Districs and Municipalities	
EPP	EPP_E	0.42 (SD = 0.17)	0.32 (SD = 0.18)
	EPP_S	0.42 (SD = 0.16)	0.32 (SD = 0.18)
Main Indicator	PP	0.43 (SD = 0.25)	0.30 (SD = 0.27)
	RA	0.16 (SD = 0.32)	0.14 (SD = 0.29)
	PM	0.57 (SD = 0.31)	0.39 (SD = 0.38)
	CM	0.55 (SD = 0.32)	0.43 (SD = 0.22)
	E	0.38 (SD = 0.22)	0.31 (SD = 0.25)

The participating districts show a different level of preparation. Districts with more inhabitants achieve a higher EPP (Figure 7). The range of EPP increases with the number of inhabitants, so that the largest districts show the greatest difference in the level of emergency preparedness within a size group. The differences in the mean values by size of the districts are significant in both cases ($p < 0.05$).

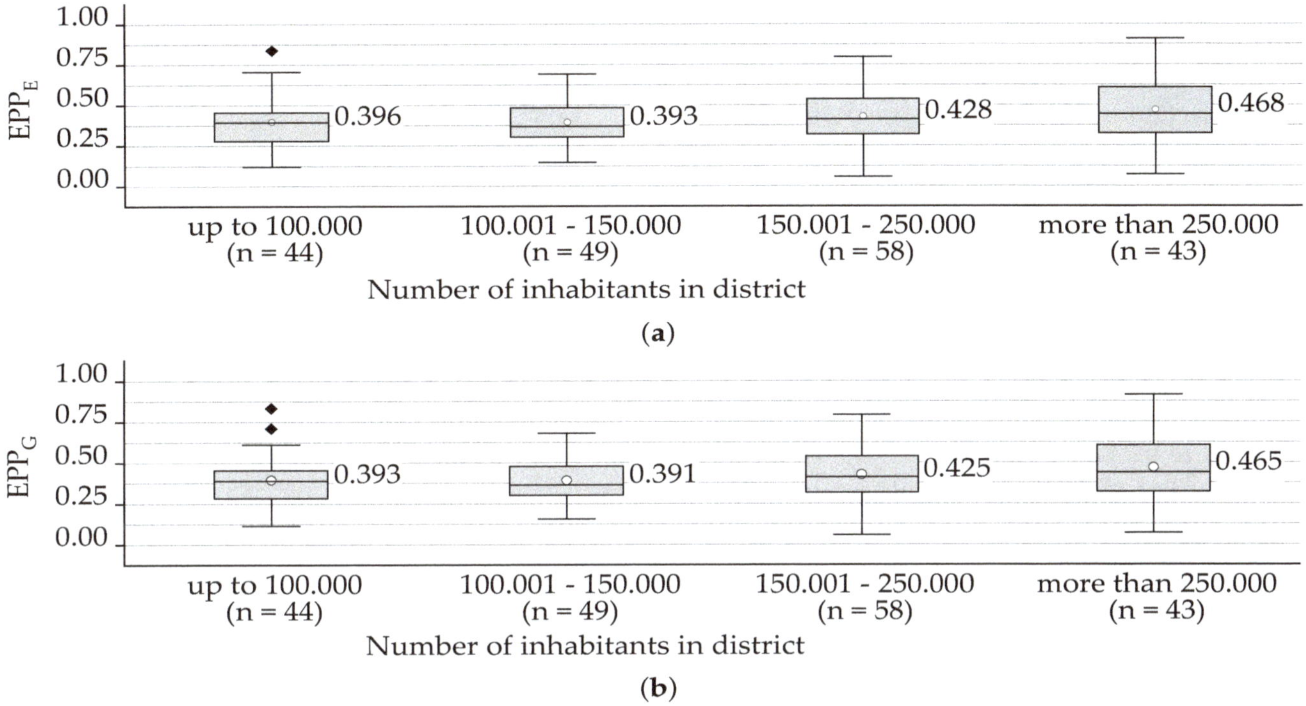

Figure 7. EPP according to the size of the districts. (**a**) Expert-based weighting of the main and sub-indicators; (**b**) Equally distributed weighting of the main and sub-indicators.

The mean values of the EPP_E and EPP_S for municipalities are 0.32. Some municipalities have thus already implemented certain aspects of emergency preparedness planning. However, these implementations are still in their beginnings. Differences between the EPP_E and EPP_S are only evident in a few cases (Figure 8), but do not show statistical significance ($p > 0.05$).

Municipalities with an increasing number of inhabitants achieve higher results in the EPP_E as well as in the EPP_S. The differences in the mean values between the size of the municipalities are significant ($p < 0.05$). However, the range of the EPP_E does not increase with a growing number of inhabitants in the municipality, which can be seen at the level of districts.

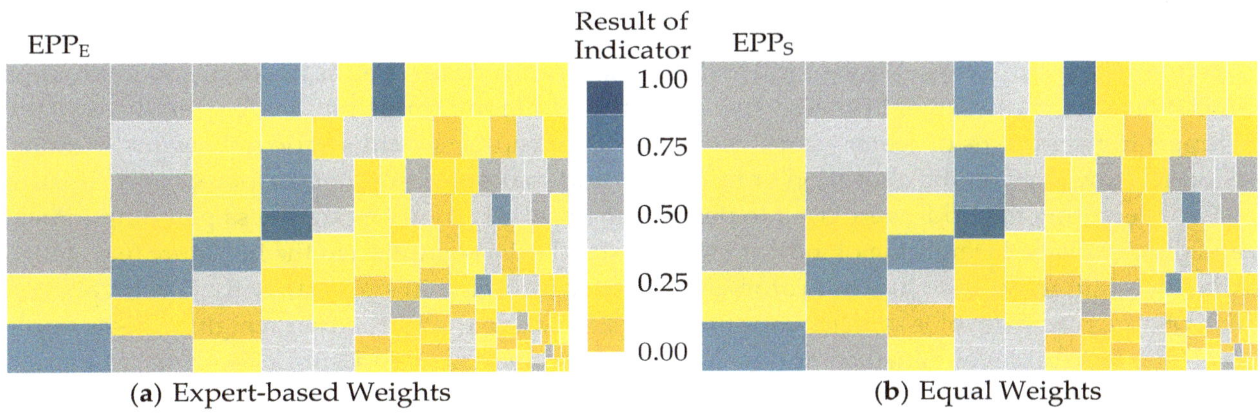

Figure 8. Emergency preparedness planning indicator by size of municipalities.

The Figure 9 shows the differences of the EPP_E and EPP_S between expert-based and equally distributed weighting. The colored variance of the rectangles shows that the different weightings affect the results of the EPP_E and EPP_S. In addition, the figure shows that the difference between EPP_E and EPP_S is in the range of ± 0.018 and is therefore only noticeable in a few cases when the result is rounded to the second decimal place.

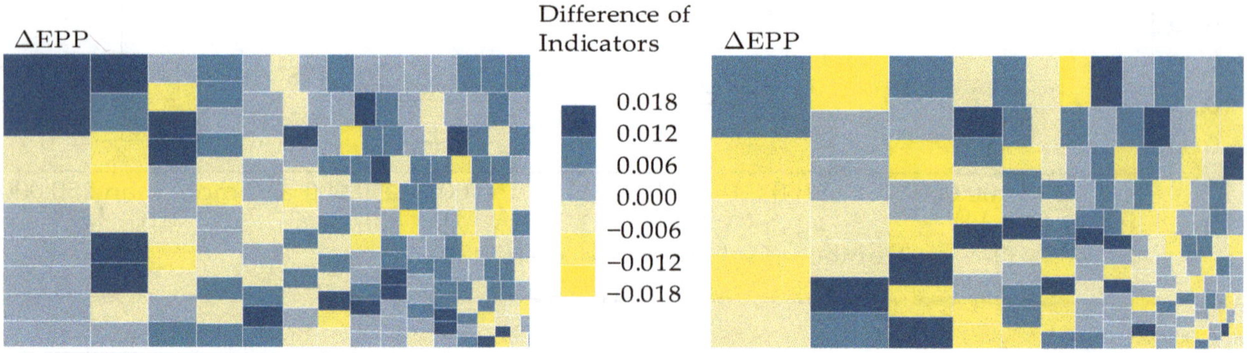

(a) Districts (b) Municipalities

Figure 9. Difference between the emergency preparedness planning indicators EPP_E and EPP_S according to the size of the data sets taken into account.

4. Discussion

4.1. Discussion of the Applied Methods

For effective planning and implementing of measures to increase the resilience of water supply systems, it is necessary to assess the status of emergency preparedness. The Emergency Preparedness Planning Indicator was developed to increase transparency by quantifying this assessment. The EPP was tested on the basis of the case study for its applicability and significance. The determination of the status of emergency preparedness planning was implemented by means of a data set of the research project NoWa I which is representative for Germany.

The composite indicator developed in this study enables a measurable assessment of the status of emergency preparedness planning. The main and sub indicators included are based on scientific publications (e.g., [12,14,17,23]), so that they reflect the current state of research on emergency preparedness planning. The development and application of the composite indicator is based on two main motivations. Firstly, the indicator can serve as a tool for self-assessment of emergency preparedness planning by asking specific questions. The self-assessment can be used by water utilities, regional or national authorities and municipalities to improve the prevention measures. The result of the indicator can also raise awareness of the relevance of emergency preparedness planning and show the need for action.

Secondly, the indicator supports local and regional authorities as well as national and international organisations in the assessment process, by comparing different municipalities, e.g., in the context of benchmarking processes of water supply systems. The results should support these institutions in decision-making, e.g., on the allocation of resources, and make them more transparent and consistent.

Two weighting methods were used to determine the emergency preparedness planning indicator. An equally distributed weighting of indicators is the standard assumption in the literature (e.g., [40,41]). If equal weightings are used, the indicators are either constructed in such a way that each variable or branch of a hierarchy level is equally weighted. To determine the EPP, equal weighting was applied to each hierarchical level. Furthermore, a weighting of the main and sub-indicators was applied based on expert knowledge. However, no strict participatory method has been applied here, where all weightings included are based on expert opinion [39]. This was only used for the weighting of the main and sub-indicators, but not for the individual indicators. For the individual indicators, aggregation at each level by arithmetic means was applied. Due to the different number of partial and individual indicators, they have a different weight despite their apparent equal weighting [42]. This also applies to the evaluated data set of the NoWa I project and must be taken into account when deriving the need for action.

The results show only minor differences with the two different weighting methods, both for the data set of the NoWa I project and the case study. Consequently the experts' opinions confirm the relevance of all five process steps of risk and crisis management according to [13,14]. In order to increase the acceptance of the indicator and to simplify the calculation, it is therefore recommended that the weighting be applied by using statistically equally distributed weights.

4.2. Discussion of the Indicator and Assessment Results

The results of the status of emergency preparedness planning for the case study show that some measures have already been implemented. An advanced state of implementation can be seen, particularly in the preliminary planning (1) and preventive measures (3). However, since the status of the risk analysis (2) still needs to be improved, the appropriate identification and implementation of preventive measures cannot be in a targeted manner. For this reason, the evaluation of the preventive measures (3) is necessary following the complete implementation of the risk analysis (2). Further action is needed in the area of crisis management (4). The sub-indicator results of this process step refer to the lowest level of implementation in the case study. However, since the crisis management (4) measures are based on the risk analysis (2) and the preventive measures (3), the implementation of a systematic approach step-by-step is an important prerequisite. Nevertheless, the individual process steps must still be evaluated and updated regularly.

The results of the composite indicator show a very heterogeneous picture with regard to the implementation status of emergency preparedness planning in the German water supply sector. The heterogeneity of the emergency preparedness planning indicator exists both in the districts and at the municipal level. Furthermore, the results of the respective five process steps are very diverse. Thus, some aspects of emergency preparedness planning have already been implemented. Nevertheless, implementation is still insufficient in some districts and municipalities.

The differentiation of districts or municipalities according to their number of inhabitants indicates that in both cases, larger municipalities have on average better emergency preparedness planning than smaller ones. Nevertheless, both groups contain outliers in both directions. Reasons for a more sophisticated emergency preparedness planning in larger municipalities may be, on the one hand, an extensive staffing or optimized structural conditions. On the other hand, the water supply in larger municipalities in Germany often lies in the responsibility of larger supply utilities, which often devote themselves more intensively to this task due to their corporate structure.

Indicator methods can reduce their usefulness for policy-makers or even lead to disadvantageous decision-making due to over-simplification of complex concepts and the use of aggregation procedures that are difficult to understand [43]. Although the answers to the questions used to determine the EPP are checklist-based self-assessments, the scope of the questions could lead to little attention being paid to the individual answers. The result of the case study shows that the procedure is applicable and the self-assessment questionnaire with 74 questions is appropriate. A shorter list of questions would lead to a less meaningful result.

The emergency preparedness planning indicator enables a quantitative comparison between municipalities or water supply utilities as well as the five process steps and the identification of the need for action. In the German water supply sector, the implementation of risk analysis should be emphasized. Preventive measures that have already been taken have to be checked for their appropriateness following the successful implementation of a risk analysis. Threshold values for sufficient or improvable emergency preparedness planning have to be defined. However, this cannot be achieved by science alone. This requires in particular a discourse between scientists, technical experts and political decision-makers.

5. Conclusions

Effective emergency preparedness planning is characterised, among other things, by the fact that its process steps can be carried out with foresight and the defined measures can be effectively put into practice in emergency situations. The five process steps of risk and crisis management have to be systematically taken into account.

The status of emergency preparedness planning in Germany was determined using a composite indicator. The data basis of the indicator system is formed by the case study of a water supply company and a survey of the NoWa I research project, which is representative for Germany. The results indicate a need for action in the different processes of emergency preparedness planning, because the process steps (1–5), especially risk analysis (2) are carried out rarely or insufficiently. However in the area of preliminary planning (1), numerous water supply companies and municipalities are already well positioned, and several preventive measures (3) are also being implemented. The regular evaluation (5) of these measures could be improved.

A need for action is especially identified in the development of practicable tools for implementation of an integrated risk and crisis management process in order to intensify the exchange of the relevant actors. Furthermore training in the area of risk and crisis management with the emphasis on extraordinary or extreme events should be conducted by water utilities and local authorities.

Author Contributions: Conceptualization: L.B., S.K., and I.W.; methodology: L.B. validation: S.K. and I.W.; formal analysis: S.K. and I.W.; investigation: L.B., I.W., and S.K.; resources: S.K. and I.W.; data curation: L.B.; writing—original draft preparation: L.B.; writing—review and editing: L.B., S.K., I.W.; visualization: L.B.; supervision: S.K. and I.W.; project administration: S.K. and I.W.; funding acquisition: S.K. All authors have read and agreed to the published version of the manuscript.

Acknowledgments: The authors would like to thank all those involved in the survey for their commitment and support. Furthermore, the authors would like to thank Salomé Parra and Christian Platschek, who laid the foundation for further work through their preliminary work within the framework of the NoWa I project, as well as Renate Solmsdorf, Sybille Rupertseder and Karolina Eggersdorfer, who helped to digitise the data sets. This study was supported by the Research Center RISK and the Bundeswehr University Munich.

Abbreviations

The following abbreviations are used in this manuscript:

CM	Crisis Management
E	Evaluation
EPP	Emergency Preparedness Planning Indicator
EPP_S	Emergency Preparedness Planning Indicator with statistical weights of main indicators
EPP_E	Emergency Preparedness Planning Indicator with weights based on expert knowledge
PM	Preventive Measures
PP	Preliminary Planning
RA	Risk Analysis
E	Evaluation

Appendix A

Table A1. Survey sheet to assess the Emergency Preparedness Planning Indicator—Part 1.

ID	Question	Reply Options	Source	Individual Indicator
	Main Indicator PP—Preliminary Planning			
	Sub Indicator PP_1—Awareness Raising			
1	Is it known how the supply zone is divided into municipalities or neighbourhoods?	Yes, partially, no	[14]	$VP_{1,1}$
2	Does the possible amount of water discharge correspond to the defined protection goals?	Yes, partially, no	[14]	$VP_{1,2}$
3	Is the technically maximum possible discharge quantity from the own extraction plant known?	Yes, partially, no	[14]	$VP_{1,3}$
4	Is the technically maximum possible water supply from other water utilities known?	Yes, partially, no	[14]	$VP_{1,4}$
5	Is the capacity of your own extraction plants known?	Yes, partially, no	[14]	$VP_{1,5}$
6	Is it known which part of the supply zone is supplied by which water extraction plant?	Yes, partially, no	[14]	$VP_{1,6}$
7	Is the following known for the individual tanks for water storage?			$VP_{1,7}$
7.1	Origin of water	Yes, partially, no	[14]	$VP_{1,7,1}$
7.2	Capacity of the storage tanks	Yes, partially, no	[14]	$VP_{1,7,2}$
7.3	max. possible feed-in quantity from the storage tanks into the grid	Yes, partially, no	[14]	$VP_{1,7,3}$
8	Is there an awareness in your community that there may be a quantitative impairment of the water supply?	Yes, partially, no	[14,21]	$VP_{1,8}$
9	Is there an awareness in your community that there may be a qualitative impairment of the water supply?	Yes, partially, no	[14,21]	$VP_{1,9}$
	Sub Indicator PP_2—Definition of Responsibilities			
10	Is it known who is the contact person for emergency situations in the water supply utility/ies?	Yes, partially, no	[12,14]	$VP_{2,1}$
11	Has a crisis task force been set up?	Yes, partially, no	[12,14]	$VP_{2,2}$
12	Is the organizational and operational structure defined?	Yes, partially, no	[12,14, 44]	$VP_{2,3}$

Table 2. Survey sheet to assess the Emergency Preparedness Planning Indicator—Part 2.

ID	Question	Reply Options	Source	Individual Indicator
	Main Indicator RA—Risk Analysis			
	Sub Indicator RA_1—Hazard Analysis			
13	Has a risk analysis been carried out?	Yes, partially, no	[14,17]	$RA_{1,1}$
14	Is there a list of which hazards have already been considered and which are not yet part of the risk analysis?	Yes, partially, no	[14]	$RA_{1,1}$
15	From the point of view of the water supply utility, do the following exceptional events represent relevant hazards for the water supply?		[14,24]	$RA_{1,2}$
15.1	Natural hazards	Yes, partially, no	[14,24]	$RA_{1,2,1}$
15.2	Accidents (human failures)	Yes, partially, no	[14,24]	$RA_{1,2,2}$
15.3	Accidents (technical failures)	Yes, partially, no	[14,24]	$RA_{1,2,3}$
15.4	Terrorism	Yes, partially, no	[14,24]	$RA_{1,2,4}$
16	Does the hazard analysis include experiences from past events?	Yes, partially, no	[14]	$RA_{1,3}$
17	Have qualitative impairments of the water supply occurred in the past so that substitute supply measures were necessary?	Yes, partially, no	[12,22]	$RA_{1,4}$
18	Have quantitative impairments of the water supply occurred in the past so that substitute supply measures were necessary?	Yes, partially, no	[12,22]	$RA_{1,5}$
19	Does the hazard analysis include other potential hazards that have not yet occurred?	Yes, partially, no	[14,17]	$RA_{1,6}$
20	Have hazards been identified that need to be prioritised?	Yes, partially, no	[14,17]	$RA_{1,7}$
	Sub Indicator RA_2—Vulnerability Analysis			
21	Has a vulnerability analysis been conducted?	Yes, partially, no	[14,17]	$RA_{2,1}$
22	Was the vulnerability analysis carried out in cooperation with water supply utilities and disaster management?	Yes, partially, no	[12,14]	$RA_{2,2}$
23	Have scenarios been identified for the vulnerability analysis?	Yes, partially, no	[12,14]	$RA_{2,3}$
24	Are the components to be analysed specified?	Yes, partially, no	[14]	$RA_{2,4}$
25	Have you checked which components would be exposed to which hazards (exposure)?	Yes, partially, no	[14]	$RA_{2,5}$
26	Has the functionality of the components been checked?	Yes, partially, no	[14]	$RA_{2,6}$
27	Has the technical replaceability of the components been checked?	Yes, partially, no	[14]	$RA_{2,7}$
28	Has the organizational replaceability of the components been checked?	Yes, partially, no	[14]	$RA_{2,8}$

Table 3. Survey sheet to assess the Emergency Preparedness Planning Indicator—Part 3.

ID	Question	Reply Options	Source	Individual Indicator
	Main Indicator RA—Risk Analysis			
	Sub Indicator RA_3—Risk Identification			
29	Was the risk assessment carried out with the involvement of specialist authorities or research institutions?	Yes, partially, no	[14]	$RA_{3,1}$
30	Has the extent of damage in the scenarios considered been determined?	Yes, partially, no	[14]	$RA_{3,2}$
31	Was the assessment of the extent of damage carried out with the involvement of those responsible for civil protection in the county/city?	Yes, partially, no	[14]	$RA_{3,3}$
32	Was the probability of occurrence determined in the scenarios considered?	Yes, partially, no	[14,21,45]	$RA_{3,4}$
33	Was the probability of occurrence carried out with the involvement of specialist authorities or research institutions?	Yes, partially, no	[16]	$RA_{3,5}$
34	Was the number of inhabitants affected in the scenarios considered determined?	Yes, partially, no	[14]	$RA_{3,6}$
35	Has the probability of occurrence and the extent of damage been classified on a scale (e.g., according to [14])?	Yes, partially, no	[14]	$RA_{3,7}$
	Sub Indicator RA_4—Risk Comparison and Evaluation			
36	Were the scenarios compared using a risk matrix?	Yes, partially, no	[14]	$RA_{4,1}$
37	Were the scenarios prioritized using a risk matrix?	Yes, partially, no	[14]	$RA_{4,2}$

Table 4. Survey sheet to assess the Emergency Preparedness Planning Indicator—Part 4.

ID	Question	Reply Options	Source	Individual Indicator
	Main Indicator PM—Preventive Measures			
	Sub Indicator PM_1—Structural Redundancies			
38	Are the extraction plants designed redundantly?	Yes, partially, no	[14]	$PM_{1,1}$
39	Are the storage tanks designed redundantly?	Yes, partially, no	[17]	$PM_{1,2}$
39.1	quantitatively redundant?	Yes, partially, no	[14]	$PM_{1,2,1}$
39.2	structurally redundant?	Yes, partially, no	[14]	$PM_{1,2,2}$
	Sub Indicator PM_2—Interrelation of Supply			
40	Are there supply links with other water utilities?	Yes, partially, no	[14,26]	$PM_{2,1}$
	Sub Indicator PM_3—Grid Construction			
41	Are there supply links with other water utilities?	Yes, partially, no	[17,28]	$PM_{3,1}$
42	Have grid development measures, which are necessary to ensure security of supply, been implemented?	Yes, partially, no	[27]	$PM_{3,2}$
	Sub Indicator PM_4—Remote Monitoring, Control Systems			
43	Is the supply system connected to a remote monitoring system?	Yes, partially, no	[17,29,30]	$PM_{4,1}$
44	Is the supply system equipped with a state-of-the-art control system?	Yes, partially, no	[14]	$PM_{4,2}$
	Sub Indicator PM_5—General Measures			
45	Have renewal measures necessary to ensure security of supply been implemented?	Yes, partially, no	[17,32]	$PM_{5,1}$
46	Have maintenance measures necessary to ensure security of supply been implemented?	Yes, partially, no	[17,32]	$PM_{5,2}$
47	Have physical protection measures, which are necessary to ensure security of supply, been implemented?	Yes, partially, no	[14,31]	$PM_{5,3}$

Table 5. Survey sheet to assess the Emergency Preparedness Planning Indicator—Part 5.

ID	Question	Reply Options	Source	Individual Indicator
	Main Indicator CM—Crisis Management			
	Sub Indicator CM_1—Organisation and Coordination			
48	Does the water utility develop contingency plans in addition to the action plans according to the Drinking Water Ordinance?	Yes, partially, no	[14,35]	$CM_{1,1}$
49	Are contingency plans for emergency situations in the water supply developed by the civil protection authority?	Yes, partially, no	[14,35]	$CM_{1,2}$
50	Are you familiar with the content of these plans?	Yes, partially, no	[14,34]	$CM_{1,2}$
51	Are the contact details of the following contact persons known?	Yes, partially, no		$CM_{1,3}$
51.1	Water utility	Yes, no	[17,23]	$CM_{1,3,1}$
51.2	Emergency management / civil protection	Yes, no	[17,23]	$CM_{1,3,2}$
51.3	Principal administrator	Yes, no	[14]	$CM_{1,3,3}$
51.4	Fire department	Yes, no	[12]	$CM_{1,3,4}$
51.5	Federal Agency for Technical Relief	Yes, no	[12]	$CM_{1,3,5}$
51.6	Red Cross	Yes, no	[12]	$CM_{1,3,6}$
51.7	Civil-Military Cooperation	Yes, no	[12]	$CM_{1,3,7}$
51.8	National Command	Yes, no	[12]	$CM_{1,3,8}$
51.9	Other authorities (e.g., health, environment, police)	Yes, no	[12]	$CM_{1,3,9}$
51.10	Press	Yes, no	[12]	$CM_{1,3,10}$
52	Are sensitive facilities available in the supply area?		[14]	$CM_{1,4}$
52.1	Hospital	Yes, no		$CM_{1,4,1}$
52.2	Nursing home	Yes, no		$CM_{1,4,2}$
52.3	Kindergarten/School	Yes, no		$CM_{1,4,3}$
52.4	Dialysis centers	Yes, no		$CM_{1,4,4}$
53	Are sensitive facilities in the supply area included?		[14]	$CM_{1,5}$
53.1	Hospital	Yes, partially, no		$CM_{1,5,1}$
53.2	Nursing home	Yes, partially, no		$CM_{1,5,2}$
53.3	Kindergarten/School	Yes, partially, no		$CM_{1,5,3}$
53.4	Dialysis centers	Yes, partially, no		$CM_{1,5,4}$
54	Are the telephone number, location and capacity of the following facilities in the district/district free city recorded?		[12]	$CM_{1,6}$
54.1	Brewery/beverage manufacturer	Yes, partially, no		$CM_{1,6,1}$
54.1.1	telephone number	Yes, partially, no		$CM_{1,6,1,1}$
54.1.2	location	Yes, partially, no		$CM_{1,6,1,2}$
54.1.3	capacity	Yes, partially, no		$CM_{1,6,1,3}$
54.2	Beverage suppliers (beverage market)			$CM_{1,6,2}$
54.2.1	telephone number	Yes, partially, no		$CM_{1,6,2,1}$
54.2.2	location	Yes, partially, no		$CM_{1,6,2,2}$
54.2.3	capacity	Yes, partially, no		$CM_{1,6,2,3}$
54.3	Carriers			$CM_{1,6,3}$
54.3.1	telephone number	Yes, partially, no		$CM_{1,6,3,1}$
54.3.2	location	Yes, partially, no		$CM_{1,6,3,2}$
54.3.3	capacity	Yes, partially, no		$CM_{1,6,3,3}$
54.4	Neighbouring Utilities			$CM_{1,6,4}$
54.4.1	telephone number	Yes, partially, no		$CM_{1,6,4,1}$
54.4.2	location	Yes, partially, no		$CM_{1,6,4,2}$
54.4.3	capacity	Yes, partially, no		$CM_{1,6,4,3}$

Table 6. Survey sheet to assess the Emergency Preparedness Planning Indicator—Part 6.

ID	Question	Reply Options	Source	Individual Indicator
	Main Indicator CM—Crisis Management			
	Sub Indicator CM_2—Provision of Resources			
55	Are the resources required for the substitute water supply (mobile treatment plants, mobile pipelines, transport vehicles) kept available or is access to them ensured?	Yes, partially, no	[14]	$CM_{2,1}$
56	Are the materials required for the substitute water supply (pressure increasing systems, hose connections, etc.) kept in stock or is access ensured?	Yes, partially, no	[14]	$CM_{2,2}$
	Sub Indicator CM_3—Exercises			
57	Was the interaction with the authorities and organisations involved in the event of a crisis in the water supply discussed?	Yes, partially, no	[14,17,23]	$CM_{3,1}$
58	Has the interaction with the authorities and organisations involved been practised for crisis situations in the water supply?	Yes, partially, no	[14,17,23]	$CM_{3,2}$
	Sub Indicator CM_4—Communication			
59	Is access to communication media ensured in the event of a crisis?	Yes, partially, no	[14,17,36]	$CM_{4,1}$

Table 7. Survey sheet to assess the Emergency Preparedness Planning Indicator—Part 7.

ID	Question	Reply Options	Source	Individual Indicator
	Main Indicator E—Evaluation			
	Sub Indicator E_1—Evaluation Preliminary Planning			
60	Are the awareness raising aspects regularly evaluated?	Yes, partially, no	[14,17]	$E_{1,1}$
61	Are the definitions of responsibilities regularly evaluated?	Yes, partially, no	[14,17]	$E_{1,2}$
	Sub Indicator E_2—Evaluation Risk Analysis			
62	Is the hazard analysis regularly evaluated?	Yes, partially, no	[14,17]	$E_{2,1}$
63	Is the vulnerability analysis regularly evaluated?	Yes, partially, no	[14,17]	$E_{2,2}$
64	Is the risk identification regularly evaluated?	Yes, partially, no	[14,17]	$E_{2,3}$
65	Are the risk comparison and evaluation regularly evaluated?	Yes, partially, no	[14,17]	$E_{2,4}$
	Sub Indicator E_3—Evaluation Preventive Measures			
66	Are the structural redundancies regularly evaluated?	Yes, partially, no	[14,17]	$E_{3,1}$
67	Are the interrelations of supply regularly evaluated?	Yes, partially, no	[14,17]	$E_{3,2}$
68	Are the grid construction measures regularly evaluated?	Yes, partially, no	[14,17]	$E_{3,3}$
69	Are the remote monitoring and control systems regularly evaluated?	Yes, partially, no	[14,17]	$E_{3,4}$
70	Are the general measures regularly evaluated?	Yes, partially, no	[14,17]	$E_{3,5}$
	Sub Indicator E_4—Evaluation Crisis Management			
71	Are the organisation and coordination measures regularly evaluated?	Yes, partially, no	[14,17]	$E_{4,1}$
72	Is the provision of resources regularly evaluated?	Yes, partially, no	[14,17]	$E_{4,2}$
73	Are the exercised regularly evaluated?	Yes, partially, no	[14,17]	$E_{4,3}$
74	Are the communication measures regularly evaluated?	Yes, partially, no	[14,17]	$E_{4,4}$

References

1. Sowby, R.B. Emergency preparedness after COVID-19: A review of policy statements for the U.S. water sector. *Util. Policy* **2020**, *64*, 101058. [CrossRef] [PubMed]
2. Haakh, F.; Merkel, W. Die Wasserversorgung im COVID-19 Krisenmanagement: Systemanalyse und Szenarienplanung. *Energie Wasser-Praxis* **2020**, *71*, 34–41.
3. Mays, L.W. *Water Supply Systems Security*; McGraw-Hill Professional Engineering Civil Engineering; McGraw-Hill: New York, NY, USA, 2004.
4. States, S. *Security and Emergency Planning for Water and Wastewater Utilities*; American Water Works Association: Denver, CO, USA, 2010.
5. Gopalakrishnan, K.; Peeta, S. *Sustainable and Resilient Critical Infrastructure Systems: Simulation, Modeling, and Intelligent Engineering*; Springer: Berlin/Heidelberg, Germany, 2010. [CrossRef]
6. Grigg, N.S. Water Utility Security: Multiple Hazards and Multiple Barriers. *J. Infrastruct. Syst.* **2003**, *9*, 81–88. [CrossRef]
7. Spellman, F.R. *Water Infrastructure Protection and Homeland Security*; Government Institutes: Lanham, MD, USA, 2007.
8. Mendonça, D.; Wallace, W.A. Impacts of the 2001 World Trade Center Attack on New York City Critical Infrastructures. *J. Infrastruct. Syst.* **2006**, *12*, 260–270. [CrossRef]
9. Mendonça, D.; Wallace, W.A. Adaptive Capacity: Electric Power Restoration in New York City following the 11 September 2001 Attacks. In Proceedings of the 2nd Symposium on Resilience Engineering, Juan-les-Pins, France, 8–10 November 2006.
10. Nelson, D.R.; Adger, W.N.; Brown, K. Adaptation to Environmental Change: Contributions of a Resilience Framework. *Annu. Rev. Environ. Resour.* **2007**, *32*, 395–419. [CrossRef]
11. World Health Organization. *Environmental Health in Emergencies and Disasters: A Practical Guide*; World Health Organization: Geneva, Switzerland, 2002.
12. Bross, L.; Wienand, I.; Krause, S. *Sicherheit der Trinkwasserversorgung: Teil 2: Notfallvorsorgeplanung*; Praxis im Bevölkerungsschutz; Bundesamt für Bevölkerungsschutz und Katastrophenhilfe: Bonn, Germany, 2019; Volume 15.
13. Bundesministerium des Innern, für Bau und Heimat. *Schutz Kritischer Infrastrukturen—Risiko- und Krisenmanagement · Leitfaden für Unternehmen und Behörden*; Bundesministerium des Innern, für Bau und Heimat: Bonn, Germany, 2011.
14. Wienand, I.; Hasch, M. *Sicherheit der Trinkwasserversorgung: Teil 1: Risikoanalyse*; Praxis im Bevölkerungsschutz, Bundesamt für Bevölkerungsschutz und Katastrophenhilfe: Bonn, Germany, 2016; Volume 15.
15. Bundesamt für Bevölkerungsschutz und Katastrophenhilfe. *Schutz Kritischer Infrastruktur: Risikomanagement im Krankenhaus*; Praxis im Bevölkerungsschutz; Bundesamt für Bevölkerungsschutz und Katastrophenhilfe: Bonn, Germany, 2008; Volume 2.
16. Bundesamt für Bevölkerungsschutz und Katastrophenhilfe. *Risikoanalyse im Bevölkerungsschutz: Ein Stresstest für die Allgemeine Gefahrenabwehr und den Katastrophenschutz*; Bundesamt für Bevölkerungsschutz und Katastrophenhilfe: Bonn, Germany, 2015.
17. AWWA. *M19 Emergency Planning for Water and Wastewater Utilities*, 5th ed.; American Water Works Association: Denver, CO, USA, 2018.
18. Organisation for Economic Co-operation and Development. *Handbook on Constructing Composite Indicators: Methodology and User Guide*; Organisation for Economic Co-operation and Development: Paris, France, 2008.
19. Bollin, C.; Hidajat, R. Community-Basded Risk Index: Pilot Implementation in Indonesia. In *Measuring Vulnerability to Natural Hazards. Towards Disaster Resilient Societies*; Birkmann, J., Ed.; United Nations University Press: Tokyo, Japan; New York, NY, USA, 2006; pp. 271–289.
20. Joerin, J.; Shaw, R.; Takeuchi, Y.; Krishnamurthy, R. The adoption of a climate disaster resilience index in Chennai, India. *Disasters* **2014**, *38*, 540–561. [CrossRef] [PubMed]
21. DIN EN 15975-2. *Sicherheit der Trinkwasserversorgung—Leitlinien für das Risiko- und Krisenmanagement—Teil 2: Risikomanagement*; Springer Vieweg: Berlin/Heidelberg, Germany, 2013.

22. Bross, L.; Krause, S.; Wannewitz, M.; Stock, E.; Sandholz, S.; Wienand, I. Insecure Security: Emergency Water Supply and Minimum Standards in Countries with a High Supply Reliability. *Water* **2019**, *11*, 732. [CrossRef]
23. AWWA. *G440 Emergency Preparedness Practices*; AWWA: Singapore, 2017.
24. AWWA. *J100 Risk and Resilience Management of Water and Wastewater Systems*; AWWA: Singapore, 2010.
25. DIN ISO 31000. *Risikomanagement*; Walter de Gruyter GmbH & Co KG: Berlin, Germany, 2018.
26. Boyle, D.B. Interagency Connections: Insurance Against Interruptions in Supply. *J. Am. Water Works Assoc.* **1980**, *72*, 192–195. [CrossRef]
27. Hoch, W. Planungsgrundsätze für das Bemessen von Wasserverteilungsnetzen unter Berücksichtigung der Löschwasserversorgung. In *Wassertransport und -Verteilung*; Sattler, R., Hirner, W., Eds.; DVGW Lehr- und Handbuch Wasserversorgung, Oldenbourg: München, Germany, 1999; pp. 85–123.
28. Baur, A.; Fritsch, P.; Hoch, W.; Merkl, G.; Rautenberg, J.; Weiß, M.; Wricke, B. *Mutschmann/Stimmelmayr Taschenbuch der Wasserversorgung*, 17th ed.; Springer Vieweg: Wiesbaden, Germany, 2019. [CrossRef]
29. Mehlhorn, H.; Weiß, M. Fernleitungssysteme. In *Wassertransport und -Verteilung*; Sattler, R., Hirner, W., Eds.; DVGW Lehr- und Handbuch Wasserversorgung, Oldenbourg: München, Germany, 1999; pp. 123–169.
30. Grombach, P.; Haberer, K.; Merkl, G. *Handbuch der Wasserversorgungstechnik*, 3rd ed.; Oldenbourg-Industrieverlag: München, Germany, 2000.
31. DVGW W 1050. Objektschutz von Wasserversorgungsanlagen. 2012. Available online: http://www.dwa.de/dwa/sitemapping.nsf/literaturvorschau?openform&bestandsnr=57260 (accessed on 1 September 2020).
32. Schlicht, H. Instandhaltung von Wasserverteilungsnetzen. In *Wassertransport und -Verteilung*; Sattler, R., Hirner, W., Eds.; DVGW Lehr- und Handbuch Wasserversorgung, Oldenbourg: München, Germany, 1999; pp. 373–403.
33. Morley, K.; Riordan, R. *Utilities Helping Utilities: An Action Plan for Mutial Aid and Assistance Networks for Water and Wastewater Utilities*; American Water Works Association: Singapore, 2006.
34. Doe, S.R.K.; Whitman, B.E. *Security and Emergency Management for Water Systems*, 1st ed.; Bentley Institute Press: Exton, PA, USA, 2011.
35. DVGW W 1020. Empfehlungen und Hinweise für den Fall von Abweichungen von Anforderungen der Trinkwasserverordnung; Maßnahmeplan und Handlungsplan. 2018. Available online: https://shop.wvgw.de/var/assets/leseprobe//510186_lp_W%201020_2018_03.pdf (accessed on 1 September 2020).
36. United States Environmental Protection Agency. *Effective Risk and Crisis Communication during Water Security Emergencies: Summary Report of EPA Sponsored Message Mapping Workshops*; United States Environmental Protection Agency: Washington, DC, USA, 2007.
37. Bundesministerium des Innern, für Bau und Heimat. *Leitfaden Krisenkommunikation*, 5th ed.; Bundesministerium des Innern, für Bau und Heimat: Bonn, Germany, 2014.
38. AWWA. *G430 Security Practices for Operation and Management*; AWWA: Singapore, 2015.
39. Asadzadeh, A.; Kötter, T.; Salehi, P.; Birkmann, J. Operationalizing a concept: The systematic review of composite indicator building for measuring community disaster resilience. *Int. J. Disaster Risk Reduct.* **2017**, *25*, 147–162. [CrossRef]
40. Islam, M.S.; Swapan, M.S.H.; Haque, S.M. Disaster risk index: How far should it take account of local attributes? *Int. J. Disaster Risk Reduct.* **2013**, *3*, 76–87. [CrossRef]
41. Lazarus, N.W. Coping capacities and rural livelihoods: Challenges to community risk management in Southern Sri Lanka. *Appl. Geogr.* **2011**, *31*, 20–34. [CrossRef]
42. Beccari, B. A Comparative Analysis of Disaster Risk, Vulnerability and Resilience Composite Indicators. *PLoS Curr.* **2016**, *8*. [CrossRef] [PubMed]
43. Balica, S. Approaches of understanding developments of vulnerability indices for natural disasters. *J. Environ. Eng.* **2012**, *11*, 963–974. [CrossRef]
44. DIN EN 15975-1. Sicherheit der Trinkwasserversorgung—Leitlinien für das Risiko- und Krisenmanagement—Teil 1: Krisenmanagement. 2016. Available online: https://www.boutique.afnor.org/standard/din-en-15975-1/security-of-drinking-water-supply-guidelines-for-risk-and-crisis-management-part-1-crisis-management-german-version-en-15975-120/article/852388/eu139819 (accessed on 1 September 2020).
45. AWWA. *Planning for an Emergency Drinking Water Supply*; U.S. Environmental Protection Agency's National Homeland Security Research Center: Manila, Philippines, 2011.

5

Is "Perceived Water Insecurity" Associated with Disaster Risk Perception, Preparedness Attitudes and Coping Ability in Rural China? (A Health-EDRM Pilot Study)

Janice Ying-en Ho [1], Emily Ying Yang Chan [1,2,*], Holly Ching Yu Lam [2], May Pui Shan Yeung [1], Carol Ka Po Wong [2] and Tony Ka Chun Yung [2]

1 Division of Global Health and Humanitarian Medicine, Jockey Club School of Public Health and Primary Care, The Chinese University of Hong Kong, Hong Kong; janice.ho@link.cuhk.edu.hk (J.Y.H.); may.yeung@cuhk.edu.hk (M.P.S.Y.)

2 Collaborating Centre for Oxford University and CUHK for Disaster and Medical Humanitarian Response, The Chinese University of Hong Kong, Hong Kong; hollylam@cuhk.edu.hk (H.C.Y.L.); wongcarol@cuhk.edu.hk (C.K.P.W.); yungtony@cuhk.edu.hk (T.K.C.Y.)

* Correspondence: emily.chan@cuhk.edu.hk

Abstract: Water security is essential for maintaining health and well-being, and for reducing a population's vulnerability in a disaster. Among resource-poor villagers in China, water-related disasters and climate change may increasingly affect people's water security. The purpose of this study was to explore the relationship between perceived water security and disaster risk perception in a rural ethnic minority community. A cross-sectional household survey was conducted in 2015 in Xingguang village, Chongqing, China, examining the association between villagers' perceptions of household water security, disaster risk, and sociodemographic variables. Among 52 household representatives, 84.6% relied on rainwater as their main water source and 63.5% reported having insufficient water on a regular basis. Only 32.7% perceived themselves to be living in a high-risk area, of which climate-related disasters such as storms (44.4%) and droughts (38.9%) were the most frequently reported disasters in their area. Insufficient water quantity, previous disaster experience, and household members on chronic disease medication were found to be associated with higher disaster risk perception. Perceived water security indicators were not found to be predictors of preparedness attitudes and coping ability. Addressing water sufficiency in both disaster risk reduction strategies and long-term water management will be necessary to improve the health and livelihood of rural villagers in the coming decades.

Keywords: water security; disaster risk; risk perception; rural; China; Health-EDRM

---

1. Introduction

Water is a basic necessity of life and health, with communities requiring the provision of accessible safe drinking water at an affordable cost to meet their basic needs [1]. Lack of access to clean adequate water supplies is an indirect contributing risk factor of disaster through poorer hygiene and water-related diseases that diminish health and increase a population's vulnerability. On the contrary, adequate water supplies enable households to not only have enough for personal consumption and hygiene but also to build livelihoods, invest in opportune projects, and facilitate community development and poverty eradication [2] (pp. 5, 22). This capacity "to safeguard sustainable access to adequate quantities of acceptable quality water for sustaining livelihoods, human well-being and socio-economic development" is also known as water security [1]. Maintaining water security in communities not only protects health and sustains development but can also help reduce a population's vulnerability and increase the resilience of households when disaster inevitably strikes. Water-related disasters comprise 90% of the world's natural disasters [3]. Disasters such as floods, droughts, and storms can greatly affect communities in their development, livelihoods, and health. At the intersection of health and disaster risk reduction is the emerging field of Health Emergency Disaster Risk Management (Health-EDRM), which emphasizes the need to understand the direct and indirect health risks of hazards and to use multisectoral approaches to strengthen evidence-based guidelines and build community health resilience [4]. Health risks in emergencies and disasters should be minimized through a systematic analysis and management of risks across the entire disaster cycle, which should include considerations of the following aspects: "(1) hazard and vulnerability reduction to prevent and mitigate risks, (2) preparedness, (3), response, and (4) recovery measures" [5]. In terms of water, if a community already experiences water insecurity prior to a disaster, this problem will be magnified when sudden or slow-onset disastrous events occur, thus affecting the vulnerability status, preparedness, response, and recovery in a disaster. Inadequate water security and unreliable water systems could compound disaster risk [6–8] and have a direct effect on disaster response if water systems fail when they are most needed for survival after a disaster [8] and for emergency healthcare and infrastructural services [9]. A community's water security is also vulnerable to disaster impacts, as water systems or sources may be damaged by the disasters [6]. Especially with climate change, which will disrupt the hydrological cycle and heighten the frequency and intensity of hydro-meteorological hazards [10], the water security of many communities will be left increasingly at risk unless they take adaptation measures.

Disaster risk perception is an intuitive judgement made by lay persons and may be divergent from objective scientific assessments of disaster risk [11]. In terms of water-related disaster risks such as floods, risk perception research is still in its infancy and many studies take on a non-theoretical approach to risk perception, although measures such as risk characteristics, coping abilities, and preparedness attitudes are often assessed [12]. Research has found risk perception to be affected by prior disaster experience and trust in authorities, with less consistent associations with socio-demographic characteristics, cultural factors, and the influence of media [12,13]. However, environmental conditions and external physical factors have rarely been assessed in relation to a person's risk perception, and water security has not been suggested amongst such contextual factors.

As securing water at the household level is a cornerstone and foundation to water security [2], there is a need to understand the water insecurity and disaster risk perception at the household and community level. This is particularly true in the context of a rural village, where water systems may be decentralized, thus leaving room for variability amongst different households. Increased reliability and provision of water service can increase the adaptive capacity of a household in the face of disaster impacts and improve household resilience [2]. By understanding the linkage between communities' water security and disaster risk perception, this can empower the development of water resources management with a consideration towards disaster risk reduction and climate adaptation, contributing to the emergency resilience of the communities [2,14].

As water insecurity problems in a community could be magnified in the occurrence of disasters, this paper seeks to explore the current state of perceived household water security and disaster risk among an ethnic minority village community in Chongqing, China. Perceived water security is measured in this study through self-reported responses adapted from WHO 2011 Guidelines for drinking water quality, 4th Ed. Vol 1 [15]. The aim of this study is to assess the associations of disaster risk perception with perceived water security indicators and socio-demographic characteristics. The study hypothesized that in a rural water-scarce area, perceived water insecurity would be associated with greater disaster risk perception, preparedness attitudes, and coping ability.

Our study was conducted during a health needs assessment trip to Xingguang village in Lutang Township, Pengshui Miao and Tujia Autonomous County, Chongqing Direct-Controlled Municipality, China. In a recent climate change impact assessment, Chongqing was identified as highly vulnerable to future climate change impacts, especially in terms of its water resources [16]. Located in a disaster-prone region, the local community has had frequent exposure to hydro-meteorological risks such as drought, landslides, floods, and storms. The rural village has a largely decentralized water system, and individual households often rely on rooftop collection of rainwater. The village is administratively divided into nine sub-villages and has a total population of approximately 2000 villagers, with average incomes around the international poverty line ($1.90 USD per day per person). It is also ethnically diverse, with minorities such as the Miao (苗族) and Tujia (土家族) ethnicities, as well as the majority ethnicity of Han Chinese.

2. Materials and Methods

A pilot cross-sectional stratified sample household survey was conducted in the Xingguang village community in Lutang Township, Chongqing China in February 2015. Households were stratified according to their sub-village and surveys were completed in all nine sub-villages. Within each cluster, we aimed to reach a 10% representation of each sub-village population by simple random sampling. This sampling format is similar to other studies conducted elsewhere [17,18] and enables a representative understanding of different locations throughout the village, limiting the over-accumulation of household surveys from one or two sub-villages. However, this method only takes characteristics of the individual village into account, thus limiting generalizability to other villages. Trained interviewers conducted the face-to-face surveys with each household representative, with the language support of local translators. Each interview took approximately 20–30 minutes. Verbal consent was obtained from all participants. Ethics approval was obtained from the Survey and Behavioural Research Ethics Committee of the Chinese University of Hong Kong. All data were double entered and cleaned by trained staff.

The survey questionnaire of the health needs assessment consisted of 10 sections, with this analysis focusing on the data provided from three sections, namely, (1) respondent background and household characteristics, (2) water and sanitation, and (3) disaster risk perception. The respondent background and household characteristics section included sociodemographic measures such as ethnicity, gender, position as household head, age, education level, occupation, main source of income, annual household income, migrant workers in family, household members with chronic disease, and household members on chronic disease medication. Annual income per capita was calculated by dividing the annual household income by the total number of household members. The water and sanitation section was comprised of general indicators (main source of drinking water, storage of water) and self-reported water security indicators adapted from WHO 2011 Guidelines for drinking-water quality [15]: quality (measured as protection of water source, and boiling of drinking water), quantity (sufficiency of water), accessibility (time needed to fetch water), affordability (money spent on water), and reliability of water (stability of water supply). The outcomes assessed in the disaster risk perception section included the following measures: risk perception (perception of living in a high-risk disaster area), preparedness attitudes (measured as importance of keeping extra medication for a disaster [19], and the necessity of a disaster bag [20]), and coping ability (perceived ability to protect their family's health and safety in the case of a disaster). The measure of previous personal disaster experience, which was also from this section, was included in the analyses as an exposure.

Descriptive analyses were conducted on the perceptions of water security, disaster risk, and sociodemographic variables. Variables were simplified into binary categorical variables for the univariate analysis. Univariate analyses were conducted using Chi-squared test on the disaster risk perception variables, as associated with subjective water security indicators and sociodemographic variables. A backward stepwise multivariable logistic regression was conducted for each of the disaster risk perception outcomes, which included sociodemographic variables of age, gender, education, and annual per capita income, and variables with $p < 0.2$ in the univariate analyses. After the significant variables were identified in the backward models, the models were re-run while controlling for age and gender. These final models, inclusive of significant variables from the backward logistic regressions and controlled for age and gender, are reported in this paper. Significance level for the multivariable analyses was set at $p \leq 0.05$. All statistical analyses used SPSS version 20.0 (SPSS Inc., Chicago, IL, USA).

3. Results

3.1. Descriptive Analyses

Around the time of the survey, Xingguang village was reported to include 540 households and approximately 2300 residents [21]. Our final study sample was comprised of 52 household representatives from the village community. The sociodemographic characteristics of the surveyed households are shown in Table 1. The median household size was five members, and the median annual household income was 20,000 RMB (equivalent to ~$2940 USD). After calculations, the median annual income per capita was 3571 RMB (equivalent to ~$525 USD).

Table 1. Sociodemographic characteristics of participants and their households in Xingguang village, Chongqing, China ($N = 52$).

Participants	n	%	Households	n	%
Gender			**Main source of household income**		
Male	36	69.2	Farming	25	48.1
Female	16	30.8	Working	25	48.1
Age			Others	2	3.8
16–24	6	11.5	**Annual income per capita ($N = 43$)**		
25–44	16	30.8	≤2500 RMB (≤$1 USD/day)	18	41.9
45–64	23	44.2	2501–5000 RMB (≤$2 USD/day)	10	23.3
≥65	7	13.5	5001–7500 RMB (≤$3 USD/day)	7	16.3
Ethnicity			>7500 RMB (>$3 USD/day)	8	18.6
Miao	11	21.2			
Tujia	4	7.7	**Household members who are ...**		
Han	37	71.2	**Migrant workers**		
Household Head			None	5	9.6
Yes	32	61.5	1	25	48.1
No	20	38.5	2	13	25.0
Education			3–5	9	17.3
No Schooling	7	13.5	**With chronic disease**		
Primary School	21	40.4	Yes	35	67.3
Middle School	16	30.8	No	17	32.7
High School	5	9.6	**On chronic disease medication ($N = 47$)**		
College or Higher	3	5.8	Yes	22	46.8
Occupation [1]			No	25	53.2
Farmer	21	40.4			
Employee	15	28.8			
Others	16	30.7			

[1] Other occupations included the following: business person, teacher, student, household work, unemployed, and retired.

Indicators of perceived water security among the surveyed households are shown in Figure 1. Most of the participants used rainwater as their main source of drinking water (84.6%) and reported having an unreliable (37.3% often no water or 54.9% occasionally no water) and insufficient (63.5%) quantity of water. Only 5.8% of respondents had a protected water source and, although half of the households stored their water, less than half of those that stored their water kept the water container covered (38.4%, $N = 10/26$). However, over 70% of the households did not need to use money to buy water (76.9%), had access within 5 minutes (76.9%, $N = 48$), and boiled their water (73.1%).

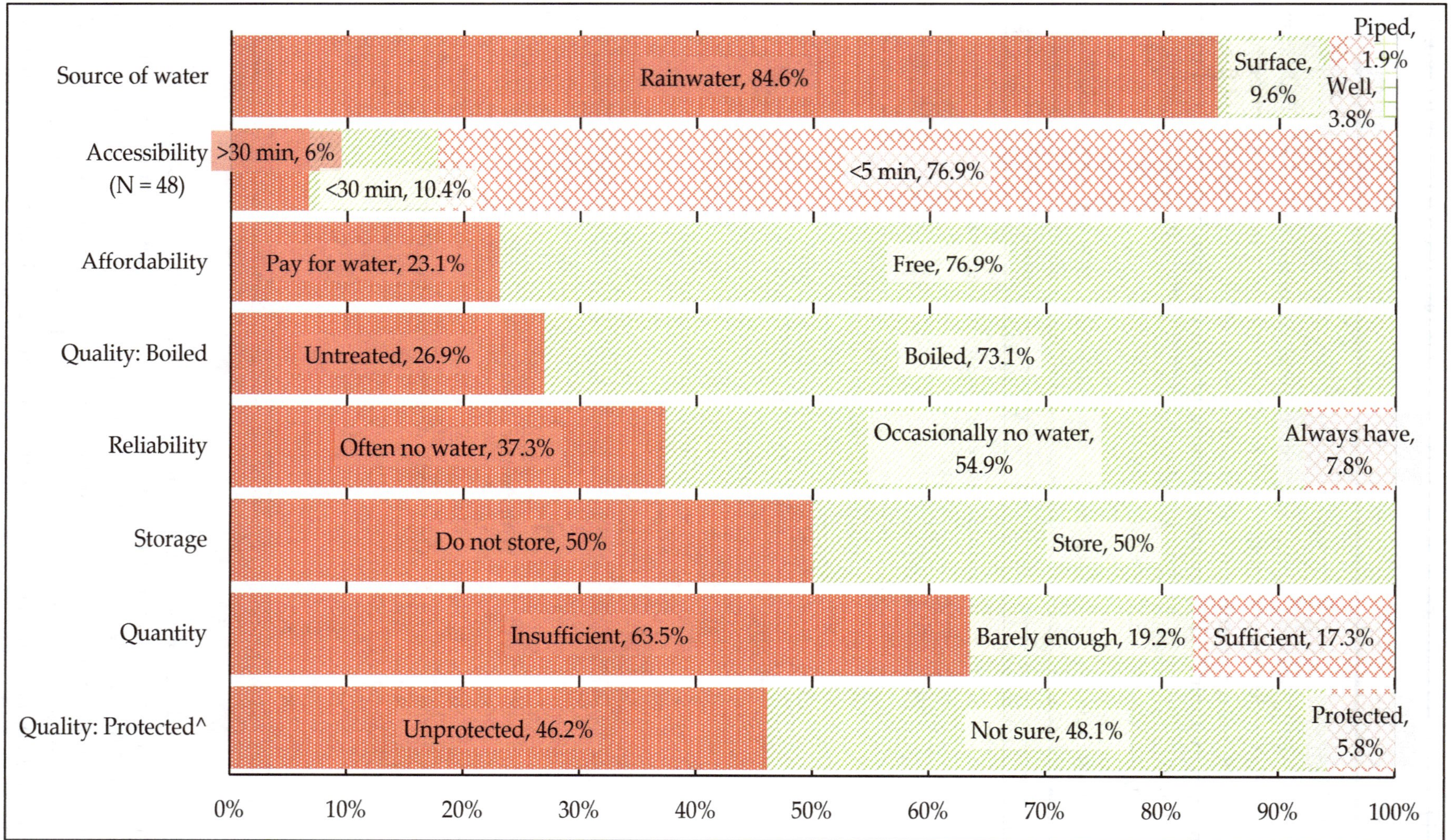

Figure 1. Descriptive statistics of water security indicators adapted from WHO guidelines [15] among households in the Xingguang village community, Chongqing, China (N = 52). ^ Protection indicates that the water source quality was protected from runoff water, bird droppings, and animals with a well-lining or casting, and a cover.

In terms of disaster risk perception indicators, over half of the respondents (60.8%) reported to have personally experienced a disaster during their lifetime, namely, floods (25.8%), storms (25.8%), snowstorms (22.6%), or droughts (12.9%), among others. However, only 32.7% of respondents believed they were living in a high-risk disaster area, of which storms (44.4%), droughts (38.9%), floods (22.2%), and snowstorms (11.1%) were the most frequently reported disasters in their area. In terms of disaster preparedness attitudes, 47.7% out of 44 respondents agreed to the importance of keeping extra medications for a disaster. Only 34.6% reported the necessity of a disaster bag, although most reported having the following emergency items at home: a flashlight (98.1%), lighter (100%), and emergency blanket (86.5%), with the exception of a whistle (3.8%). Finally, only 34.6% believed they had the ability to protect their family's health and safety in the case of a disaster.

3.2. Multivariable Analyses

Results from the multivariable analyses are shown in Table 2. Perception of living in a high-risk disaster area was found to be associated with insufficient quantity of water (Adjusted Odds Ratio, AOR = 30.48, 95% CI: 1.79–520.47), previous personal disaster experience (AOR = 37.17, 95% CI: 1.44–957.29), and household members on chronic disease medication (AOR = 23.68, 95% CI: 1.49–377.65), after adjusting for gender, age, and annual per capita income. Perceived importance of keeping extra medication for a disaster, as an indicator of disaster preparedness attitudes, was found to be associated with household members with chronic disease (AOR = 4.66, 95% CI: 1.08–20.04), after adjusting for gender, age, and annual per capita income. However, the preparedness attitude of disaster bag necessity was not found to be significantly associated with any predictors. Coping ability, as demonstrated through the perceived ability to protect their family's health and safety in the case of a disaster, also was not observed to have any significant associations in the backward logistic regression model.

Other perceived water security indicators were not found to be associated with the disaster risk outcomes. Although some perceived water security indicators (such as drinking water source, water storage, and water affordability) were associated with disaster risk outcomes in our univariable analyses, they were no longer associated with disaster risk outcomes in the multivariable analyses.

Table 2. Multivariable analyses of disaster risk outcomes in Xingguang village, Chongqing, China.

Outcome	Variable	Adjusted Odds Ratio (95% CI)	*p*-Value
Risk perception: Living in a high-risk disaster area (*N* = 46) [1]			
	Female	0.51 (0.05, 5.76)	0.584
	45 or older	2.39 (0.24, 24.32)	0.462
	Insufficient quantity water	30.48 (1.79, 520.47)	0.018 *
	Personal disaster experience	37.17 (1.44, 957.29)	0.029 *
	Household member on chronic disease medication	23.68 (1.49, 377.65)	0.025 *
	Per capita income (Ref: >5000 RMB)		
	≤5000 RMB	16.03 (0.92, 278.92)	0.057
	Refuse to answer	1578.1 (6.65, 374,389.16)	0.008 *
Preparedness attitude: Importance of keeping extra medication for a disaster (*N* = 44) [2]			
	Female	0.96 (0.21, 4.34)	0.954
	45 or older	0.48 (0.12, 1.88)	0.289
	Household member with chronic disease	4.66 (1.08, 20.04)	0.039 *
	Per capita income (Ref: >5000 RMB)		
	≤5000 RMB	0.81 (0.17, 3.81)	0.79
	Refuse to answer	0.07 (0.01, 0.98)	0.048 *
Preparedness attitude: Necessity of disaster bag (*N* = 50) [3]			
	Nil		
Coping ability: Perceived ability to protect in disaster (*N* = 52) [4]			
	Nil		

The following variables had $p < 0.2$ in the univariate analyses and were included in the backward stepwise logistic regression models: [1] main source of drinking water, water quantity, previous personal disaster experience, and household members on chronic disease medication (or, alternately, household members with chronic disease); [2] water storage, ethnicity, occupation, and household members with chronic disease; [3] education, previous personal disaster experience, and household members on chronic disease medication; [4] water affordability. Each backward logistic regression analysis included age, gender, education, and annual per capita income. * Statistically significant at $p < 0.05$.

4. Discussion

Overall, our study found that Xingguang village in Chongqing, China, faced vulnerabilities in their perceived water security. The Xingguang village has been obligated to rely on the collection of rainwater as their main source of drinking water despite the low quantity, relatively low reliability, and potential risks of poor quality reported among the majority of the respondents in the village. This indicates a water-scarce context where there is no better alternative source of water resources available. Our findings support the premise that some aspects of perceived water insecurity could further exacerbate the village's disaster risk perception. Although only one-third of respondents perceived themselves to be in a high-risk disaster area, our findings showed that perceived insufficient water quantity was positively associated with higher disaster risk perception. This demonstrates that within a community that regularly experiences insufficient water quantities, the awareness of their disaster risk is influenced by this external circumstance.

Consistent with previous research, prior disaster experience was found to be associated with a higher perceived disaster risk [12,13,22], while sociodemographic variables, such as age and gender, were not found to be associated [12,13]. Moreover, those on chronic disease medications were more likely to feel at risk of disasters than those who do not take medications, although the preparedness attitude for supplying extra medications was associated with chronic disease persons in general. These results indicate that those who have had relevant experiences related to their vulnerabilities (such as previous disasters or chronic diseases) seem to have greater risk awareness and express more willingness to protect themselves. By enabling more community members to identify their health-related disaster risks and corresponding preparedness actions, this would help lower the vulnerability of the community.

Preparedness attitude (perceived necessity of a disaster bag) and coping ability (perceived ability to protect one's family in a disaster) were relatively low, with only one-third of respondents in agreement. However, we could not identify any water security or sociodemographic predictors for these two outcomes among a rural population. This indicates that the ability to prepare or cope with disasters is not impaired or impacted by the community's frequent issues of water insecurity. These two outcomes were also not associated with age or gender, although education might potentially have some effect on coping ability, as it was found to be marginally significant (p = 0.088) but did not remain in the final model. Higher risk perception, prior disaster experience, and resources-related variables, such as income, were not found to be associated with preparedness attitudes of a disaster bag, or respondents' coping ability. As this household survey was conducted during the needs assessment phase of our project, our results indicate the disaster preparedness attitudes and coping ability prior to any disaster education interventions in the community. Thus, increased awareness through a disaster education intervention may be applicable to community members and could be beneficial towards developing an appropriate attitude in regard to disaster preparedness. Additionally, respondents did report possessing common household items that would be useful in the case of a disaster. This indicates that they possess the necessary resources to respond to potential disasters but could be further guided in their awareness and educated on the applicability of their resources.

Our findings on the association between insufficient water and high-risk perception is aligned with the premise that if a community regularly experiences water insecurity then this problem may be objectively exacerbated when sudden or slow-onset disastrous events occur. As such, more should be done to develop the water supply of households in the village, to decrease their vulnerability, and increase their resilience to respond to forthcoming water-related disasters. Literature has shown that those with higher levels of perceived risk are more likely to engage in risk reduction behaviors [23,24]. Households could be guided to better harness the use of rainfall collection, such that they could collect greater quantities of water. Community development should be conducted with the awareness of the risks natural disasters pose to the water supply. Disaster risk reduction activities could be carried out to address this association [25], such as spatial hazard mapping of water insecure households. This may contribute to identifying a vulnerable group in the village that may be more exposed to water insecurity or disaster hazards. Risk assessments can be further conducted to prevent or mitigate the effect of disasters on their water supply. Early warning systems can be put into place for different types of water-related disasters (such as droughts, floods, etc.), such that the villages can ensure a timely response and collect or prepare their water resources sufficiently in the case of emergencies.

Other water security indicators were not found to be associated with disaster risk perception, which supports the argument that adequate water quantity is of greater importance than water quality in water-scare conditions [26]. However, despite the non-significant associations, care should be taken to ensure that the increase of water quantity does not come at the cost of other water security indicators that would further increase the vulnerability of the villagers. Appropriate storage containers could be identified that can maintain the quality of water and protect it from potentially hazardous elements. These actions would in turn not only reduce the disaster risk of the community, but also further enhance the community's water security.

Our study faced limitations in terms of its cross-sectional study design, small sample size, and missing data. We were unable to include objective assessments of water security indicators, such as water quantity measures or measures of chemical or microbiological contaminants. Additionally, we had no information on respondents' actual disaster preparedness or coping ability and were only able to assess their attitudes towards it. Our findings cannot be attributed as causation. Excessive amounts of predictor variables would have reduced the power of the analysis, nevertheless we tried to standardize our findings by adjusting for gender and age in the final models. As this was only a pilot study with limited sample size, future research could help tease out possible relationships between water security and disaster risk perception or further identify any associations.

5. Conclusions

As far as we know, our study is the first to examine the relationship between water security and disaster risk perception and responses, and our results identified a relationship between insufficient water quantity and disaster risk perception. These findings support the hypothesis that external physical factors, namely inadequate water quantity, can be a contextual factor which affects disaster risk perception. If a community already experiences water insecurity prior to a disaster, its vulnerability will be magnified when affected by sudden or slow-onset disastrous events. With rapid socioeconomic development in China, water security will be challenged and exacerbated. Our study identifies that in a water insecure rural village, perceived insufficient water quantity is associated with higher disaster risk perception, but not preparedness attitudes and coping ability. Water security, particularly sufficiency of water quantity, is an important consideration not only in objective disaster risk assessments but also among disaster risk perceptions and disaster risk management. Particularly in a rural decentralized context, it is essential to consider and develop long-term water management in the lens of disaster risk reduction, as well as disaster risk reduction strategies with an awareness of water sufficiency levels. Such a two-pronged Health-EDRM approach would be valuable to combat future water security challenges and improve the health and livelihoods of disaster-prone rural villages.

Author Contributions: Conceptualization: E.Y.Y.C. and J.Y.H.; Methodology: E.Y.Y.C., J.Y.H., and M.P.S.Y.; Formal Analysis: J.Y.H.; Investigation: M.P.S.Y. and T.K.C.Y.; Resources: E.Y.Y.C.; Data Curation: H.C.Y.L.; Writing—Original Draft Preparation: J.Y.H.; Writing—Review and Editing: J.Y.H., E.Y.Y.C., H.C.Y.L., M.P.S.Y., C.K.P.W., and T.K.C.Y.; Visualization: J.Y.H.; Supervision: E.Y.Y.C.; Project Administration: H.C.Y.L. and C.K.P.W.; Funding Acquisition: E.Y.Y.C.

Acknowledgments: The authors would like to acknowledge the EMHP-CCOUC team members who participated in the 2015 Xingguang field trip and collected the data to make this study possible: Kelvin WK Ling, Carman KM Mark, Chun Wai Yee, Chung Po Lam, Lucille C But, Chaoqin Chen, Pui Yee Tina Cheng, On Wa Ng, and Wing Yi To.

References

1. United Nations University Institute for Water Environment & Health. *Water Security & the Global Water Agenda: A UN-Water Analytical Brief*; United Nations University: Hamilton, ON, Canada, 2013.
2. Asian Development Bank; Asia-Pacific Water Forum. *Asian Water Development Outlook 2013: Measuring Water Security in Asia and the Pacific*; Asian Development Bank: Mandaluyong, Philippines, 2013.
3. World Water Assessment Programme (WWAP). *Managing Water under Uncertainty and Risk*; United Nations Educational, Scientific and Cultural Organization (UNSECO): Paris, France, 2012.
4. Lo, S.T.T.; Chan, E.Y.Y.; Chan, G.K.W.; Murray, V.; Abrahams, J.; Ardalan, A.; Kayano, R.; Yau, J.C.W. Health Emergency and Disaster Risk Management (Health-EDRM): Developing the Research Field within the Sendai Framework Paradigm. *Int. J. Disaster Risk Sci.* **2017**, *8*, 145–149. [CrossRef]
5. World Health Organization; Public Health England; United Nations Office of Disaster Risk Reduction (UNISDR). *Emergency Risk Management for Health: Overview*; World Health Organization: Geneva, Switzerland; Public Health England: London, UK; United Nations Office of Disaster Risk Reduction (UNISDR): Geneva, Switzerland, 2013.
6. Schipper, L.; Pelling, M. Disaster risk, climate change and international development: Scope for, and challenges to, integration. *Disasters* **2006**, *30*, 19–38. [CrossRef] [PubMed]
7. Shi, W.; Xia, J.; Gippel, C.J.; Chen, J.; Hong, S. Influence of disaster risk, exposure and water quality on vulnerability of surface water resources under a changing climate in the Haihe River basin. *Water Int.* **2017**, *42*, 462–485. [CrossRef]
8. Phan, H.L.; Winkler, I.T. Water Security. In *Research Handbook on Disasters and International Law*; Breau, S.C., Samuel, K.L.H., Eds.; Edward Elgar Publishing: Cheltenham, UK, 2016.
9. Centers for Disease Control and Prevention (CDC). Water, Sanitation, & Hygiene (WASH)-Related Emergencies & Outbreaks. Available online: https://www.cdc.gov/healthywater/emergency/index.html (accessed on 5 November 2018).
10. Asian Development Bank. *Disaster Risk Assesment For Project Preparation: A Practical Guide*; Asian Development Bank: Mandaluyong, Philippines, 2017.
11. Ho, M.C.; Shaw, D.; Lin, S.; Chiu, Y.C. How do disaster characteristics influence risk perception? *Risk Anal.* **2008**, *28*, 635–643. [CrossRef] [PubMed]
12. Kellens, W.; Terpstra, T.; De Maeyer, P. Perception and communication of flood risks: A systematic review of empirical research. *Risk Anal.* **2013**, *33*, 24–49. [CrossRef] [PubMed]
13. Wachinger, G.; Renn, O.; Begg, C.; Kuhlicke, C. The risk perception paradox—Implications for governance and communication of natural hazards. *Risk Anal.* **2013**, *33*, 1049–1065. [PubMed]
14. Asian Development Bank. *Water-Related Disasters and Disaster Risk Management in the People's Republic of China*; Asian Development Bank: Mandaluyong, Philippines, 2015.
15. World Health Organization. *Guidelines for Drinking-Water Quality*, 4th ed.; World Health Organization: Geneva, Switzerland, 2011.
16. Asian Development Bank. 24: Climate Change Impact Assessment. In *Chongqing Urban-Rural Infrastructure Development Demonstration II Project (RRP PRC 45509): Linked Documents*; Asian Development Bank: Mandaluyong, Philippines, 2013.
17. Chan, E.Y.Y.; Lam, H.C.Y.; Chung, P.P.W.; Huang, Z.; Yung, T.K.C.; Ling, K.W.K.; Chan, G.K.W.; Chiu, C.P. Risk Perception and Knowledge in Fire Risk Reduction in a Dong Minority Rural Village in China: A Health-EDRM Education Intervention Study. *Int. J. Disaster Risk Sci.* **2018**, *9*, 306–318. [CrossRef]
18. Thorogood, M.; Connor, M.D.; Hundt, G.L.; Tollman, S.M. Understanding and managing hypertension in an African sub-district: A multidisciplinary approach. *Scand. J. Public Health Suppl.* **2007**, *69*, 52–59. [PubMed]
19. Chan, E.Y.; Sondorp, E. Medical Interventions following Natural Disasters: Missing out on Chronic Medical Needs. *Asia-Pac. J. Public Health* **2007**, *19*, 45–51. [CrossRef] [PubMed]
20. Pickering, C.J.; O'Sullivan, T.L.; Morris, A.; Mark, C.; McQuirk, D.; Chan, E.Y.; Guy, E.; Chan, G.K.; Reddin, K.; Throp, R.; et al. The Promotion of 'Grab Bags' as a Disaster Risk Reduction Strategy. *PLoS Curr. Disasters* **2018**. [CrossRef]

21. Wu Zhi Qiao (Bridge to China) Charitable Foundation. *Investigation Report on the Village of Xingguang Village, Lutang Township, Pengshui County, Chongqing (Chinese)*; Wu Zhi Qiao (Bridge to China) Charitable Foundation: Hong Kong, China, 2014.
22. Chan, E.Y.; Kim, J.H.; Lin, C.; Cheung, E.Y.; Lee, P.P. Is previous disaster experience a good predictor for disaster preparedness in extreme poverty households in remote Muslim minority based community in China? *J. Immigr. Minor. Health* **2014**, *16*, 466–472. [CrossRef] [PubMed]
23. Lepesteur, M.; Wegner, A.; Moore, S.A.; McComb, A. Importance of public information and perception for managing recreational activities in the Peel-Harvey estuary, Western Australia. *J. Environ. Manag.* **2008**, *87*, 389–395. [CrossRef] [PubMed]
24. Martin, W.E.; Martin, I.M.; Kent, B. The role of risk perceptions in the risk mitigation process: The case of wildfire in high risk communities. *J. Environ. Manag.* **2009**, *91*, 489–498. [CrossRef] [PubMed]
25. Baas, S.; Ramasamy, S.; de Pryck, J.D.; Battista, F. *Disaster Risk Management Systems Analysis: A Guide Book*; 1684 8241; Food and Agriculture Organization of the United Nations: Rome, Italy, 2008.
26. Bostoen, K.; Kolsky, P.; Hunt, C. Improving Urban Water and Sanitation Services: Health, Access and Boundaries. In *Scaling Urban Environmental Challenges: From Local to Global and Back*; Marcotullio, P.J., McGranahan, G., Eds.; Earthscan: London, UK, 2007; pp. 106–131.

6

"Share Your Tools"—A Utility Study of a Norwegian Wildland-Fire Collaboration Exercise

Jarle Løwe Sørensen [1,*], Carina Halvorsen [1], Jens Petter W. Aas [1] and Eric Carlström [1,2]

[1] USN School of Business, University of South-Eastern Norway, P.O. Box 235, 3603 Kongsberg, Norway; car-halv@online.no (C.H.); wergelandaas@outlook.com (J.P.W.A); eric.carlstrom@usn.no (E.C.)

[2] Sahlgrenska Academy, University of Gothenburg, 413 90 Göteborg, Sweden

* Correspondence: jarle.sorensen@usn.no

Abstract: Based on the assumption that crisis collaboration exercises lead to better team-integration and more efficient problem solving, the aim of this study is to test whether there is a relationship between exercise participation and perceived levels of learning and utility. Online survey data was collected from participants in a 2018 two-day, full-scale, wildland-fire collaboration exercise in southeastern Norway. The instrument of choice was the collaboration, learning, and utility (CLU) scale. Findings indicate a strong covariation between participation in Norwegian wildland-fire collaboration exercises and the perceived level of learning, with a medium to small covariation between perceived learning and utility. The results indicate the importance of giving clear instructions, focus on collaboration, and sufficient forms of discussion during and after the exercise in order to gain learning. However, learning had a limited impact on utility. The study indicates joint evaluations, improvising, and testing of new and alternative strategies across sectors are important when exercises are constructed. The data was retrieved from a questionnaire, observations and interviews can add more and comprehensive insight into the studied phenomenon.

Keywords: crisis management; collaboration; exercises; learning; utility

1. Introduction

In 1996, Karl Weick [1] published his allegory of organizational studies "Drop your Tools." In his paper, Weick points to 10 possible reasons why 27 wildland firefighters lost their lives when they failed to follow orders to drop their tools and run when overrun by exploding fires. His study is based on values developed by James D. Thompson [2] and data collected from two main wildland fire disasters: Mann Gulch in Montana (1949) and South Canyon in Colorado (1994). Weick shows that the willingness of endangered firefighters to leave equipment behind and run was overdetermined due to deeply rooted routines and identity. An important conclusion was that fighting wildland-fires requires skills in cross-sectional collaboration to break familiar and iterative routines during extra-ordinary situations. Such skills develop through collaboration exercises. There exists an assumption in emergency preparedness that exercises lead to better team-integration and more efficient problem solving. However, though few in number, all relevant international studies indicate that the perceived effects of exercises by participants are rather limited [3–7].

As the effects of collaboration exercises and specially wildland-fire collaboration exercises are little researched, this should be considered a gap in the collaboration literature. As a contribution to closing this gap, this study focuses on the perceived effects of such exercises with an emphasis on learning and usefulness. Further, this study has a practical utility value, as it defines perceived problem areas, which can help exercise organizers and managers to further develop collaboration learning and usefulness. The following research questions were developed: (1) To what extent is there a relationship between participation in Norwegian wildland-fire collaboration exercises and perceived level of learning? (2) To what extent is there a relationship between participation in Norwegian wildland-fire collaboration exercises and perceived level of utility? A collaboration exercise is here defined as an exercise where multiple emergency stakeholders come together to develop preparedness, team-integration, and behavioral response [8]. In Norway, where this data is collected, collaboration is one out of four national emergency preparedness principles. The principle imposes on all relevant emergency stakeholders the commitment to ensure the best possible collaboration with other relevant actors across all phases of emergency preparedness [9]. The three other principles of responsibility, equality, and proximity are also formalized in the other Scandinavian countries, but thus far Norway is the only country that has adopted collaboration by law. This paper first starts out by reviewing literature on collaboration, learning, and utility. Second, it outlines the study's materials and methods, before summarizing and presenting the study's results. The discussion section then describes and interprets the findings, with the final section summarizing the answers to the stated research questions, outlining the theoretical and practical implications, and making recommendations.

1.1. Collaboration

Collaboration is here defined as a horizontal process where stakeholders, both at the organizational and individual level, share competences, unite resources, and unprestigiously work together towards a common goal. [10]. Compared with coordination and cooperation, collaboration calls for more frequent interaction, higher embeddedness, and a larger will of risk sharing [11]. There are multiple motives for engaging in collaborative processes, but possible explanations include an overall assessment of advantages vs. disadvantages [3], a desire for individual or social benefits [12], and the sharing of risks [13]. As a working form, it has over the years become popular across multiple fields and branches and received considerable attention, especially in management literature [14–17]. Well-functioning collaboration processes are often presented as a solution to task allocation and regulatory fragmentation [18], thus they represent the leading perspectives within fields such as team-development, coaching, and integration [19]. In the field of crisis management, collaboration is viewed as a key success criterion [20–22] and has been found to positively affect the overall outcome of a crisis [23]. We define a crisis as a situation or incident that outsources available resources [24] and is not confined within administrative, geographical, or physical boundaries [25]. Collaboration, or more specifically cross-sector collaboration, which is the main focus of this study, is viewed in the crisis literature as a core concern as it helps both crisis managers and societies to effectively deal with adverse consequences [23] and meet societal expectations [26]. On the contrary, if managers fail in their quest, a lack of collaboration may lead to less resilience, flexibility, and efficiency [27]. While there are examples of sudden, informal collaboration processes during major disasters such as Hurricane Katrina [28] and the 2011 terrorist attacks in Norway [29], collaboration is something that, in most cases, needs to be learned, developed, and exercised. Thus, there exists an assumption that cross-sector collaboration exercises develop, train, and test joint preparedness efforts and response [8]. The problem, however, is that recent studies have found that such exercises tend to have limited perceived levels of learning and utility [30–35]. Sources today are conflicting as to why this perceived limitation occurs, but cited reasons include a lack of focus on variation [36], lack of trust [37], and insufficient focus on collaboration learning and utility enhancing elements [3,6,7,38]. Collaborative strategies can, however, differ depending on the current situation. On a scale of less to more collaboration sequential, parallel, and synchronous types of collaboration have been identified. Sequential strategies are often used when it is optimal to go through official channels and stick to routines. Parallel routines are when tasks are carried out simultaneously, while acting "on their own". Such a subtle type of collaboration is used when members do not go in and help each other across. It is characterized by the standardization of developed roles and established procedures. Synchronous collaboration means stepping over the boundary into the unfamiliar and flexibly covering for others where needed, even if this does not lie within a specific area of competence. Synchronous collaboration is the idealized seamless form of collaboration referred to when governing bodies stress their ability to interact, but it is also a challenging and exhausting type of collaboration. These types of collaboration have been identified as useful depending on the current situation. The synchronous type of collaboration is seldom used in everyday practice, but merely when there is a lack of resources such as during mass casualty scenarios [3].

1.2. Learning and Utility

The goal of learning is to acquire new knowledge [39]. The idea of collaboration learning during exercises is, in this study rooted in, and limited to, Johan Stein's [40] and Klabber's [41] perspectives on how institutions learn, hence the differences between first- and second-order learning. First-order learning is when participants learn new things during the exercise but are unable or unwilling to transfer knowledge to practice. Second-order learning, on the other hand, is when participants manage to acquire new knowledge and apply that knowledge in real situations [31]. While the goal of obtaining new collaboration skills and understanding during exercises may seem obvious, Berlin and Carlström [3] found that while it was considered theoretically and socially correct to support collaboration engaging processes, participants, in practice, prefer their everyday, standardized working patterns, which results in a decoupling between theoretical structures and practice [42]. To increase exercise utility, planners should focus more on integrating collaboration-learning elements, hence creating new configurations of thoughts that bridge exercise learning and real life practice [43]. Bourgeois et al. [44] discovered that the promotion of collaboration enhancing factors increased the sense of team-belonging and the ability to learn, thus substantiating Borell and Eriksson's [36] later argument on how perceived crisis learning is greatly dependent on the design and applied exercise model. When designing an exercise, there are multiple ways to enhance both collaboration learning and exercise utility. Firstly, the exercise needs to have a purpose and primary objective [45], hence the exercise needs a clearly defined training content with associated learning outcomes [46]. Participants must be informed that the main goal is collaboration development, not only complex scenario solving. Secondly, the organizers need to provide clear collaborative instructions and ensure that the exercise participation feels relevant and is free from long or unnecessary waiting periods [31]. Thirdly, it is important that all participants at all times have an overview of the ongoing scenario development [45] and feel that their opinions matter. Moreover, they must be included in formative assessment and collective reflection processes throughout all stages of the exercise [39]. On that note, organizers and managers also need to take into consideration that collaboration learning processes are not always either black or white. Some professional boundaries are, and will always be non-negotiable due to e.g., jurisdiction or complexity of task [47].

2. Materials and Methods

This study reports on data collected from a 2018, two-day, full-scale, wildland-fire collaboration exercise in southeastern Norway. The main goal of the exercise was collaboration development, but included also technical, logistical and managerial elements. Participants included the Norwegian Civil Defense, County Wildland-Fire troops, local fire and rescue personnel, the Norwegian Directorate for Civil Protection, and local fire planes and helicopters. The exercise scenario ran from alarm to completion and included air- and land-based fire extinguishing, controlling of fires, and establishment of fire ditches. Logistical exercise elements included crew reception, parking, and housing/catering establishment. The exercise planning and directing staff was composed of senior representatives from the participating organizations. There were no performed joint evaluations following the exercise. The exercise was conducted in May, and data was collected in early fall. The exercise had 184 participants (N = 184) representing local full-time and part-time fire and rescue services, regional wildland-fire troops, civil defense, and wildland-fire planes and helicopter personnel.

The sample included both the operational and tactical level personnel. The selection of sample participants was based on an assumption that relevant personnel in need of collaboration exercise participated, and that the exercise had a relevant and clearly defined collaborative purpose and primary objective.

2.1. Data Collection and Procedures

A G*Power 3.13 analysis [48] calculated the appropriate sample size to be 82 participants. A *t*-test, linear bivariate regression—one group, two-tailed, with an alpha significance level of 0.05 [49], a statistical power of 0.80, and an effect size of 0.3—was applied. The collection of data occurred through the use of a validated online survey instrument. The collaboration, learning, and utility scale (CLU-scale) [31] became the instrument of choice as it is especially designed to measure the perceived effects of collaboration exercises, with an emphasis on learning and usefulness (Table 1). Also, as the CLU has been applied in similar studies [7,31,32], a comparison with other collaboration exercises are made possible. CLU is a Swedish developed survey tool. An expert group of five academic instrument-developing experts together with three emergency practitioners, representing blue-light response organizations, developed it. The instrument was developed in different stages based on Meyer and Rowan's 1977 decoupling theory [42], Berlin and Carlström's theories on sequential, parallel, and synchronous collaboration [50], and Stein's [40] learning theories, which have their outspring from Klabber's [41] perspectives on how institutions learn, hence the differences between first- and second-order learning. Before completion, the CLU-scale was tested in multiple pilot-studies. The final product consisted of 17 items measuring the three dimensions collaboration (C), learning (L), and utility (U). The C dimension measures the perceived collaboration characteristics, the L dimension emphasizes collaboration related lessons, and the U concerns transfer of value to real-life scenarios. The CLU-scale is based on a 5-point Likert scale with the values 1 (strongly disagree), 2 (mildly disagree), 3 (neutral), 4 (mildly agree), and 5 (strongly agree). The instrument's homogeneity was tested through a calculation of Cronbach's alpha, showing an alpha of 0.88 [51]. Analysis stems from descriptive data and bivariate and multiple regressions. Means and standard deviations were included for descriptive purposes. The instrument has earlier been applied in multiple, similar studies [7,30–33,52]. To ensure appliance with ethical research standards, the researchers sought permission from the Norwegian Center for Research Data (NSD) prior to data collection.

Table 1. The collaboration, learning, utility scale (CLU-scale).

C	The exercises were focused on collaboration
C	Sufficient forms of discussions were provided
C	There were opportunities to improvise
C	Personnel in need of exercise participated
C	I performed well-known activities
C	Collaboration was initiated immediately
C	Clear instructions of collaboration were presented
C	My points of view were regarded
L	I learned new things during the exercise
L	I learned about other's organizational aspects
L	I learned about other's communication patterns
L	I learned about other's prioritizing of activities
L	I learned other's concepts and abbreviations
U	Based on what I learned, the exercises were useful to real-life activities
U	Based on what I learned, the exercises were useful to command officers
U	Based on what I learned, the exercises were useful to ordinary operative staff
U	Based on what I learned, the experiences from the exercises impact my daily work

Dimensions: Collaboration (C), Learning (L), Usefulness (U). Source: Berlin and Carlström [31].

Prior to contacting the defined sample population, permission was sought from the participating organizations. The email contained information about the study, methods, instrument, and purpose. The letter emphasized volunteerism and assurance of anonymity. After obtaining written permissions and email addresses from the organizations, an invitation to participate was sent out to the population sample. Apart from a hyperlink to the survey designed in the online survey platform "Nettskjema" [online-form] hosted by the University in Oslo, the invitation contained information about the study, data handling, and how to contact the researchers. Volunteerism and anonymity were highlighted, as well as the option to at any time withdraw from the study without facing consequences. To ensure further anonymity, only demographical questions related to gender, age, professional experience, and professional affiliation were asked. Age and experience were divided into groupings, and affiliation was limited to public or NGO sectors. Age groupings were 1 = 18–26, 2 = 27–35, 3 = 36–44, 4 = 45–53, 5 = 54–62, and 6 = 62+. Choice of affiliation was 1 = private, 2 = public, and 3 = volunteer. Years of professional experience was divided into 1 = 0–5, 2 = 6–11, 3 = 12–15, 4 = 16–20, and 5 = 21+. Number of collaboration exercises attended over the last five years were divided into 1 = 1–3, 2 = 4–7, 3 = 8–11, and 4 = 11+. The participants were asked to complete the survey within three weeks. During this period, two reminders were sent out. After collection, all data was uploaded into Statistical Package for the Social Sciences (SPSS) and analyzed. Identifiable information in the data set was removed and replaced with a number. The scrambling key was stored on a safe drive at the University of South-Eastern Norway accessible only to the research team. The key and identifiable information were deleted after the completion of this research project.

2.2. *Analysis*

The analysis process commenced with the exploration of demographical information, followed by an analysis of the collaboration, learning, and usefulness (CLU) characteristics (Table 2). Here means and standard deviations were identified for describing data distribution variations [53]. The empirical relationship between the CLU variables were tested by performing two bivariate regression analyses, where the first one tested the relationship between collaboration (C) and learning (L), and the second tested the relationship between learning (L) and usefulness (U). Demographical data was collected exclusively for description purposes, thus not integrated into the regression analysis. The working assumption was that focusing on collaboration enhancing elements during a collaboration exercise leads to collaboration learning, which again leads to usefulness [50]. In this first test, collaboration was defined as an independent variable relative to learning (dependent), while in the second test, learning was the independent variable to usefulness (dependent). Pearson correlation coefficients (Pearson's r) were calculated to measure the linear dependence between the variables. Coefficients of determination (r2) were calculated to determine what proportions of the variance in the dependent variables could be considered predictable from the independent variables [54]. To test the difference in parameters between the observed results and the stated hypotheses, standard errors and F-values were calculated. Further, the significance level (p-value) was calculated to determine the probability of rejecting the null hypothesis. Statistical significance was set to $p < 0.05$, and all tests were two-tailed [49]. In the next step, the relevant predictor and criterion variables that were found significant were tested in multiple regression analysis [48]. Here collaboration and learning were used as integrated independent variables relative to usefulness (dependent variable). The standardized coefficient values (beta), and the differences between them, were calculated both for the bivariate and multiple regression analyses to analyze the strength of the effects of each CLU variable. Towards the end, p-values were calculated together with the performance of a Shapiro-Wilk test [55]. The last was done to ensure that the CLU variables met normal assumptions for regression analysis.

Table 2. Mean values—CLU-dimensions.

	Mean Values	Standard Deviation
Collaboration	4.12	0.547
Learning	3.97	0.850
Utility	3.68	0.543

Note: n = 71, sign = $p < 0.05$.

3. Results

3.1. Demographics

Seventy-one persons participated in the study; 90.1% percent were males and 9.9% were females. The overall response rate was 38.6%. Most age groups were represented, besides the 62+ group. Most respondents belonged to the 45–53 group (52.1%), while the mean age group was 36–44. Ninety-seven percent of the participants belonged to a public organization, and the number of years of professional experience ranged from the 0–5 group to the 21+ group. Most (38%) belonged to the 0–5 group. The number of collaboration exercises attended over the last five years ranged from the 1–3 group to the 11+ group. The majority (57%) had participated in 1–3 exercises during the last five years.

3.2. Collaboration

In total, 84.3% of the sample population either strongly or mildly agreed that the exercise focused on collaboration; none strongly disagreed (M = 4.43, SD = 0.791). On the question regarding whether sufficient forms of discussions were provided, 14.1% strongly agreed and 35.2% mildly agreed. Further, 15.5% mildly disagreed, while 1.4% strongly disagreed (M = 3.47, SD = 0.985). Over half of the sample population (60.6%) either strongly or mildly felt that there were opportunities to improvise, while 21.1% remained neutral (M = 3.74, SD = 1.112). When it came to perceptions of whether the collaboration had been immediately initiated, most mildly (42.3%) or strongly (36.6%) agreed. None of the participants strongly disagreed (M = 3.93, SD = 1.10). In total, 53.5% strongly agreed that they had performed well-known activities. Nobody mildly or strongly disagreed (M = 4.37, SD = 0.790). A total of 85.9% either strongly (64.8%) or mildly (21.1%) agreed that personnel in need of exercise participated, while 11.3% remained neutral (M = 4.55, SD = 0.697). Of the respondents, 77.5% either mildly or strongly agreed that instructions about collaborative practice were presented during the exercises (M = 4.28, SD = 0.922). Finally, when it came to whether the population perceived that their points of view were regarded, 42.3% strongly agreed, 16.9% mildly agreed, and 40.8% remained neutral (M = 4.01, SD = 0.918). The overall mean for the collaboration dimension was 4.12 (SD = 0.547).

3.3. Learning

Most of the respondents either strongly (69.0%) or mildly (18.3%) agreed that they had learned new things during the exercise (M = 4.51, SD = 0.980). A total of 74.6% either strongly (39.4%) or mildly (35.3%) agreed that they had learned about others' organizational aspects (M = 4.07, SD = 1.041), while more than half (71.8%) had learned about others' communication patterns. Here, 19.7% remained neutral (M = 4.03, SD = 1.021). As to whether the exercise participants felt that they had learned about how collaborating organizations prioritized their activities, 7.0% mildly disagreed while 2.8% strongly disagreed (M = 3.77, SD = 1.002). Some 45.1% agreed that they had either strongly (16.9%) or mildly (28.2%) learned new concepts and abbreviations (M = 3.43, SD = 1.050). The overall mean for the learning dimension was 3.97 (SD = 0.850).

3.4. Utility

Most of the sampled population (94.4%) found the exercise useful for real-life activities (M = 4.69, SD = 0.623). While 18.3% strongly and 19.7% mildly agreed that the exercise was useful for commanding officers, 29.6% remained neutral (M = 3.17, SD = 1.248). Some 42.3% either mildly or strongly agreed that the exercises were useful for ordinary operative staff. Here, 42.3% remained neutral (M = 3.40, SD = 0.900). Finally, under half (45.1%) agreed that their experiences of the exercises would affect their daily work, while 33.8% remained neutral (M = 3.40, SD = 1.102). The overall mean for the utility dimension was 3.68 (SD = 0.543).

3.5. Bivariate and Multivariate Regression Analysis.

RQ 1: *To what extent is there a relationship between participation in Norwegian wildland-fire collaboration exercises and perceived level of learning?*

Bivariate analysis. The most pronounced significance was found between learning and the item "Clear instructions of collaboration were presented" (r = 0.501, r2 = 0.239, F = 20,761, $p \leq 0.000$). The item "The exercises were focused on collaboration" had the second highest pronounced significance (r = 0.451, r2 = 0.191, F = 16.349, $p \leq 0.000$), followed by "Sufficient forms of discussions were provided" (r = 0.421, r2 = 0.164, F = 13.564, $p \leq 0.000$). "My points of view were regarded" had an R-value of 0.398 (r2 = 0.145, F = 12.034, $p \leq 0.001$), while "there were opportunities to improvise" had an R-value of 0.282 (r2 = 0.65, F = 5.508, $p \leq 0.022$). "Collaboration was initiated immediately" had somewhat lower significance level (r = 0.255, r2 = 0.050, F = 4.439, $p \leq 0.039$). The final item with a pronounced significant was "Personnel in need of exercise participated" with an *R*-value of 0.253 (r2 = 0.049, F = 4.291, $p \leq 0.042$). The item "I performed well-known activities" was found insignificant (r = 0.06, r2 = −0.01, F = 0.30, p = 0.58) and was therefore excluded from the multiple regression analysis (Table 3).

Table 3. Bivariate regression of the collaboration dimensions of learning.

Dependent Variable: Learning. Independent Variables: Collaborative Characteristics of Exercises				
	R	R2	*F*	Sign (*p*)
The exercises were focused on collaboration	0.451	0.191	16.349	0.000
Sufficient forms of discussions were provided	0.421	0.164	13.564	0.000
There were opportunities to improvise	0.282	0.065	5.508	0.022
Personnel in need of exercise participated	0.255	0.050	4.439	0.039
I performed well-known activities	0.045	−0.014	0.124	0.726
Collaboration was initiated immediately	0.253	0.049	4.291	0.042
Clear instructions of collaboration were presented	0.501	0.239	20.761	0.000
My points of view were regarded	0.398	0.145	12.034	0.001

Note: N = 71, sig = $p \leq 0.05$.

Multivariate analysis. The joint collaborative characteristics predicted 29.3% (r2 = 0.293) of the learning variance, meaning that the remaining 70.7% of the predicted variance was unaccounted for. Still, the variables "There were opportunities to improvise," "Collaboration was initiated immediately," and "Personnel in need of exercise participated" were found to be significant (Table 4). The regression analysis indicated a 61% (r = 0.61) covariation between collaboration and learning, which is considered strong [49].

Table 4. Multiple regression of the collaboration dimensions of learning.

Dependent Variable: Learning Independent Variables: Collaboration Characteristics			
	Biv. reg. Stand.Beta	Mult.regr. Stand. Beta	Sign. (*p*)
The exercises were focused on collaboration	0.451	0.286	0.056
Sufficient forms of discussions were provided	0.428	0.203	0.129
There were opportunities to improvise	0.282	−0.049	0.722
Personnel in need of exercise participated	0.255	−0.064	0.641
Collaboration was initiated immediately	0.253	−0.025	0.839
Clear instructions of collaboration were presented	0.501	0.308	0.023
My points of view were regarded	0.398	0.101	0.469

Note: N = 71, R = 0.611, *r2* = 29.3 sig = $p \leq 0.05$

RQ 2: (2) *To what extent is there a relationship between participation in Norwegian wildland-fire collaboration exercises and perceived level of usefulness?*

Bivariate analysis (Table 5). The most pronounced significance was found between usefulness and "I learned other's concepts and abbreviations" (r = 0.436, r2 = 0.177, F = 14.755, $p \le 0.000$). This was followed by "I learned about other's organizational aspects" (r = 0.388, r2 = 0.137, F = 10,998, $p \le 0.002$) and "I learned new things during the exercise" (r = 0.343, r2 = 0.103, F = 8.259, $p \le 0.006$). The item "I learned about other's prioritizing of activities" received a R-value of 0.324 (r2 = 0.091, F = 7.290, $p \le 0.009$), and "I learned about other's communication patterns" a R-value of 0.323 (r2 = 0.090, F = 7.358, $p \le 0.009$).

Table 5. Bivariate regression of the learning dimension of usefulness.

Dependent Variable: Utility Independent Variables: Learning Characteristics of Exercises				
	R	**R2**	***F***	**Sign (*p*)**
I learned new things during the exercise	0.343	0.103	2.874	0.006
I learned about other's organizational aspects	0.388	0.137	3.316	0.002
I learned about other's communication patterns	0.323	0.090	2.713	0.009
I learned about other's prioritizing of activities	0.324	0.091	2.700	0.009
I learned other's concepts and abbreviations	0.436	0.177	3.841	0.000

Note: N = 71, sig = $p \le 0.05$.

Multivariate analysis (Table 6.). The perceived learning items predicted 17% (r2 = 0.170) of the usefulness variance, meaning that the remaining 83% of the predicted variance was unaccounted for. The only item that was found significant was "I learned about other's prioritizing of activities" ($p = -0.049$). Thus, these results indicate a medium to small [49] covariation between learning and utility.

Table 6. Multiple regression of the learning dimensions of usefulness.

Dependent Variable: Utility Independent Variables: Learning Characteristics			
	Biv. reg. Stand.Beta	**Mult.regr. Stand. Beta**	**Sign. (*p*)**
I learned new things during the exercise	0.343	−0.072	0.743
I learned about other's organizational aspects	0.388	0.256	0.277
I learned about other's communication patterns	0.323	−0.049	0.826
I learned about other's prioritizing of activities	0.324	0.078	0.649
I learned other's concepts and abbreviations	0.436	0.345	0.022

Note: N = 71, R = 0.488, $r2 = 0.170$, sig $p \le 0.05$

4. Discussion

The results from this study indicate a strong covariation between participation in Norwegian wildland-fire collaboration exercises and perceived level of learning, and a medium to small covariation between perceived learning and utility. Thus, our results support findings in past international studies, all of which indicate that participants' perceived effects of exercises are rather limited [3–7]. Initially, a significant majority of the sample population in this study (84.3%) agreed that the exercise focused on collaboration. This supports the assumption that it is considered rhetorically correct to be in support of collaboration-enhancing initiatives and exercises [3], hence contributing to maintaining the crisis management assumption that collaboration is viewed as a core concern, as it helps managers and societies to effectively deal with the adverse consequences of a crisis [22]. The results indicate the importance of giving clear instructions and sufficient forms of discussion during and after the exercise in order to gain learning. The study indicates joint evaluations, improvising and testing of new and alternative strategies across sectors as successful. An extensive crisis sometimes requires more focus on flexibility, e.g., synchronous collaboration compared to an everyday emergency, e.g., sequential and parallel collaboration. Exercises are opportunities to train horizontal and vertical working processes, either mechanistic or a more organic approach. Even non-collaborative decisions when a situation requires acts of demarcation or exclusion can be tested and evaluated [56]. The skill of choosing alternative strategies and approaches can be of special value during catastrophes and disasters [45].

Over half (53.3%) strongly agreed to whether they had performed well-known activities, while the rest mildly agreed or remained neutral. This suggests that the exercises contained elements of drilling, which have a focus on developing and repeating discipline-specific key procedures [4]. It should here be taken into consideration that putting out wildland-fires, together with flying planes and helicopters, requires specific skills and training and is thus difficult to entrust to others, something that may explain the finding that 85.9% agreed that personnel in need of exercise participated. This assumption is further supported by the fact that 97% of the participants belonged to a public organization, suggesting that these exercise participants were by and large specialists within their own fields.

A clear majority of participants (87.3%) agreed that they had learned new things. Over half agreed that they had learned about others' organizational aspects (74.6%) and communication patterns (71.8%). While these are high numbers, we argue for the need to see them in a context involving exercise participants that are highly trained, specialist professionals who already perform well-known activities. It may thus be assumed that the participants, as fire professionals, through everyday interaction and common training, already had a basic knowledge of each other's way of organizing. That under half (45.1%) agreed that they had learned new concepts and abbreviations suggests, however, that there were organizational differences and a slight lack of focus regarding cross-organizational communication development during the exercise. This, together with the high degree of familiar task performance, indicates that the exercise was dominated by sequential or parallel working patterns [19], where participants either perform their task in a defined order, similar to an assembly-line approach, or work side by side, while maintaining focus on an individual sector specific task. Even if all levels of collaboration are necessary to practice depending on the current situation, there is, according to past studies, a tendency to avoid synchronous collaboration during exercises. The reason can be a desire to avoid challenges associated with having to understand the collaborating organization's way of working or communicating [3], or as a means to reach individual professional goals [35]. However, in this study, it may also be a result of the practical need to perform tasks in a certain order, such as when to apply air vs. ground resources.

While most of the sample population (94.4%) initially found the exercise useful for real-life activities, the analysis of the other utility items suggests that there was some uncertainty related to who the exercise was for and which organizational level found it most useful. While 38% agreed that the exercise was useful for commanding officers, 42.3% agreed it was useful for ordinary operative staff. However, an interesting observation was that 29.6% and 42.3% chose to respond neutrally to the same questions. This suggests that the exercise lacked a clearly defined purpose, joint discussions, and the presentation of clear instructions. These assumptions are also supported by the fact that barely half (49.3%) agreed that sufficient forms of discussion were provided, and just above half (59.2%) perceived that their points of view were regarded. Overall, under half (45.1%) agreed that their experiences of the exercises would affect their daily work, while 33.8% remained neutral. From a learning point of view, these numbers suggest a potential of improvement. The results can be explained by the discovery that exercise participants have a tendency to distinguish between exercise and real-life behavior [57].

Limitations

First, this study was limited in scope as data was collected from a limited number of exercise participants during a short period. Second, the achieved population sample of 71 resulted in a statistical power of 0.86. Nevertheless, due to the relatively few wildland-fire collaboration exercises involving a large number of participants, data from this exercise gave good indications of the perceived levels of collaboration, learning, and utility. Also, the achieved power is, according to Cohen [49], still to be considered strong. Thirdly, the possible occurrence of a somewhat low term-validity needs to be taken into consideration, as the researchers did not pre-define the meaning of the CLU variables for the exercise participants. Fourth, the time passed between participants' participation in the exercise and time answering the survey may have led to lower response rate, as well as possible lower response validity. The data was retrieved from a questionnaire, observations and interviews can add more and comprehensive insight into the studied phenomenon.

5. Conclusions

As Karl Weick [1] found in his study, wildland-fire fighters have a strong identity and prefer keeping "their familiar tools in a frightening situation" (p. 7). Weick assumed that this was because they considered the unfamiliar alternative even more frightening. As such, the results from our study may be seen as supportive of Weick's supposition, as they indicate that the exercise population prefers working in familiar patterns. While this study found a strong covariation between participation in Norwegian wildland-fire collaboration exercises and perceived level of learning, it also found a medium-to-small covariation between perceived learning and utility. The results show that the exercise contributed positively to adding new learning. However, on the basis that the goal was to strengthen collaboration utility value, the study indicates the need to focus more on collaboration building and enhancing elements throughout all phases of the exercise. To ensure an effective and optimized use of available resources in crisis, cross-boundary tasks need to be integrated into the exercise; more room for improvising and testing of unfamiliar and alternative strategies are suggested. As this study was limited in scope and population, we recommend conducting similar studies, preferably through the use of the same instrument.

Author Contributions: Conceptualization, C.H., J.P.W.A., and J.L.S.; methodology, C.H., J.P.W.A., E.C., and J.L.S.; validation, E.C. and J.L.S.; formal analysis, C.H. and J.P.W.A.; investigation, C.H. and J.P.W.A.; writing—original draft preparation, C.H. and J.P.W.A.; writing—review and editing, C.H., J.P.W.A., E.C., and J.L.S.; visualization, C.H. and J.P.W.A.; supervision, J.L.S. All authors have read and agreed to the published version of the manuscript.

Acknowledgments: Reported data were first were first published in Halvorsen, C., & Aas, J.P.W. (2019). [Samvirke–Går vi mot felles mål? Subjektiv opplevelse av læring og nytte i en skogbrannkontekst (Master's thesis, University of South-Eastern Norway).

References

1. Weick, K.E. Drop your tools: An allegory for organizational studies. *Adm. Sci. Q.* **1996**, *41*, 301–313. [CrossRef]
2. Thompson, J.D. On building an administrative science. *Adm. Sci. Quart.* **1956**, *1*, 102–111. [CrossRef]
3. Berlin, J.M.; Carlström, E.D. Why is collaboration minimised at the accident scene? *Disaster Prev. Manag. Int. J.* **2011**, *20*, 159–171. [CrossRef]
4. Berlin, J.M.; Carlström, E.D. The three-level collaboration exercise–impact of learning and usefulness. *J. Conting. Crisis Manag.* **2015**, *23*, 257–265. [CrossRef]
5. Perry, R.W. Disaster exercise outcomes for professional emergency personnel and citizen volunteers. *J. Conting. Crisis Manag.* **2004**, *12*, 64–75. [CrossRef]
6. Magnussen, L.I.; Carlstrøm, E.; Sørensen, J.L.; Torgersen, G.-E.; Hagenes, E.F.; Kristiansen, E. Learning and usefulness stemming from collaboration in a maritime crisis management exercise in Northern Norway. *Disaster Prev. Manag.* **2018**, *27*, 129–140. [CrossRef]
7. Sørensen, J.L.; Magnussen, L.I.; Torgesen, G.-E.; Christiansen, A.M.; Carlstrom, E. Perceived usefulness of maritime cross-border collaboration exercises. *Arts Social. Sci. J.* **2018**, *9*, 1–5.

8. Rutty, G.N.; Rutty, J.E. Did the participants of the mass fatality exercise Operation Torch learn anything? *Forensic Sci. Med. Pathol.* **2012**, *8*, 88–93. [CrossRef] [PubMed]
9. Norwegian Ministry of Justice and Public Security. National Emergency Preparedness Principles 2019. Available online: https://www.regjeringen.no/no/tema/samfunnssikkerhet-og-beredskap/innsikt/hovedprinsipper-i-beredskapsarbeidet/id2339996/ (accessed on 20 May 2020).
10. Murphy, M.; Arenas, D.; Batista, J.M. Value creation in cross-sector collaborations: The roles of experience and alignment. *J. Bus. Eth.* **2015**, *130*, 145–162. [CrossRef]
11. Martin, E.; Nolte, I.; Vitolo, E. The Four Cs of disaster partnering: Communication, cooperation, coordination and collaboration. *Disasters* **2016**, *40*, 621–643. [CrossRef] [PubMed]
12. Mill, J.S. On liberty. In *A Selection of His Works*; Springer: New York, NY, USA, 1966; pp. 1–147.
13. Elkington, N.E.; Massie, D. The changing nature of international resource sharing: Risks and benefits of collaboration. *Interlend. Doc. Supply* **1999**, *2*, 95–103. [CrossRef]
14. Austin, J.E. Strategic collaboration between nonprofits and businesses. *Nonprofit Volunt. Sect. Q.* **2000**, *29*, 69–97. [CrossRef]
15. Gray, B. Collaborating: Finding common ground for multiparty problems. *Acad. Manag. Rev.* **1989**, *15*, 545–547.
16. Kourula, A.; Laasonen, S. Nongovernmental organizations in business and society, management, and international business research: Review and implications from 1998 to 2007. *Bus. Soc.* **2010**, *49*, 35–67. [CrossRef]
17. Richter, J. Public–private Partnerships for Health: A trend with no alternatives? *Development* **2004**, *47*, 43–48. [CrossRef]
18. Drucker, P.F. *Management Challenges for the 21st Century*; Routledge: Abingdon-on-Thames, UK, 2007.
19. Berlin, J.M.; Carlström, E.D. The 20-minute team—A critical case study from the emergency room. *J. Eval. Clin. Pract.* **2008**, *14*, 569–576. [CrossRef] [PubMed]
20. Brattberg, E. Coordinating for contingencies: Taking stock of post-9/11 homeland security reforms. *J. Conting. Crisis Manag.* **2012**, *20*, 77–89. [CrossRef]
21. Kapucu, N. Collaborative emergency management: Better community organising, better public preparedness and response. *Disasters* **2008**, *32*, 239–262. [CrossRef]
22. Powley, E.H.; Nissen, M.E. If you can't trust, stick to hierarchy: Structure and trust as contingency factors in threat assessment contexts. *J. Homel. Secur. Emerg. Manag.* **2012**, *9*, 1–9. [CrossRef]
23. Sawalha, I.H.S. Collaboration in crisis and emergency management: Identifying the gaps in the case of storm "Alexa". *J. Bus. Contin. Emerg. Plan.* **2014**, *7*, 312–323.
24. Van Wart, M.; Kapucu, N. Crisis management competencies: The case of emergency managers in the USA. *Public Manag. Rev.* **2011**, *13*, 489–511. [CrossRef]
25. Ansell, C.; Boin, A.; Keller, A. Managing transboundary crises: Identifying the building blocks of an effective response system. *J. Conting. Crisis Manag.* **2010**, *18*, 195–207. [CrossRef]
26. Boin, A.; Bynander, F. Explaining success and failure in crisis coordination. *Geografiska Annaler A Phys. Geogr.* **2015**, *97*, 123–135. [CrossRef]
27. Jung, K.; Song, M. Linking emergency management networks to disaster resilience: Bonding and bridging strategy in hierarchical or horizontal collaboration networks. *Qual Quant.* **2015**, *49*, 1465–1483. [CrossRef]
28. U.S. Centers for Disease Control and Prevention. *Health hazard evaluation of police officers and firefighters after Hurricane Katrina–New Orleans, Louisiana, -28 and November 30-December 5, 2005*, MMWR: Morbidity and mortality weekly report. 2006; pp. 456–458.
29. Norwegian Official Report 2012:14. Rapport fra 22. juli-kommisjonen: Oppnevnt ved kongelig resolusjon 12. august 2011 for å gjennomgå og trekke lærdom fra angrepene på regjeringskvartalet og Utøya 22. juli 2011; avgitt til statsministeren 13. august 2012. Available online: https://www.regjeringen.no/contentassets/bb3dc76229c64735b4f6eb4dbfcdbfe8/no/pdfs/nou201220120014000dddpdfs.pdf (accessed on 20 May 2020).
30. Carlström, E.; Berlin, J. Var och en på sin kant om avsaknaden av synkron samverkan på olycksplatsen. *Kommunal Ekonomi och Politik* **2009**, *13*, 3.
31. Berlin, J.M.; Carlström, E.D. Collaboration exercises: What do they contribute? —*A study of learning and usefulness. J. Conting. Crisis Manag.* **2015**, *23*, 11–23. [CrossRef]
32. Sørensen, J.L. Norwegian Maritime Crisis Collaboration Exercises: Are They Useful? Ph.D. Thesis, Northcentral University, San Diego, CA, USA, May 2017.

33. Carlström, E.; Berlin, J.; Sørensen, J.L. Collaboration exercises in emergency work: Outcomes in terms of learning and usefulness. *Disaster Divers. Emerg. Prep.* **2019**, *146*, 147.
34. Sorensen, J.L.; Kim, T.-E.; Christiansen, A.; Torgensen, G.-E. Old dogs, new tricks? A Norwegian study on whether previous collaboration exercise experience impacted participant's perceived exercise effect. *Int. J. Emerg. Serv.* **2018**, *8*, 122–136. [CrossRef]
35. Kristiansen, E.; Sorensen, J.L.; Magnussen, L.I.; Carlstrøm, E. Time to rethink Norwegian maritime collaboration exercises. *Int. J. Emerg. Serv.* **2017**, *6*, 14–28. [CrossRef]
36. Borell, J.; Eriksson, K. Learning effectiveness of discussion-based crisis management exercises. *Int. J. Disaster Risk Reduct.* **2013**, *5*, 28–37. [CrossRef]
37. Curnin, S.; Owen, C.; Paton, D.; Trist, C.; Parsons, D. Role clarity, swift trust and multi-agency coordination. *J. Conting. Crisis Manag.* **2015**, *23*, 29–35. [CrossRef]
38. Berlin, J.M.; Carlström, E.D. Collaboration exercises—The lack of collaborative benefits. *Int. J. Disaster Risk Sci.* **2014**, *5*, 192–205. [CrossRef]
39. Sommer, M.; Njå, O. Dominant Learning Processes in Emergency Response Organizations: A Case Study of a Joint Rescue Coordination Centre. *J. Conting. Crisis Manag.* **2012**, *20*, 219–230. [CrossRef]
40. Stein, J. How institutions learn: A socio-cognitive perspective. *J. Econ. Issues* **1997**, *31*, 729–740. [CrossRef]
41. Klabbers, J. *The Exercises Planners Guide*; HMSO: London, UK, 1999.
42. Meyer, J.W.; Rowan, B. Institutionalized organizations: Formal structure as myth and ceremony. *Am. J. Sociol.* **1977**, *83*, 340–363. [CrossRef]
43. Gredler, M.E. *Learning and Instruction: Theory into Practice*; Macmillan: New York, NY, USA, 1992.
44. Bourgeois, S.; Drayton, N.; Brown, A.-M. An inovative model of supportive clinical teaching and learning for undergraduate nursing students: The cluster model. *Nurse Educ. Pract.* **2011**, *11*, 114–118. [CrossRef]
45. Andersson, A.E.C.; Berlin, J. Organizing a simulated reality: On exercises with public safety organizations. *Nord. Organ. Stud.* **2013**, *15*, 34–64.
46. van Laere, J.; Lindblom, J. Cultivating a longitudinal learning process through recurring crisis management training exercises in twelve Swedish municipalities. *J. Conting. Crisis Manag.* **2019**, *27*, 38–49. [CrossRef]
47. Andersson, A. Boundaries as mechanisms for learning in emergency exercises with students from emergency service organisations. *J. Vocat. Educ. Train.* **2016**, *68*, 245–262. [CrossRef]
48. Faul, F.; Erdfelder, E.; Buchner, A.; Lang, A.-G. Statistical power analyses using G* Power 3.1: Tests for correlation and regression analyses. *Behav. Res. Methods* **2009**, *41*, 1149–1160. [CrossRef]
49. Cohen, J. *Statistical Power Analysis for the Behavioral Sciences*; Academic press: Cambridge, MA, USA, 2013.
50. Berlin, J.; Carlström, E. *Samverkan På Olycksplatsen: Om Organisatoriska Barriäreffekter*; University West: Trollhattan, Sweden, 2009.
51. Altman, D.G. *Practical Statistics for Medical Research*; CRC Press: Boca Raton, FL, USA, 1990.
52. Sørensen, J.L.; Carlström, E.; Torgensen, G.-E.; Christiansen, A.; Kim, T.-E.; Wahlstrøm, S.; Magnussen, L.I. The organizer dilemma: Outcomes from a collaboration exercise. *Int. J. Disaster Risk Sci.* **2019**, *10*, 261–269.
53. Bennett, J.; Briggs, W.; Triola, M. *Statistical Reasoning for Everyday Life*; Pearson: London, UK, 2009.
54. Trochim, W.; Donnelly, J.P. *The Research Methods Knowledge Base Mason*; Atomic Dog: Cincinnati, OH, USA, 2008.
55. Shapiro, S.S.; Wilk, M.B. An analysis of variance test for normality (complete samples). *Biometrika* **1965**, *52*, 591–611. [CrossRef]
56. Burns, T.; Stalker, G. Mechanistic and organic systems. *Organ. Behav.* **2005**, *2*, 214–225.
57. Berlin, J.M.; Carlström, E.D. The 90-second collaboration: A critical study of collaboration exercises at extensive accident sites. *J. Conting. Crisis Manag.* **2008**, *16*, 177–185. [CrossRef]

7

Regional Flexible Surge Capacity—A Flexible Response System

Viktor Glantz [1], Phatthranit Phattharapornjaroen [1,2], Eric Carlström [3,4] and Amir Khorram-Manesh [1,5,*]

1 Institute of Clinical Sciences, Department of Surgery, Sahlgrenska Academy, Gothenburg University, 40010 Gothenburg, Sweden; viktor.glantz@vgregion.se (V.G.); phatthranit.pha@mahidol.edu (P.P.) ;
2 Department of Emergency Medicine, Ramathibodi Hospital, Mahidol University, Bangkok 10400, Thailand
3 Institute of Healthcare Sciences, Sahlgrenska Academy, Gothenburg University, 40010 Gothenburg, Sweden eric.carlstrom@gu.se
4 USN School of Business, University of South-Eastern Norway, P.O. Box 235, 3603 Kongsberg, Norway
5 Department of Research and Development, The Swedish Armed Forces Center for Defense Medicine, 40010 Gothenburg, Sweden
* Correspondence: amir.khorram-manesh@surgery.gu.se

Abstract: Surge capacity is the ability to manage the increased influx of critically ill or injured patients during a sudden onset crisis. During such an event, all ordinary resources are activated and used in a systematic, structured, and planned way to cope with the situation. There are, however, occasions where conventional healthcare means are insufficient, and additional resources must be summoned. In such an event, the activation of existing capabilities within community resources can increase regional surge capacity in a flexible manner. These additional resources together represent the concept of Flexible Surge Capacity. This study aims to investigate the possibility of establishing a Flexible Surge Capacity response system to emergencies by examining the main components of surge capacity (Staff, Stuff, Structure, System) within facilities of interest present in the Western Region of Sweden. Through a mixed-method and use of (A) questionnaires and (B) semi-structured key-informant interviews, data was collected from potential alternative care facilities to determine capacities and capabilities and barriers and limitations as well as interest to be included in a flexible surge capacity response system. Both interest and ability were found in the investigated primary healthcare centers, veterinary and dental clinics, schools, and sports and hotel facilities to participate in such a system, either by receiving resources and/or drills and exercises. Barriers limiting the potential participation in this response system consisted of a varying lack of space, beds, healthcare materials, and competencies along with a need for clear organizational structure and medical responsibility. These results indicate that the concept of flexible surge capacity is a feasible approach to emergency management. Educational initiatives, drills and exercises, layperson empowerment, organizational and legal changes and sufficient funding are needed to realize the concept.

Keywords: capacity; community; crisis; disaster; flexible; major incident; surge; management

1. Introduction

Adequate preparedness efforts and proper contingency planning can mitigate and minimize the impact of major incidents and disasters (MID) in societies [1]. Contingency plans are the organized and coordinated courses of action that present institutional roles and resources, information processes, and operational arrangements based on scenarios of potential crises and hazard analyses [2]. Strategies for disaster management include establishing command and control, reliable and efficient communication, information, organization, warning systems, stockpiling of resources, and response plans for the mobilization and management of resources such as personnel, equipment, volunteers, and emergency facilities. The efficiency of the organizational structure is paramount for the outcome of the event [3,4]. Disaster preparedness and contingency planning involve all actors in society. However, in particular, the healthcare sector is designated to respond in a planned and efficient manner to prevent mortality and morbidity, resulting from an increasing number of global and local threats, at the lowest possible cost to society [3–5].

The initial approach to proper management of MID is to increase the management system's capacity, i.e., Surge Capacity (SC). Three broad areas of healthcare demand SC in response to a MID [6]: Firstly, Public health Surge capacity (the ability of the public health system to increase capacity for patient care, epidemiological investigation, laboratory services, mass fatality management, etc.); secondly, Healthcare Facility-Based Surge Capacity (augments the response within the healthcare facility structure, e.g., triage-tent on hospital grounds); and finally, Community-based Surge Capacity (the public effort to support and augment the healthcare system). The four essential elements of SC, i.e., Staff, Stuff, Structure, and System (4S), should rapidly and effectively be surged in the affected areas. Staff refers to available/alternative personnel, Stuff refers to available/alternative equipment, Structures refer to hospitals, clinics and Alternate Care Facilities (ACF), and systems are procedures and guidelines that govern the emergency management process [7,8].

The expansion of MID necessitates a new surge capacity (secondary SC), which underlines the need for increased effort to obtain additional resources still available within the management system [9–11]. A further expansion of incidences demands new approaches, policies, and adjustable preparedness within the community to scale up and down resources in a quick and seamless manner, i.e., "flexible surge capacity" (FSC) [12]. The concept of FSC is concordant with the new paradigm of proactivity in disaster management and emphasizes risk reduction rather than focusing on pure relief operations to reduce vulnerability and increase resilience within communities [13]. Therefore, risk assessment and focus on all four elements of SC is necessary for achieving a FSC. The disaster management cycle should incorporate, recognize, and value the participation of affected communities [14], and it is therefore necessary that adequate infrastructure is in place to ensure access to emergency services [15]. In this perspective, the readiness of community-owned resources is essential and includes alternative facilities to take care of victims or to unburden hospitals [16–18].

Focus on all four elements of SC is necessary for achieving a FSC. Staff pools may be needed, and new staff categories should be considered to replace the regular staffing structure. Equipment and devices placed in different parts of a community should be registered and available for use. Buildings of opportunity, i.e., facilities with the capacity to hold a high number of people that can act as an ACF should be identified [4,6,18]. Finally, relevant systems and guidelines should be produced to link all these measures. The focus of this paper, however, is on ACFs at predesignated, strategic buildings. These untapped resources available within a community can be lifesaving and deserve recognition and support from all agencies within the emergency management network [12,16]. A more comprehensive view of the Structure component of SC includes *buildings of opportunity* and *facilities of interest* that can be designated and converted to act as an ACF. Such buildings can consist of, but are not restricted to, outpatient clinics, dental and veterinary clinics, schools, hotels, convention centers, and sports facilities [6,10,12,17,18].

In the Swedish crisis and emergency management system, the responsibility for crisis and disaster management resides at national, regional, and local levels based on the principles of Responsibility, Parity, and Proximity [19]. According to these principles, all actors retain their responsibilities during MID management while the methods and structures should be kept as similar as possible to those used in normal circumstances. The geographical responsibility to manage an event lies with those parties affected at the local level, i.e., close to the incident [19]. The Region Västra Götaland (VGR) in Sweden has about 1.6 million inhabitants in 49 municipalities in its 300 km long and 250 km wide area. VGR is responsible for healthcare, growth, and development within the region and is one of the largest employers in Sweden with over 50,000 employees. According to current legislation, the preparedness of Swedish healthcare should be formed in close collaboration and cooperation between primary healthcare, hospitals, municipalities, county administrative boards (CAB), ambulance dispatch centers, and medical officers [19].

2. Aim

This study aims to investigate the possibility of implementing a FSC response system to MIDs by examining the feasibility and the potential need for additional resources and barriers in ACFs within VGR of Sweden.

3. Method

This study uses mixed methods, has an explanatory sequential design, and is partitioned into four phases of data collection and analysis [20–22].

3.1. Sample

The potential for FSC planning regarding ACFs was investigated in five VGR cities with a population ranging from 40,000 to over 600,000 inhabitants [23]. The cities were chosen because they all have essential healthcare infrastructure. Due to limited previous research in this field, a pilot study was planned with an approximate sample size of 99 facilities (around 20 facilities in each city) to receive questionnaires and supplementary informant interviews to a point of saturation [22,24]. Sampling was performed mainly using online search engines with map services to identify facilities of interest in each city. Each facility of interest/potential ACF, defined as veterinary and dental clinics, schools, sports clubs, and hotels, was checked for suitability by using information from the actors' websites and by Google Street View© to assess the location, accessibility, size, and proximity to hospitals. The final sample was relatively well distributed across the ACF categories in the investigated cities.

3.2. Questionnaire

The questionnaire (Appendix A) was developed by using the Nominal Group Technique [25]. Three academically skilled experts with extensive experience in instrument development and disaster and emergency management (one physician, one prehospital nurse, and one hospital nurse) developed the tool and tested it for face validity based on logic, relevance, comprehension, legibility, clarity, usability, and consensus. The questionnaires contained a vignette where the facility of interest faces a fictitious scenario of a mass casualty incident and is asked to help the healthcare sector to respond. It included both open-ended and close-ended questions to capture and generate relevant data [26,27 Questionnaires were sent out January–March 2020 to 99 primary healthcare centers, dental and veterinary clinics, schools, sports facilities, and hotels during the first phase of this study.

3.3. Interviews

Qualitative data collection was performed through semi-structured interviews with 12 key informants [26,27]. The interview framework was constructed from the same general questions as the ones used in the questionnaire, but more in-depth. Before each interview, the actor's previous answers from the questionnaire were reviewed for content. The questionnaire and review notes were brought to the interview to allow for follow-up questions to written answers and comments. The interview framework contained open-ended questions to enable the conversation to capture all content of interest. The interviewees were allowed to diverge from the interview guide and explore other areas related to the subject. No more interviews were held after reaching the point of data saturation [22,26,27].

3.4. Data Processing

The data was analyzed for results, discussion, and conclusion. Sequential analysis was performed [21,27] to determine what the qualitative data added to the questionnaire data. The qualitative analysis consisted of coding for thematic content to identify capabilities, barriers, and interest to partake in a FSC-response system.

3.5. Statistical Analysis

Cronbach's alpha was measured on the finalized tool and showed internal consistency of 0.739 [28].

4. Results

The results are presented in four sections. All conclusions about capabilities and barriers that pertain to a specific category of facilities of interest are presented in Section 4.4.

4.1. Central Measurements, Phase One

Roughly 42% of respondents answered the questionnaire (41/97). The response rate was higher in a smaller city than in a larger city (86% vs. 34%, respectively). Reliability analysis was performed on the 14 items of questionnaire data. The value for Cronbach's alpha was acceptable at 0.739 [28], and the questionnaire could be deemed a valid instrument. All returned questionnaires had comments and notes written on them. About half of the respondents answered several questions in the comment section. Some respondents did not answer all the items in the questionnaire. Two questionnaires, both belonging to sports facilities, were not returned due to absent mailboxes.

4.2. Central Measurements, Phase Two

Several interviews had to be rescheduled due to the social distancing strategy implemented to counter the COVID-19 outbreak. Three face-to-face interviews were conducted with one Primary Health Care Center (PHCC) physician, two school nurses (from one school), and one chief veterinary surgeon from a major veterinary clinic. Nine more interviews were conducted via telephone: with one PHCC physician, three chief dentists, one manager for dental care development in the regional council for dental care, two more chief veterinary surgeons, one school nurse, one sports facility administrator, and two hotel managers. The average duration of an interview was approximately 28 min. The face-to-face interviews were notably longer than telephone interviews. They were more beneficial to this study because the meetings took place at the potential ACFs, allowing for visual inspection of facilities.

4.3. General Results

The majority of interview respondents from investigated facilities of interest indicated that their workplace could be converted into an ACF to care for affected persons from a MID. Some could also accept patients not affected by the emergency to alleviate pressure on the nearest hospitals. Many respondents had materials in limited amounts for minor surgery, while some facilities only had small first aid kits. Many respondents indicated that additional resources were needed for a further developed capacity and preparedness. The most common materials missing for an increased capability were suture kits and first aid packages (basic and advanced). Many potential ACFs would accept a package or cache with more advanced medical equipment (e.g., tracheal tube, thoracic drainage system, etc.) if proper education was provided and the FSC-response system managed maintenance of the cache. Many respondents and interviewees expressed enthusiasm for the ACF concept; however, they also mentioned a need for an overarching organization governing the planning processes for the FSC response system and a need for educational exercises and drills to further develop their capabilities as well as a clear legal definition of the role they may have during a MID response [29]. The suggested educational initiatives were CPR, first aid, advanced first aid, basic trauma care, ATLS-based courses, disaster management, scene management and task-specific training (e.g., cast appliances, intubation techniques). Most respondents indicated a need for financial support and reimbursement for any invested time and effort into the FSC-response system.

4.4. ACF Specific Results

The following section presents a summary of ACF-specific results. The triage colors mentioned in the text are standard triage models used in MID and are widely used in many countries. The colors define the type of injury and the acuity of medical management. Red stands for immediate management (life-threatening injuries), yellow for delayed management (non-life-threatening injuries) and green for minimal supervision (minor injuries) [30].

4.4.1. Primary Healthcare Centers (PHCCs)

Eight out of 11 sampled PHCCs answered the questionnaire, and two key informant physicians were interviewed before the point of saturation. One interview was conducted in person and another over telephone. All eight clinics indicated an interest in taking part in a FSC-response system, and various levels of involvement were suggested in both questionnaire comments and notes and interviews. All clinics reported capability to receive green patients, and one clinic indicated the ability to stabilize yellow patients before transport to a major hospital. Three clinics stated that they could receive patients from a hospital, unrelated to the type of MID, to alleviate emergency departments. Half of the PHCCs could offer psychosocial support to people affected by a major incident.

4.4.2. Dental Clinics

Ten out of 12 questionnaires were returned with answers outlining capabilities useful to SC planning. Two interviews were conducted with chief dental officers at two clinics before the point of saturation was reached. All responding dental clinics reported both interest and a type of ability to participate in a FSC-response system. Nonetheless, some significant barriers were also reported regarding missing competence to care for injuries other than dental. Three clinics indicated that they could care for green patients from a major incident to alleviate hospital emergency wards. One clinic did not want to fully answer the questionnaire because it was perceived to obligate competency that was absent at the clinic and instead referred the issue to the regional level. At the regional level, one key informant was identified and interviewed. This key informant confirmed the data from both questionnaires and interviews but also shed new light on possible implementation procedures to involve the public dental care resources in a FSC-response system. The results from the interview with the regional informant contextualized and corroborated findings from both phases one and two of this study that pertain to all components of SC.

4.4.3. Veterinary Clinics

All responding veterinary clinics reported interest in participating to some extent in a FSC-response system. All clinics offered to make equipment and facilities available to the FSC-response system, and five out of six indicated capability to receive green patients from a MID. Two clinics also reported the ability to receive yellow patients and other patients from hospitals, unrelated to the type of emergency. Most clinics indicated the ability to treat minor surgical injuries, clean and suture wounds, administer intravenous fluids, and diagnose acute conditions. Many clinics reported to house diagnostic resources that can be useful during a disaster or major incident, such as ultrasonography and radiology, and capabilities to monitor patients for respiratory distress or other somatic deterioration. One clinic indicated that they could not provide healthcare to humans without having to close their veterinary operations. Barriers for veterinary clinics to partake in a FSC-response include the lack of competence to care for humans, legal hindrances for providing healthcare to humans, and the degree of difference between human and veterinary medicine in terms of beds, materials, and equipment. Some veterinarians had different views on how they can be involved in a FSC-response system. One interviewee expressed the belief that similar anatomy amongst all mammals makes trauma surgery similar for both human and veterinary medicine.

Another veterinarian expressed his concerns about the legal aspects and emphasized the need for clear and transparent legislation to enable their participation in a FSC-response system.

4.4.4. Schools

Nine out of 14 questionnaires were returned answered by a school dean, principal, or nurse. All responding schools reported capabilities and interests to be included in a FSC-response system, and all but one school indicated the ability to receive green patients from a MID. Some schools reported limited healthcare resources as school nurses have many students to care for during often limited office hours. One school reported hesitance to receive injured persons for care and treatment and preferred to distribute food and water and administer psychosocial support exclusively. One interviewee questioned having injured persons at the school at all. The reported barriers to partaking in a FSC-response system included the lack of personnel and medical expertise, lack of beds and healthcare materials, and the priority of keeping the school open.

4.4.5. Hotels

Five out of the ten questionnaires were returned answered, and all respondents indicated interest and ability to partake in a FSC-response system. One hotel reported the capacity to receive green patients from a major incident, and the remaining four reported the ability to prepare food, water, and shelter for over 40 persons. All responding hotels indicated that they could house evacuees or injured for treatment by healthcare professionals. Both interviewees expressed an enthusiastic interest in partaking in the proposed FSC-response system. A lack of competency and material were reported as barriers.

4.4.6. Sports Facilities

It was difficult to establish contact with sports facilities. From the twelve distributed questionnaires, two envelopes were returned due to missing mailboxes and only three questionnaires were answered. Two sports facilities indicated a capacity to participate in a FSC-response system. One facility did not answer the questions in the questionnaire but informed that they have no beds, no material, and no regular staff to contribute. Another informant responded that they could help, but they were limited in terms of what they could do. Multiple sites were contacted for interviews, but neither the owners nor managers were available for discussion or interested in being interviewed because nobody could answer for the whole facility. One sports facility administrator was briefly interviewed via telephone. The sports facilities that did report a capability to be included in a FSC-response system indicated that they could provide shelter and water for many people and distribute food. An important caveat regarding the mapping of sports facilities' capabilities is that they are often owned by the public and are managed by a municipal sport and association board. The power of decision making over daily operations often lies in municipal political councils that are disconnected from the day-to-day work at the facility.

5. Discussion

The study's results emphasize the importance of inter-organizational collaboration and the willingness of other stakeholders to participate in the management of MIDs. These findings also demonstrate the feasibility of the FSC-concept and enable all contingency planners to approach this concept fairly. A FSC-plan may offer the crisis management system another tier of resources, resulting in a regionally increased capacity to safely treat many victims. However, before any attempts to retrofit facilities of interest into functional ACFs are undertaken, a range of issues must be considered carefully. The following sections discuss the proposed FSC-concept concerning the four main components of surge capacity.

5.1. *Staff*

The required staffing of a FSC-response system is crucial. Those who are supposed to operate the ACFs must have both the necessary competencies and be readily available when the need arises. Some facilities of interest, such as PHCCs and veterinary clinics, have the capacity and ability to care for a few patients with minor injuries from a MID. Nonetheless, if they are to care for a group of patients or to deliver a higher level of care, they must be reinforced with additional staff. Other facilities, such as dental and veterinary clinics, lack competent staff to care for injured patients. Hotels and sports arenas may not have staff resources that are appropriately trained to care for even patients with minor injuries [12]. Establishing a dynamic personnel base between competencies and across disciplines could solve some issues of staffing. Staff can, to some extent, be reassigned from ambulatory or home-service care and from hospital wards not under severe pressure from the MID. Emergency staff, including physicians, will likely have a prominent role in managing the care at ACFs, as their competency is required at the center of all responses to MIDs [31]. Volunteers with appropriate skills and competencies (e.g., from the Red Cross or other volunteer civil defense organizations) can also report to an established ACF and help healthcare professionals to deliver appropriate care. There have been exciting developments regarding the use of immediate responders and initiatives such as CITIZENAID and Stop the bleed that educate the public in simple and lifesaving techniques that can be used in a MID [32]. A recent publication from Sweden indicated a high willingness among civilians to participate in the management of MIDs [32]. Civilian defense conscription can be activated by the government without declaring heightened alert and can potentially contribute (at least in part) to staffing ACFs [33–36].

5.2. *Stuff (Healthcare Equipment and Materials)*

Ensuring the adequate distribution of sufficient critical equipment is a significant task for the proposed FSC-response system. Many respondents indicated that the amount of material and equipment present at their facilities are among the most constricting factors on their capability and capacity. Distributing a material cache to potential ACFs appears to be an efficient and viable way of stocking and equipping a functional FSC response system [18]. The content of the proposed material cache should be adapted to the size and assigned task. Stockpiling used to be a convenient method to secure the provision of essential goods, but the contemporary strategy is generally built on "just-in-time delivery" and access to international markets and imports [34,35]. Altogether, the purveyance of healthcare goods and materials to countries such as Sweden has become more vulnerable than previously recognized [34–37]. To compensate for resource scarcity, many county administrative boards have developed and should develop creative solutions for supplemental reinforcement, including networking with other committees for shared resource pools and infrastructure for improved response.

5.3. *Structure*

Many of the investigated facilities (PHCC, veterinary, and dental clinics) are suitable for utilization in a FSC-response system. Some are operational presently, while others require a retrofitting effort such as preparing bed space, ensuring utilities and wraparound services, and clearing the facility from other operations. Hotels and sports arenas demand a more extensive retrofitting process to ensure adequate operational facility standards for healthcare provision. Countries such as Sweden have historically had little experience of domestic healthcare provision in nonconventional or standardized facilities. Nonetheless, as part of the response to the COVID-19 pandemic, several areas have been explored to increase the capacity of Swedish healthcare [35,37]. In line with the total defense structure, civilian-military collaboration has also increased, and military field hospitals have been deployed to house additional beds outside of major hospitals. The transportation of critical patients has been performed with military helicopters. However, to avoid misunderstanding and to smooth the pace of collaboration, these efforts should be planned and trained [35].

5.4. System

The responsibility for and management of the proposed FSC-concept must be carefully considered before implementation into a crisis management system. To rapidly deploy and operate ACFs, the logistics and transportation of material, equipment, and patients must be swift and well-coordinated. The efficiency of communication structures and the distribution of resources are of paramount importance. The command and control of the FSC is one of the most critical factors in achieving a successful response. In any context, leadership and decision-making are two critical factors that determine an event's outcome. Besides having a central coordinator, such as a public health agency, the ACF should be operating locally, close to the incident scene, with regional operational guidance and possible material reinforcement distributed from the regional and/or national levels and related agencies [12,19].

The importance of correct and efficient triage during a MID cannot be stressed enough, and selection of the patients for treatment at an ACF is crucial. Over-triage could lead to an unnecessary overflow of patients to hospitals, which could result in the depletion of precious resources, and under-triage may endanger the lives of the victims [30]. Readiness and competence to conduct simple and vital maneuvers, including ventilating a patient until transport to the definitive care, should be presented, and necessary materials must be available. Triage should also give particular concern to vulnerable populations.

Exercises are crucial to create a coherent system that allows for practicing in a FSC and efficient deployment and operation of ACFs. Broad collaborative exercises involving all actors in the crisis management system should be held regularly to streamline efforts from all parties. Appropriate educational initiatives can increase the motivation to help. Educational initiatives should be adapted to the level of care in the assigned task and existing competencies at the facilities of interest [38]. Further studies should determine the content of educational initiatives suitable for professionals and civilians involved in MID management. Findings from a recent study in Sweden indicate a need for new public education initiatives to enable nonprofessionals to become immediate responders [32,36]. There is also the potential to incorporate volunteer resources in some of the ACF operations. All MIDs are likely to affect the mental health of victims, which must be considered and treated alongside their physical injuries and trauma. Mental health preparedness has been deemed insufficient in most countries and must improve [39].

Preserving a network of concurrent material provision and maintenance with education, training, and exercise initiatives continuously running requires significant financial resource allocation, which must be prioritized. Without necessary resources a FSC-response system is toothless. Insufficient program duration has been identified as an essential factor that explains the considerable ineffectiveness of many community-based health and safety programs. Having a long-term program view, active planning against conflicting missions, and mobilizing sufficient resources are necessary to establish, deliver, and sustain the system over time [7].

6. Implications and Recommendations

Integrated participatory and sustainable planning can increase resilience and is closely related to some of the World Health Organization's (WHO) sustainable development goals [40]. If optimally implemented, the FSC-concept can lead to a safer and more resilient society by encouraging increased civil engagement and educational initiatives [12,32]. However, a successful implementation of FSC depends on some essential factors:

1. Mapping capabilities, resources, and networks in the community as part of contingency planning. While decentralizing forces and resources can benefit the independence of communities, they still need support from higher levels. Smaller cities had a higher response rate in this study, which might reflect a higher willingness to engage in their community.

2. Empowering communities, nonprofessionals, and professional individuals to create pools of resources to utilize ACFs, as shown in recent studies and projects.
3. Changing legal and organizational rules and norms necessary to implement the concept into any crisis management system.
4. Financial investment from municipalities, regions, and, ultimately, the state, which might prompt policy and budget changes.
5. Avoiding political interference in public health-related issues to limit crippling the healthcare apparatus more than necessary. The simplicity of disaster plans should be maintained and no excessive changes to the organization, staffing, or supply-chains should occur during a MID.
6. Ethical, safety, and security aspects of using ACFs in response to MIDs should also be considered as the system is implemented.
7. Regulation regarding monitoring and evaluating the initiative is also crucial for the improvement of the response system. Once implemented in policy, the involved parties must exercise and train the FSC-concept in real life for the response system to be efficient and effective.
8. Further research is needed to explore possible use of ACFs and the FSC-concept. FSC can be a reasonable way to increase regional surge capacity, not only within the fields of trauma and surgery but also in other medical emergencies, e.g., CBRNE (Chemical, Biological, Radiological, Nuclear, Explosive)-related events.

7. Limitations and Strengths

The small number of investigated facilities, especially sports facilities, did not allow any statistical analysis of the results. However, the descriptive results confirm that the FSC-concept can be applied in more contexts than the Swedish one and has transferability to other settings in Europe and possibly to other regions as well [41].

The lack of previous studies in this field did not allow any comparison of results with other publications.

8. Conclusions

Management of MID is a multi-professional approach in a chain of reactions. A chain is not stronger than its weakest link. The flexible surge capacity concept is a feasible approach to emergency management that involves all stakeholders within the community. Educational initiatives, drills and exercises, nonprofessionals' empowerment, professional alternatives, organizational and legal changes, and sufficient funding are needed to realize the concept. This response system can also increase societal resilience through community participation and may advance nations' fulfillment of some of the WHO's Sustainable Development Goals. Components that explore possibilities of an attainable increased regional flexible preparedness are novel to the Swedish as well as other contexts. They could lead to a change in the crisis management system. The mobilization of sufficient resources to establish, deliver, and sustain programs over time will be essential to effective implementation of the FSC-concept. This study has found ample will residing in civil society to help the healthcare sector respond to MIDs. It is now up to the crisis management system to channel this will to help in a smart, safe, and efficient way.

Author Contributions: Conceptualization, A.K.-M.; formal analysis, V.G., P.P., E.C., and A.K.-M.; investigation, V.G.; methodology, E.C. and A.K.-M.; project administration, V.K.; resources, A.K.-M.; supervision, A.K.-M.; writing—original draft, V.G.; writing—review and editing, P.P., E.C., and A.K-M. All authors have read and agreed to the published version of the manuscript.

Acknowledgments: The authors would like to thank Associate Professor Yohan Robinson for his support to this project.

Appendix A

Information Sheet, Questionnaire and interview guide (English Translation for review only)

Flexible Surge Capacity Questionnaire

All resources within a community need to be used to combat a major incident or disaster. This puts high demands on a healthcare system in close collaboration with other partners and authorities. Such collaboration requires both knowledge, planning and practice and must be based on mutual understanding and respect for areas of activity and related responsibilities. In the event of many injured persons needing urgent care, can the need for resources exceed the capacity of the hospitals near your centre/clinic/working place. We would like to investigate how different healthcare players/institutions/organizations can work together in specific events (scenario). Below are several questions that could provide guidance on how such collaboration can be built up in a given scenario. After reading the scenario carefully, please mark the answers that corresponds to the ability of your centre/clinic/working place. It is possible to select several options on the same question.

Participation in this study is voluntary, data would be handled confidentially and the answers will be de-identified. We hope you take the short time needed to answer our questions. This study is part of a PhD program at the University of Gothenburg/Sweden and Mahidol University/Thailand.

On behalf of the research group
Name: xxxxxxxxxxxxxxxxxxxxx, Date: xxxxxx

Scenario

After an accident near your centre, there are 120 injured at the site. A sum of 40 severely injured victims require all emergency resources at the major hospital's surgery and intensive care units. Another 40 people are at immediate risk of inhalation injuries and must be under observation with intubation readiness (creating free airways by inserting a tube through the mouth and then into the airway) for the next few hours. Some people also have burn and splinter injuries. The last 40 patients have minor injuries and can be treated either at a hospital or at another unit.

A. Primary care/Health

If your centre is staffed adequately when the event occurs, how can you help?

You can receive the less injured from the incident.

You can receive serious injured from the event for physiological stabilization pending further transport to major hospitals.

You can relieve the hospital emergency departments by receiving other emergency cases, not related to the incident.

Your health care staff can connect to the hospital for reinforcement.

You can can offer resources, e.g., space, instrument, material.

Your centre can handle minor surgical procedures, suture wound injuries, plaster uncomplicated fractures, etc.

Your centre can handle medical patients.

Your centre can offer psychosocial support to patients and staff.

Your centre can coordinate transport for patients to the home.

Your centre cannot help.

Other?

Prerequisites for Healthcare to be able to help.

Equipment/Material:

You have sufficient equipment and materials for the desired ability to assist in special events.

You lack equipment/materials for increased ability. For increased ability, you need ____________________.

Other?

Local Supply:

You have adequate facilities for the desired ability to assist in specific events

You do not have adequate facilities for the desired ability to assist in specific events. For increased ability, you need?

Other?

Staffing:

What kind of resource or knowledge your staff need to increase their ability in to take care of injured people?

Other?
Competences:
Do you have the skills required for what you would like to do in the event of a major incident when the needs exceed the available resources?
Yes, absolutely.
Yes, but we need more training/practice.
No, but we can after a directed training/exercise. Suggestion?
Other comments and extensions?

B. Veterinary Clinic
If your centre is staffed adequately when the event occurs, how can you help?
You can receive the less injured from the incident.
You can receive seriously injured from the event for physiological stabilization pending further transport to major hospitals.
You can relieve the hospital emergency departments by receiving other emergency cases not related to the incident.
Your health care staff can connect to the hospital for reinforcement.
You can can offer resources, e.g., space, instrument, material.
Your centre can handle minor surgical procedures, suture wound injuries, plaster uncomplicated fractures, etc.
Your centre can handle medical patients.
Your centre can offer psychosocial support to patients and staff.
Your centre can coordinate transport for patients to the home.
Your centre cannot help.
Other?
Prerequisites for Healthcare to be able to help.
Equipment/Material:
You have sufficient equipment and materials for the desired ability to assist in special events.
You lack equipment/materials for increased ability. For increased ability, you need?
Other?
Local Supply:
You have adequate facilities for the desired ability to assist in specific events
You do not have adequate facilities for the desired ability to assist in specific events. For increased ability, you need?
Other?
Supply of competence:
Do your veterinary clinic have the skills required for what you would like to do in the event of greatly increased care needs?
Yes, absolutely.
Yes, but we need more training/practice.
No, but we can after a directed training/exercise. Suggestions?
Other comments and extensions?

C. Dentistry
If your centre is staffed adequately when the event occurs, how can you help?
You can receive the less injured from the incident.
You can receive seriously injured from the event for physiological stabilization pending further transport to major hospitals.
You can relieve the hospital emergency departments by receiving other emergency cases, not related to the incident.
Your health care staff can connect to the hospital for reinforcement.
You can can offer resources, e.g,. space, instrument, material.
Your centre can handle minor surgical procedures, suture wound injuries, plaster uncomplicated fractures, etc.
Your centre can handle medical patients.
Your centre can offer psychosocial support to patients and staff.
Your centre can coordinate transport for patients to the home.
Your centre cannot help.
Other?

Prerequisites for Healthcare to be able to help.
Equipment/Material:
You have sufficient equipment and materials for the desired ability to assist in special events.
You lack equipment/materials for increased ability. For increased ability, you need?
Other?
Local Supply:
You have adequate facilities for the desired ability to assist in specific events
You do not have adequate facilities for the desired ability to assist in specific events. For increased ability, we need?
Other?
Supply of competence:
Do you have the skills required for what you would like to do in the event of a significant increase care needs?
Yes, absolutely.
Yes, but we need more training/practice. Suggestions?
No, but we can after a directed training/exercise. We suggest?
Other comments and extensions?

D. Schools
How can you help in the urgent care of those affected?
We can stop bleeding, repair wounds, and administer cardiac resuscitation and other emergency procedures.
We can receive the minor injured from the incident.
We can receive shocked people and administer psychosocial support.
We can prepare sleeping accommodation for homeless, evacuated or otherwise afflicted people.
We can prepare food and water for the needy.
We can take care of children so that parents can help elsewhere.
We can send staff to help other authorities.
No, we can't help.
Other?
Do you have the skills for what you would like to do?
Yes, absolutely.
Yes, but we need more education. Suggestions?
No, but we can after a targeted education. Suggestions?
Other?
Prerequisites for your reception to help.
Equipment/Material:
We have enough equipment and materials for the desired ability to help in special cases events.
We lack equipment/materials for increased ability. For increased ability, we need?
Other?
Local Supply:
We have adequate facilities for the desired ability to assist in specific events
We do not have adequate facilities for the desired ability to assist in specific events. For increased ability, we need?
Other?
Supply of competence:
Do you have the skills required for what you would like to do in the event of a significant increase care needs?
Yes, absolutely.
Yes, but we need more training/practice. Suggestions
No, but we can after a directed training/exercise. We suggest?
Other comments and free text?

E. Gym /Sports clubs / Hotel
How can you help in the urgent care of those affected?
We can stop bleeding, repair wounds, and administer cardiac resuscitation and other emergency procedures.
We can receive the minor injured from the incident.
We can receive shocked people and administer psychosocial support.
We can prepare sleeping accommodation for homeless, evacuated or otherwise afflicted people.

We can prepare food and water for the needy.
We can take care of children so that parents can help elsewhere.
We can send staff to help other authorities.
No, we can't help.
Other?
Do you have the skills for what you would like to do?
Yes, absolutely.
Yes, but we need more education. Suggestions?
No, but we can after a targeted education. Suggestions?
Other?
Prerequisites for your reception to help.
Equipment/Material:
We have enough equipment and materials for the desired ability to help in special cases events.
We lack equipment/materials for increased ability. For increased ability, we need?
Other?
Local Supply:
We have adequate facilities for the desired ability to assist in specific events
We do not have adequate facilities for the desired ability to assist in specific events. For increased ability, we need?
Other?
Supply of competence:
Do you have the skills required for what you would like to do in the event of a significant increase care needs?
Yes, absolutely.
Yes, but we need more training/practice. Suggestions
No, but we can after a directed training/exercise. Suggestions
Other comments and free text?

References

1. Skliarov, S.; Kaptan, K.; Khorram-Manesh, A. Definition and General Principles of Disasters. In *Handbook of Disaster and Emergency Management*; Khorram-Manesh, A., Ed.; Kompendiet: Göteborg, Sweden, 2017; Chapter 1; pp. 17–22.
2. Jacobsen, K. *Introduction to Global Health*, 3rd ed.; Jones & Bartlett: Burlington, MA, USA, 2019.
3. Vitalii, S.; Khorram-Manesh, A.; Nyberg, L. Disaster Cycle and Management. In *Handbook of Disaster and Emergency Management*; Khorram-Manesh, A., Ed.; Kompendiet: Göteborg, Sweden, 2017; Chapter 2; pp. 23–29.
4. United Nations International Strategy for Disaster Reduction, (UNISDR). *Terminology on Disaster Risk Reduction*; United Nations: Geneva, Switzerland, May 2009. Available online: https://www.unisdr.org/files/7817_UNISDRTerminologyEnglish.pdf (accessed on 25 June 2020).
5. Stikova, E.; Lazarevski, P.; Gligorov, I. Global public health threats and disaster management. *Health Promot. Dis. Prev.* **2017**, *5*, 746–772.
6. Hick, J.; Christian, M.; Sprung, C. Surge Capacity and Infrastructure considerations for mass critical care. *Intensive Care Med.* **2010**, *36*, 11–20. [CrossRef] [PubMed]
7. Barbich, D.; Koenig, K. Understanding Surge Capacity: Essential Elements. *Acad. Emerg. Med.* **2006**, *6*, 1098–1102. [CrossRef] [PubMed]
8. Kaji, A.; Koenig, K.L.; Bey, T. Surge capacity for healthcare systems: A conceptual framework. *Acad. Emerg. Med.* **2006**, *13*, 1157–1159. [CrossRef]
9. Bonnet, C.; Peery, B.; Cantrill, S.; Pons, P.; Haukoos, J.; McVaney, K.; Colwell, C. Surge capacity: A proposed conceptual framework. *Am. J. Emerg Med.* **2007**, *25*, 297–306. [CrossRef]
10. Runkle, J.D.; Brock-Martin, A.; Karmus, W.; Svendsen, E.R. Secondary Surge Capacity: A framework for understanding long-term access to primary care for medically vulnerable populations in disaster recovery. *Am. J. Public Health.* **2012**, *102*, 24–32. [CrossRef]
11. Adams, L.M. Exploring the concept of surge capacity. *Issues Nurs.* **2009**, *14*, 2. [CrossRef]
12. Khorram-Manesh, A. Flexible Surge Capacity - Public Health, Public Education, and Disaster Management. *Health Promot. Perspect* **2020**, *10*, 175–179. [CrossRef]
13. The Lancet Editorial. Disaster prevention should be equal. *Lancet Glob. Health* **2017**, *5*, 1047. [CrossRef]

14. Krolik, M. Exploring a rights-based approach to disaster management. *Aust. J. Emerg. Manag.* **2013**, *28*, 44–48. Available online: https://knowledge.aidr.org.au/resources/ajem-oct-2013-exploring-a-rights-based-approach-to-disaster-management/ (accessed on 30 June 2020).
15. Rice, K.; Felizzi, M.V.; Hagelgans, D. Human Rights-Based Approach to Disaster Management: Valparaiso, Chile. *J. Hum. Rights Soc. Work* **2017**, *2*, 117–127. [CrossRef]
16. Marston, C.; Hinton, R.; Kean, S.; Baral, S.; Ahuja, A.; Costello, A.; Portela, A. Community participation for transformative action on women's, children's and adolescents' health. *Bull. World Health Org.* **2016**, *94*, 376–382. [CrossRef] [PubMed]
17. Bayram, J.; Zuabi, S.; Subbarao, I. Disaster Metrics: Quantitative Benchmarking of Hospital Surge Capacity in Trauma-Related Multiple Casualty Events. *Disaster Med. Public Health Prep.* **2011**, *5*, 117–124. [CrossRef] [PubMed]
18. Agency for Healthcare Research and Quality (AHRQ). Disaster Alternate Care Facilities. In *Report and Interactive Tools*; Chapter 4; Rockville: Montgomery, MD, USA, 2018. Available online: https://www.ahrq.gov/research/shuttered/acfselection/chapter4.html. (accessed on 25 June 2020).
19. Khorram-Manesh, A.; Hedelin, A.; Örtenwall, P. Regional coordination in medical emergencies and major incidents; plan, execute and teach. *Scand. J. Trauma Resusc. Emerg. Med.* **2009**, *17*, 32. [CrossRef] [PubMed]
20. Szostak, R. Interdiciplinary and Transdiciplinary Multimethod and Mixed Methods Research. In *The Oxford Handbook of Multimethod and Mixed Methods Research Inquiry*; Oxford University Press: Oxford, UK, 2015. [CrossRef]
21. Bowen, P.; Rose, R.; Pilkinton, A. Mixed Methods-Theory and Practice. Sequential, Explanatory Approach. *Int. J. Quant. Qual. Res. Methods* **2017**, *5*, 10–27.
22. Saunders, B.; Sim, J.; Kingstone, T.; Baker, S.; Waterfield, J.; Bartlam, B.; Burroughs, H.; Jinks, C. Saturation in qualitative research: Exploring its conceptualization and operationalization. *Qual. Quant.* **2018**, *52*, 1893–1907. [CrossRef] [PubMed]
23. Sweden, S. Population by Region and Year. 2019. Available online: http://www.statistikdatabasen.scb.se/pxweb/sv/ssd/START__BE__BE0101__BE0101A/BefolkningNy/table/tableViewLayout1/ (accessed on 25 June 2020).
24. Sofaer, S. Qualitative research methods. *Int J. Qual. Health Care* **2002**, *14*, 329–336. [CrossRef]
25. Harvey, N.; Holmes, C.A. Nominal group technique: An effective method for obtaining group consensus. *Int. J. Nurs. Pract.* **2012**, *18*, 188–194. [CrossRef]
26. Brinkmann, S. Unstructured and Semi-Structured Interviewing. In *The Oxford Handbook of Qualitative Research*; Leavy, P., Ed.; Oxford University Press: Oxford, UK, 2014. [CrossRef]
27. Tracy, S. Interview planning and design. In *Qualitative Research Methods–Collecting Evidence, Crafting Analysis, Communicating Impact*; Wiley-Blackwell: Hoboken, NJ, USA, 2013.
28. Tavakol, M.; Dennick, R. Making sense of Cronbach's alpha. *Int. J. Med. Edu.* **2011**, *2*, 53–55. [CrossRef]
29. Ashkenazi, M.; Liebiediev, D. Legal aspects in disasters. In *Handbook of Disaster and Emergency Management*; Khorram-Manesh, A., Ed.; Kompendiet: Göteborg, Sweden, 2017; Chapter 26; pp. 44–47.
30. Khorram-Manesh, A.; Lennquist Montán, K.; Hedelin, A.; Kihlgren, M.; Örtenwall, P. Prehospital triage, discrepancy in priority-setting between emergency medical dispatch centre and ambulance crews. *Eur. J. Trauma Emerg. Surg.* **2011**, *37*, 73–78. [CrossRef]
31. Phattharapornjaroen, P.; Glantz, V.; Dahlén Holmqvist, L.; Carlström, E.; Khorram-Manesh, A. Alternative Leadership in Flexible Surge Capacity—The Perceived Impact of Tabletop Simulation Exercises on Thai Emergency Physicians Capability to Manage a Major Incident. *Sustainability* **2020**, *12*, 6216. [CrossRef]
32. Khorram-Manesh, A.; Plegas, P.; Peyravi, M.; Carlström, E. Immediate Response to Major Incidents: Defining an immediate responder! *Eur. J. Trauma Emerg. Surg.* **2019**. [CrossRef] [PubMed]
33. Khorram-Manesh, A.; Robinsson, Y.; Boffard, K.; Örtenwall, P. The History of Swedish Military Healthcare System and Its Path Toward Civilian-Military Collaboration From a Total Defense Perspective. *Mil. Med.* **2020**, usaa071. [CrossRef] [PubMed]
34. Blimark, M.; Örtenwall, P.; Lönroth, H.; Mattsson, P.; Boffard, K.D.; Robinson, Y. Swedish emergency hospital surgical surge capacity to mass casualty incidents. *Scand. J. Trauma Resusc. Emerg. Med.* **2020**. [CrossRef] [PubMed]
35. Khorram-Manesh, A.; Lönroth, H.; Rotter, P.; Wilhelmsson, M.; Aremyr, J.; Berner, A.; Nero Andersson, A.; Carlström, E. Non-medical aspects of civilian-military collaboration in management of major incidents. *Eur. J. Trauma Emerg. Surg.* **2017**, *43*, 595–603. [CrossRef] [PubMed]

36. Khorram-Manesh, A.; Carlström, E. Civilmilitär samverkan behövs för att Klara masskadelägen. *Lakartidningen* **2019**, *116*. FRZE.
37. Goniexicz, K.; Khorram-Manesh, A.; Hertelendy, A.J.; Goniewicz, M.; Naylor, K.; Burkle, M.B. Current response and management decisions of the European Union to the COVID-19 outbreak: A review. *Sustaianability* **2020**, *12*, 3838. [CrossRef]
38. Khorram-Manesh, A.; Berlin, J.; Carlström, E. Two validated ways of improving the ability of decision-making in emergencies; Results from a literature review. *Bull. Emerg. Trauma* **2016**, *4*, 186–196.
39. Roudini, J.; Khankeh, H.; Witruk, E. Disaster mental health preparedness in the community: A systematic review study. *Health Psychol. Open* **2017**, 1–12. [CrossRef]
40. World Health Organization (WHO). *Sustain. Dev. Goals.* Available online: https://sustainabledevelopment.un.org/?menu=1300 (accessed on 25 June 2020).
41. Franklin, M. Doing Research-Gathering data. In *Understanding Research: Coping with the Quantitative-Qualitative Divide*; Taylor & Francis Group: New York, NY, USA, 2013; Volume 6, pp. 167–210.

8

Food-Related Health Emergency-Disaster Risk Reduction in Rural Ethnic Minority Communities: A Pilot Study of Knowledge, Awareness and Practice of Food Labelling and Salt-Intake Reduction in a Kunge Community in China

Emily Ying Yang Chan [1,2,3,*], Holly Ching Yu Lam [1], Eugene Siu Kai Lo [1], Sophine Nok Sze Tsang [1], Tony Ka Chun Yung [1] and Carol Ka Po Wong [1]

1 Collaborating Centre for Oxford University and CUHK for Disaster and Medical Humanitarian Response (CCOUC), JC (Jockey Club) School of Public Health and Primary Care, Faculty of Medicine, Chinese University of Hong Kong, Hong Kong, China; hollylam@cuhk.edu.hk (H.C.Y.L.); euglsk@cuhk.edu.hk (E.S.K.L.); sophinetsang@cuhk.edu.hk (S.N.S.T.); yungtony@cuhk.edu.hk (T.K.C.Y.); wongcarol@cuhk.edu.hk (C.K.P.W.)

2 Nuffield Department of Medicine, University of Oxford, Oxford OX3 7BN, UK

3 François-Xavier Bagnoud Center for Health & Human Rights, Harvard University, Boston, MA 02138, USA

* Correspondence: emily.chan@cuhk.edu.hk

Abstract: Food safety and unhealthy dietary pattern are important global health problems. Understanding food-related health needs and providing corresponding support are important to health risk reduction. A needs assessment, education intervention for food labelling, and another intervention for salt-intake reduction were conducted in a rural Kunge community in Yunnan, China in 2014, 2015 and 2016, respectively. Not checking the expiry date of packaged food (37.1%) and a high salt diet (53.9%) were the most common problems in the community. Both topics were selected for education intervention. Pre- and post-intervention questionnaires were used to evaluate the effectiveness. Education interventions were found effective in improving food-health-related knowledge, changing attitudes toward behaviors such as willingness to read food labels before buying and consuming packaged food. However, no significant improvements were found for the attitudes toward not consuming expired food, controlling salt-intake, and decreasing the consumption of cured food. Health education was shown to be effective in promoting food-health-related knowledge but was limited in changing relevant behaviors in a rural ethnic minority community.

Keywords: food-related health; risk reduction; rural; ethnic minority; food label; salt; food safety; education intervention; Health-EDRM

1. Introduction

Globally, food safety and unhealthy dietary have always been major health concerns for societies. According to World Health Organization (WHO) [1], food safety is the "assurance that food will not cause harm to the consumer when it is prepared and/or eaten according to its intended use". It has been a persistent problem in China and has caused different foodborne illnesses and food poisoning incidents over-time [2]. In addition, inappropriate dietary behavior is also prevalent in China, leading to significant rates of non-communicable diseases. For example, high salt consumption is associated with hypertension, cardiovascular disease and strokes [3]. This study focuses on two food-related health topics: food labelling and salt consumption in rural China population with education intervention.

Food safety issues are often multifaced. For example, suboptimal food safety system (for example regulation violations during transportation or storage) could lead to large scale food-borne disease outbreaks in a community. On the individual level, insufficient food safety knowledge could lead to incorrect food-process or consumption and to food-borne illness eventually [4,5]. Relevant food-related knowledge, awareness, and practices vary from place to place and were shown to be different between urban and rural [6]. A study from Nigeria [6] found that the practices of checking food labels and expiry date were significantly different between rural and urban population. More rural respondents thought that checking food labels and expiry dates did not have a significant impact on health than urban respondents. The lower awareness of food safety among rural population might contribute to their vulnerability, especially among ethnic minorities. In China, selling expired and rotten food has been reported to be prevalent in rural villages [7–9]. In the Food Safety Situation Investigation Report of China 2008 [10], expired food, no food labelling and hygiene of packaged food were the top food safety concerns listed by the rural villagers.

In terms of unhealthy food consumption, high salt intake has been recognized as a critical problem due to its association with hypertension [3]. Hypertension is a major public health problem and the leading disease among populations aged 40 or above in China [11–13]. According to the China Statistical Yearbooks Database data [14], the 2013 prevalence of hypertension in China's rural regions was 12.31%, which was about three-fold greater than the prevalence data previously collected in 2008 (3.85%). Furthermore, it was found that Yunnan was one of the regions with the highest prevalence of hypertension in China [15]. Hence, salt intake reduction is considered as one of the preventive measures against the increase in non-communicable diseases in China [16]. Moreover, a study [17] that investigated the salt consumption habits among 21 countries found China has the highest rate of salt consumption; 80 percent of the population in China had a mean sodium intake higher than 5 g/day (the recommended maximum salt intake for adults by the WHO [3]). In particular, hypertension prevalence in rural regions was found higher than those in urban regions [18,19]. This might be due to the suboptimal medication [20] and inadequate knowledge [21] in rural regions. Therefore, salt intake-related health issues need to be emphasized, especially health interventions to reduce salt consumption and the risk of hypertension. During disasters, a high proportion of chronic diseases such as hypertension would further increase the health vulnerability of the community [22]. Furthermore, food safety would be an important health determinant for resilience. Therefore, ensuring food safety and enhancing dietary knowledge and practices are non-negligible for health-related emergency and disaster risk management (Health-EDRM) in the household level [23].

To tackle health risk-associated food safety and high salt intake problems among China's rural villagers, understanding villagers' practices and promoting relevant knowledge are essential. The authors and the team have developed a 1.5-year project to: 1) understand the current practices regarding food safety and salt intake of China rural villagers, 2) to promote food safety and salt intake knowledge through delivering education interventions to China rural villagers and 3) to evaluate the effectiveness of the education interventions. The target population of this project was a subgroup of an ethnic minority group in rural Yunnan, China—the Kunge. Yunnan is an earthquake-prone province in China. Keeping reserves of packaged food is a common practice in disaster-prone communities [24,25]. This project not only aimed to enhance the food-related health status of the community, but also to increase their capacity for Health-EDRM in rural community. This case study presents the background, methods, and findings of the project.

Project Background and Study Context: Kunge People in Xishuangbanna Dai Autonomous Prefecture in Yunnan

In 2009 the Ethnic Minority Health Project (EMHP) was established in China by the authors and the team, with a core mission to develop and evaluate effective interventions of bottom-up Health-EDRM for vulnerable populations in remote areas of the country. One of the 14 project sites, Xishuangbanna Dai Autonomous Prefecture in Yunnan, was chosen to be one of the study areas on the basis of studying the risk of disaster and health situation which affected the ethnic minority group. The Yunnan ethnic minority health project was initiated in 2014.

The Kunge people reside in Kunge Mountain, Mengyang township, Jinghong city, Xishuangbanna Dai Autonomous Prefecture in Yunnan. It is one of the Xishuangbanna's ethnic groups, officially classified as a branch of the Bulang ethnic group by the People's Republic of China (PRC), and accounts for no more than 2500 residents in China [26]. There are total six Kunge groups in a Mengyang township with a total population of around 1600 [27]. To the authors' knowledge, there were only a few articles exploring the Kunge population and those all were related to the language [26,27]. Bulang people have their own dialogue and religious beliefs. Males and females made up a similar proportion of the village population. Most of the population were farmers, mainly growing rice, sweet corns, tea, and rubber. The average annual household income was approximately RMB 3000–4000 (approximately USD 1.34–1.79 per day, which is lower than the official poverty line of USD 1.90 per day, defined by the World Bank 2015 [28]). Their income mainly comes from exporting agricultural products to other areas in the region. The villagers generally had a regular pattern of life and spent most of their daytime working on farms. In the estimation from our team field visit, there were 140 households with 608 residents living in ManBangTang Village in 2016.

A total of three visits were made in 2014, 2015 and 2016, respectively. A needs assessment was performed in 2014. Although agricultural activity provides the main food source for the Kunge people, as per our interviews in the 2014 visit, all villagers reported the practice of purchasing packaged food, supplied from the local food companies and markets in Mengyang township. Besides packaged food, consumption of salt-cured food, pickled vegetables, and salted meat were also reported. During the needs assessments in ManBangTang, villagers were found to use a generous amount of salt during cooking.

Based on the findings in the literature review and needs assessment conducted in November 2014, two interventions, targeting food labelling in January 2015 and salt-intake reduction in March 2016, were conducted in the same population.

2. Methodology

This was an 18 months serial cross-sectional survey-based study. A total of three research visits were done throughout the project period from November 2014–March 2016.

2.1. Sampling and Study Subject

Representatives of village households (age 18 years or older) were invited for the needs assessment (2014) and the interventions (2015 and 2016). Only one participant was invited from each household. Due to the lack of community information such as household maps, convenience sampling was used for recruiting respondents for the needs assessment and interventions in the village. Recruitment was promoted through household visits, broadcasting promotion messages by the village head, delivering leaflets, and poster distribution. There were 140 registered households with 608 residents in the ManBangTang village during the study period. There were 52 respondents (37.41% of all households) in the needs assessment (2014); 40 (25.15% of all households) participated in the first intervention in 2015 and 45 (28.13% of all households) participated in the second intervention in 2016.

2.2. Evaluation Tool and Data Collection

The 2014 health needs assessment tool was a questionnaire combining eight health topics (including chronic disease management, food and cooking safety (including food labelling and salt intake), personal hygiene, water supply and quality, waste management, disaster risk reduction, first-aid training, and local climate change), sociodemographic details and environmental assessments were surveyed to collect the perception and practices of the villagers. The needs assessment were developed based on the guidance report from the WHO for building a healthy village [29].

For the food labelling (2015) and salt-intake reduction intervention (2016), pre- and post-intervention questionnaires assessing knowledge, attitude, and practices (intention to practice) (KAP) of the relevant topics and sociodemographic information were used for intervention evaluations. The needs assessment results were intended to also be used to design intervention. Thus the questionnaires also included the messages delivered in the interventions (knowledge, attitude and practice (KAP)). Interventions content were adopted from relevant sources: for the salt intake standard, it was adopted from the Chinese Nutritional Society [30]; the food label standard was referenced to the Standard for the Labeling of Prepackaged Food of the China Food and Drug Administration [31]. Table 1 shows the food-related health questions in this study.

Table 1. Questions used in assessing food labelling and salt consumption awareness, attitude and behaviour in the visits (2014, 2015 & 2016).

2014 Visit: Needs Assessment	2015 Visit: Food Labelling	2016 Visit: Salt Consumption
Food labelling related information	Pre- & post- intervention question	Pre- & post- intervention question
Have you ever brought package food before? (exclude rice, oil, and salt) (Answer: Yes/ No)	Do you agree: "I understand that consuming expired food will affect my health."? (Answer: Yes/ No)	Do you think you consume enough salt per day? (Answers: Not enough, enough, more than enough)
What kinds of packaged food you usually buy? (Answers: multiple choice with various food type)	Do you agree "I can distinguish whether the food is expired or not."? (Answer: Yes/ No)	Do you think high salt consumption will cause hypertension? (Answer: Yes/ No)
How often do you read the food label on packaged food before consuming it? (Answer: Always, sometimes and never)	Is the following packaged food expired? (3 Yes/No questions with their local food package images)	Do you think cure food is high in salt? (Answer: Yes/ No)
Why don't you check food labels on packaged foods? (Answer: Multiple choices)	Do you agree "I will check the food label before purchasing the packaged food."? (Answer: Yes/ No)	Do you think hypertension causes cardiovascular disease? (Answer: Yes/ No)
What information on the food label will you usually pay attention to? (Answer: Multiple choices)	Will you check the food label before consuming the packaged food? (Answer: Yes/ No)	Do you think hypertension causes stroke? (Answer: Yes/ No)
Have you ever encountered any food label that you didn't understand? (Answer: Yes/ No)	Do you agree "I will not purchase and consume any expired packaged food."? (Answer: Yes/ No)	Do you know the recommended daily salt consumption level for adults? (Answer: Yes/ No with an open answer on the salt amount)
If you encounter a food label that you don't understand, what will you do? (Answer: Multiple choices)	I will remind my family and friends to check the food labels and pay attention to expired food. (Answer: Yes/ No)	Do you know the function of a salt restriction spoon? (Answer: Yes/ No)
Salt-consumption related question	Post-intervention only question	Do you know the function of a salt restriction bottle? (Answer: Yes/ No)
Please estimate your daily salt consumption. (3 answers: less than, approximately and more than 1 teaspoon)	Do you agree "I am confident to build a habit of checking the food labels on packaged food."? (Answer: Yes/ No)	Can you control your daily salt consumption at less than 6 g in the next month? (Answer: Yes/ No)

Table 1. *Cont.*

2014 Visit: Needs Assessment	2015 Visit: Food Labelling	2016 Visit: Salt Consumption
Food safety related questions Have you experienced any food safety problem before? (Answer: Yes/ No)		Can you consume less cure food in the next month? (Answer: Yes/ No)
Have you got sick or suffered from food poisoning after experiencing the above food safety problem? (Answer: Checklist)		
Which factor will you consider to determine whether the food has gone bad or not? (Answer: Multiple choices)		

Translators were recruited to facilitate communication with the study respondents who could not speak Mandarin (6.25% out of the attendees in the second visit). Verbal consent was obtained from all study respondents prior to administering the questionnaire. All questionnaires were administered face-to-face by field researchers and local translators.

2.3. Statistical Analysis

The data were double entered by trained research staff. Descriptive analysis of sociodemographic information of study subjects was generated and compared to the 2010 Yunnan population census. Chi-squared test was used to compare results from pre- and post-intervention questionnaires for the effectiveness of health interventions. The significant level of this study was set at $p < 0.05$. All statistical analyses were conducted using SPSS version 21.0 (IBM Corp., Armonk, NY, United States). Ethics approval was obtained from the Joint Chinese University of Hong Kong- New Territories East Cluster Clinical Research Ethics Committee.

3. Results

Results are presented in three sections. The first section describes the sociodemographic characteristics of the respondents. The second part presents the results of 2014 needs assessment which included perception and practice of food labelling, general salt intake, and other food safety issues were described. The third section examines the effectiveness of the education intervention in 2015 and 2016 which targeted food labelling and salt reduction respectively.

3.1. Sociodemographic Characteristics of the Sample among the Three Visits

A total of 52 (37.41%), 26 (18.57%) and 34 (24.29%) households were recruited in the 2014 needs assessment, 2015 food labelling intervention and the 2016 salt-intake reduction intervention, respectively (Table 2). The sample in 2015 was younger than the population recruited in 2014 and 2016 ($p < 0.05$), while the proportion of respondents with lower education level was higher in the 2014 sample. The ethnic minority samples were not comparable to the general Yunnan population ($p < 0.05$). The study sample had a high proportion of female and people with lower education level.

Table 2. Sociodemographic characteristics of the households participating in the 2014 to 2016 field visits in ManBangTang Village, Yunnan, China.

	ManBangTang Village			Yunnan [a]
	2014	2015	2016	2010
N	52	26	34	NA
Age *	30.0 (24.25–40.0)	20.0 (18.0–37.25)	35.0 (24.0–48.0)	NA
Female	20 (38.5%)	13 (43.3%)	11 (34.4%)	48.11%
Male-to-female ratio	1:0.63	1:0.76	1:0.52	1:0.9273
Education level *				
Illiterate/Non-formal Education	7 (13.7%)	3 (11.5%)	9 (26.5%)	14.97%
Primary school	30 (58.8%)	6 (23.1%)	10 (29.4%)	43.39%
Junior secondary	13 (25.5%)	17 (57.7%)	14 (41.2%)	27.48%
Senior secondary	1 (2.0%)	2 (7.7%)	1 (2.9%)	8.38%
Tertiary	0 (0.0%)	0 (0.0%)	0 (0.0%)	5.78%

[a] Sources: the Sixth National Population Census report in 2010 [32]; * $p < 0.05$.

3.2. General Food-Health-Related Practices and Experiences

3.2.1. Food Labelling

Among the 52 respondents, 36 of them (69.23%) reported the practice of buying packaged food. Snacks (52.8%, 19/36) and meat (33.3%, 12/36) were the most commonly brought packaged foods. As for the practice of reading the food labels before consuming packaged food, 60.0% (21/35) reported that they would read the food label. Among this group, 37.1% (13/21) claimed they always read the labels. The expiry date was the type of information on food labels that most respondents paid attention to; 95.2% among those that would read food labels would pay attention to expiration dates. Among those who did not practice reading food labels (14/35), about half of them (6/14) stated that they did not understand the label. Among respondents who practiced reading food labels on packaged food ($n = 21$), half of them (11/21) reported seeing confusing food labels before. About half (10/21) would ignore the label if they could not understand it.

3.2.2. Salt Consumption

Out of 52 respondents, 39 had reported their daily salt consumption. Among these, 56.8% (21/39) claimed they consumed one teaspoon or more of salt per day, only 27.0% (10/.39) claimed they consumed less than one teaspoon of salt per day.

3.2.3. Food Safety Problems

Out of the 52 respondents, 42 answered the question "had you encountered any food safety problem before" (Table 3). Among them, 23.8% (10/42) had encountered food safety problems before. Among those had encountered food safety problems, 40% were related to expired food (4/10) while 50% were associated with food quality problems (5/10). Thirty percent (3/10) had reported feeling sick or suffering from food poisoning as a result of the food quality problem.

Table 3. Needs assessment results related to food labelling, salt consumption, and food safety problems.

Questions (*N*)	Items/Choices	*N* (%)
Food Labelling [a]		
Type of food packages they bought ($n = 36$)		
	Fish	2 (5.6%)
	Meat	12 (33.3%)
	Fruit	6 (16.7%)
	Cereal	5 (13.9%)
	Milk/Product	3 (8.3%)
	Egg	2 (5.6%)
	Snacks	19 (52.8%)
	Others	4 (11.1%)
Check the food label before consuming the packaged food ($n = 35$)		
	Always	13 (37.14%)
	Sometimes	8 (22.86%)
	Never	14 (40 %)
Reasons for not checking the food labels on the packaged food ($n = 14$) [b]		
	Do not know there is a food label on the packaged food	1 (7.1%)
	Do not understand	6 (42.9%)
	Never thought about this before	2 (14.3%)
	Don't know	1 (7.1%)
	Rejected Answer	4 (28.6%)
Types of food labels subject pay attention to ($n = 21$)		
	Nutrition **	4 (19.0%)
	Expiration date	20 (95.2%)
	Way of Storage	2 (9.5%)
	Manufacture location	3 (14.3%)
Had you met the confusing food labels ($n = 21$)		
	Always	4 (19.0%)
	Sometimes	7 (33.3%)
	Never	5 (23.8%)
	Don't Know	3 (14.3%)
	Refuse to answer	2 (9.5%)
What will you do if you meet any un-understandable food label ($n = 21$)		
	Ignorance	10 (47.6%)
	Ask others for information	2 (9.52%)
	Not to purchase/eat	6 (28.57%)
	Don't know	2 (9.52%)
	Refuse to answer	1 (4.76%)
Salt consumption		
Daily Salt intake($n = 39$)		
	1 teaspoon or above	21 (53.85%)
	Less than 1 teaspoon	10 (25.64%)
	Cannot estimate the salt intake	8 (20.51%)
Food safety related problem		
Encountered any Food safety problem ($n = 52$)		
	Yes, usually	2 (4.76%)
	Yes, but not often	8 (19.05%)
	Never	32 (76.19%)

Table 3. *Cont.*

Questions (*N*)	Items/Choices	*N* (%)
Encountered what kinds of food safety problem (n = 10) [c]		
	Food expired	4 (40%)
	Counterfeit food	1 (10%)
	Food spoilage	5 (50%)
	Usage of illegal additive	1 (10%)
	Would you get any food poisoning due to food safety problem	3 (30.0%)
Factors to define whether the food is gone bad or not (n = 44)		
	Taste	8 (16.3%)
	Smell	6 (12.2%)
	Appearance	21 (42.9%)
	Feeling	6 (12.2%)
	Date/Food Label	3 (6.1%)

** One respondent specifically mentioned protein and fat; [a] Respondents were also asked if they had bought Cereal and Beans, but none replied they had; [b] No respondent replied "No label on the packaged food" and "not important" as the reason for not checking the food label; [c] No respondents report they had encountered "wrong/misleading instruction" as a food safety problem.

The most common methods used by the respondents to determine whether the food had gone bad or not were checking the appearance (42.9%, 21/44), followed by tasting (16.3%, 8/44), smelling (12.2%, 6/44), personal feeling (12.2%, 6/44) and reading the food label (6.1%, 3/44).

3.2.4. Associating Factors of the Food-Health-Related Practices (Food Labelling and Salt-Intake Reduction)

The association between sociodemographic characteristics and the practice of reading food labels and salt consumption were explored using the needs assessment data (2014). The chi-squared test showed that higher education level was associated with more frequent use of reading food label (p = 0.046), where 80% of those with secondary education; 59.1% of those with primary education and 0.0% of those receiving no formal education would always or sometimes read the label. Age and gender were not shown to be associated with the practices of reading food labelling or salt consumption related behavior.

3.3. Evaluation of Health Education Intervention Effectiveness

There were 26 (81.25%) valid pre-and post-intervention questionnaires in the 2015 health intervention on food labeling topic and 40% (N = 18) valid pre- and post-intervention questionnaires in the 2016 health intervention on the salt-intake reduction topic. The dropout rate was due to the open-to-public format of the interventions. Some respondents left before completing the post-questionnaire or arrived after the intervention had started. Only those who had completed a pre- and a post-questionnaire were considered attending the whole intervention. This group of respondents could reflect the interventions' effect better and therefore were considered in the evaluations. The pre- and post-questionnaires were compared using pairwise McNemar's test to evaluate the changes in knowledge, awareness, and behaviors on both topics after the intervention. Table 4 shows the evaluation results of both interventions.

Table 4. Key findings on the effectiveness of pre-and post-intervention in the 2015 Food Labelling.

2015 Health Intervention on Food Labelling ($N = 26$)			
	Pre- (%)	Post- (%)	*p* value
Food Labelling awareness and knowledge			
Understand that eating expired package food will affect health	73.1%	100.0%	0.004 *
Able to distinguish if the food is expired	46.2%	88.5%	<0.001 *
Question sample 1 (Able to distinguish if the food is expired)	36.0%	72.0%	0.012 *
Question sample 2 (Able to distinguish if the food is expired)	44.0 %	48.0%	0.780
Question sample 3 (Able to distinguish if the food is expired)	24.0%	54.0%	0.023 *
Food Labelling behavior			
Will not eat or buy any expired food	69.1%	76.9%	0.532
Check the expiry date every time before buying	34.6%	80.8%	0.001*
Check the expiry date every time before consuming	30.8%	76.9%	0.001 *
Remind my family and friends keep checking the expiry date	69.2%	92.35	<0.035 *
Confident enough to cultivate the habits of reading food labels	-	100%	-

* $p < 0.05$.

3.3.1. 2015 Health Intervention on Food Labelling

In the 2015 health intervention, 26 valid sets of pre- and post- questionnaires were analyzed. Ten questions, including the food labelling awareness, knowledge, and behaviors, were asked (Table 4). Significant improvements in knowledge and awareness towards food labelling were observed after the intervention (four out of five questions). After the intervention, more respondents understood expired food could affect health (from 73.1 % to 100%, $p < 0.001$, McNemar's test). Three food label samples were presented to test if the respondents were able to tell whether the food was expired based on the information on the food label. Significant improvements were found in two out of the three questions after the interventions (Table 4). Changes in attitude towards reading food labelling were also observed after health intervention (two out of four questions). The number of respondents who indicated that they would check the expiry date before buying and consuming packaged food increased from 34.6% to 80.8% ($p = 0.002$, McNemar's test) and 30.8% to 76.9% ($p = 0.002$, McNemar's test), respectively.

3.3.2. 2016 Health Intervention on Salt-Intake Reduction

In the 2016 visit, 18 sets of valid pre- and post-questionnaires were collected (Table 5). Significant improvement was found in three out of six awareness and knowledge questions after the intervention. The proportion of respondents who knew high salt intake would cause hypertension increased from 50% to 88.9% ($p = 0.039$, Chi-square test). More respondents (from 44.4% to 88.9%) were aware that hypertension might cause heart disease ($p = 0.012$, Chi-square test). Although only half of the respondents could tell the correct suggested amount of daily salt consumption after the intervention, the improvement was statistically significant (from 11.1% to 50%, $p = 0.039$, Chi-square test).

After the intervention, the proportion of respondents who understand the function of the salt-reduction spoons and bottles increased from 11.1 % to 83.3% ($p < 0.001$, Chi-square test) and 11.1% to 72.2% ($p = 0.001$, Chi-square test), respectively. No significant changes were found for the attitude towards cutting down the daily salt-intake to the suggested standard or decreasing cured food consumption were observed.

Table 5. Key findings on the effectiveness of pre-and post-intervention in 2016 Salt Reduction.

2016 Health Intervention on Salt Reduction ($N = 18$)			
	Pre- (%)	Post- (%)	p value
Salt reduction awareness and knowledge			
Consume enough salt on a daily basis	61.1%	55.5%	1.000
High salt diet cause hypertension	50%	88.9%	0.039 *
Cured food contains high salt amount	61.1%	72.2%	0.375
Chronic hypertension cause heart disease	44.4%	88.9%	0.012 *
Chronic hypertension cause stroke	38.9%	72.2%	0.065
Understand the suggested amount of daily salt consumption	11.1%	50%	0.039 *
Salt reduction behavior			
Understand the function of salt-restriction spoon	11.1%	83.3%	<0.001 *
Understand the function of salt-restriction bottle	11.1%	72.2%	0.001 *
Control the consumption of salt below 6g daily in future month	66.7%	94.4%	0.063
Control the consumption of cured food in future month	72.2%	94.4%	0.125

* $p < 0.05$.

4. Discussion

This study examined the behavioral patterns in the 2014 needs assessment (including reading food labels and salt consumption), the effectiveness of health education interventions on food labeling (in 2015) and salt-intake reduction (in 2016) among an ethnic minority-based community (the Kunge population) in rural China. Results indicated about 60% of respondents who consumed packaged food would read the food label and most of them read the food label for expiry date information. Those who had a higher education level were more likely to read the food label. However, about half of them had found food labels confusing to comprehend. About half of the respondents also reported a daily salt intake level higher than the WHO's recommended amount [3] and about 24% of respondents reported experiencing some form of food safety problems. For both food labelling and salt-intake interventions, significant improvements in knowledge, including the health effects of consuming expired food, how to read the expiry date in a food label, the suggested amount of daily salt intake for adults, the association among high salt intake, hypertension and heart diseases, and the function of the salt-restriction-spoon and bottle, were observed after the interventions. In terms of attitude towards behaviors, more respondents indicated that they would check the expiry date before buying and eating packaged food and would control their salt consumption after the interventions, though the changes in attitude for salt consumption control was not statistically significant.

Only 60% of the respondents who had bought packaged food would pay attention to the food label. This figure was lower compared to another similar research from India. The study from Puducherry in India [33] reported that 90% of the respondents would pay attention to the food labels on packaged food. The relatively lower rate found in the Kunge respondents might be associated with the lack of relevant health education and education level in the community. As mentioned in the introduction, there are many incidents of problematic food products in rural areas [7–9]. This suggested that the awareness of food safety was insufficient in these areas, which increases the vulnerability in this population. Our needs assessment's result found that respondents with a higher education level had greater awareness of reading food labels. This supports the need, and potential value, to raise the food-health-related awareness in the community. The evaluation results showed that education interventions were effective in increasing awareness as well as their attitude towards the corresponding behaviors. A larger scale of education programmes and evaluation of the long-term impact of such programmes should be considered for the community.

High salt intake appeared to be common in the Kunge population in Yunnan. Nearly 60% of the respondents consumed one teaspoon or more per day, which exceeded the suggested standard for adults by the WHO (under one teaspoon) [3]. The result was consistent with those found in studies of other minority groups from rural China communities [16,17]. High salt intake was also found in another ethnic minority, the Yi, in Yunnan [34]. About 80% of them preferred preserved food which was suggested to be one of the underlying causes of a high prevalence of hypertension (37%) among the Yi population. Hence, salt-intake reduction should be promoted in rural community in Yunnan, in particular for ethnic minority communities, to reduce the risk of relevant health problems.

Among those who have encountered food safety problems (23.8%), food spoilage (50%) and expired food (40%) were the top two food safety problems reported. This finding is different from that of a study conducted in urbanized regions, Beijing and Nanjing, in China [35]. The greatest concerns found in the urban study were about food hygiene and food poisoning while expiry date only ranked the 4th among the food safety issues. The differences in food safety concerns between rural and urban regions may be related to the food surveillance systems as spoilage food was more commonly found in the food markets in rural areas due to the less efficient surveillance of food quality [7].

Significant improvement in knowledge and intention to practice the behavior were identified in both the salt reduction and food labelling interventions. Despite the improvements in the understanding of the effects of consuming expired food and the ability and willingness to read the food label, the proportion of respondents that claimed they would not purchase or consume expired food (76.9%) was still lower than that reported in another Chinese study conducted in 31 provinces (89.4%) [36]. This may be related to the economic status among the rural village. Our needs assessment in 2014 found that the study community was under the poverty line. For financial reasons, respondents might still consume expired food even if they understood the potential adverse health effects. Improving the quality of local food supply and encouraging the community to purchase packaged food when needed (to avoid overstocking) might help to reduce the chances for the community to consume expired food. More studies are warranted for drafting effective policies to tackle the problem. Similarly, improvement in salt intake-related knowledge did not imply a change of behavior in salt-intake and consumption of cured food. More research will be needed to understand the economic, cultural, and behavioral challenges.

There were a few limitations in this study. First, only immediate effects of the interventions could be measured due to the project nature. Evaluation of long-term effects should be considered whenever possible to assess and achieve sustainability of the knowledge transferred. Second, this study did not cover the entire food-related behavior topic. Among food safety and consumption pattern, only salt consumption and food labelling of expiration date were investigated. There are other important dietary behaviors such as sugar and oil consumption and food-safety related behavior like storage or information seeking [5] to be explored in future studies. Third, the sample size for evaluating the effectiveness of the intervention was small which may not represent the whole community, especially for the salt-intake reduction. This limited the power of analysis and did not allow subgroup analysis and special consideration should be paid when interpreting the results for scaling up of related programs. Furthermore, there is also a lack of published or official documentation about this minority group for data triangulation. Lastly, language barrier was another limitation. For that, translators were invited to assist during data collection to minimize the barrier. Yet, despite of these limitations, this article will provide information about food and diet, two important aspects of H-EDRM for this special minority group in China.

5. Conclusions

This study identified the food-related Health-EDRM issues in a rural ethnic minority (Kunge) village in Yunnan, China. Not checking expiry dates of packaged food and a high salt diet were the most common problems in the Kunge community. Education interventions were found effective in improving food-related health knowledge despite the small sample sizes. These included the adverse health effects of consuming expired food, how to read the food label for expiry date information, the association among high salt intake, hypertension and heart health, the suggested maximum amount of salt intake for adults, and the function of salt-restriction-spoon and bottle. These interventions were also shown to be effective in changing attitudes toward some behaviors, such as willingness to read the food labels before buying and consuming packaged food. However, no significant improvements were found for the attitudes toward not consuming expired food, control salt-intake and decreased consumption of cured food. This suggests that although health education was effective in raising awareness and promoting health knowledge in a rural ethnic minority community, other elements, including economic status, culture and local food policy, should be considered when promoting changes of health behavior [37]. Special attention should be paid when interpreting the results for the representativeness of the small sample size.

Author Contributions: Conceptualization, E.Y.Y.C.; Methodology, H.C.Y.L.; T.K.C.L., C.K.P.W.; Validation, H.C.Y.L.; Formal analysis, E.S.K.L., S.N.S.T.; Investigation, E.Y.Y.C., H.C.Y.L., E.S.K.L., S.N.S.T., T.K.C.L., C.K.P.W.; Data curation, E.S.K.L., S.N.S.T.; Writing-Original Draft Preparation, E.Y.Y.C., E.S.K.L., S.N.S.T.; Writing—Review & Editing, E.Y.Y.C., H.C.Y.L., E.S.K.L., S.N.S.T.; Project Administration, E.Y.Y.C., T.K.C.L., C.K.P.W.; Funding Acquisition, E.Y.Y.C.

References

1. World Health Organization. Food Safety Overview. Available online: http://www.searo.who.int/entity foodsafety/topics/overview/en/ (accessed on 11 March 2019).
2. Xue, J.; Zhang, W. Understanding China's food safety problem: An analysis of 2387 incidents of acute foodborne illness. *Food Control* **2013**, *30*, 311–317. [CrossRef]
3. World Health Organization. Salt Reduction. Available online: https://www.who.int/news-room/fact-sheets/detail/salt-reduction (accessed on 26 February 2019).
4. World Health Organization. Food Safety. Available online: https://www.who.int/news-room/fact-sheets detail/food-safety (accessed on 11 March 2019).
5. World Health Organization. Food Safety: What You Should Know. Available online: http://www.searo.who/.int/entity/world_health_day/2015/whd-what-you-should-know/en/ (accessed on 26 February 2019).
6. Adebowale, O.; Kassim, I.O. Food safety and health: A survey of rural and urban household consumer practices, knowledge to food safety and food related illnesses in Ogun state. *Epidemiol. Biostat. Public Health* **2017**, *14*, e12568-1–e12568-7.
7. Liu, J. Woguo shao shu minzz shipin anquan wenti ji qi zhìli (The food safety problem and mangement in China). *Guizhou Soc. Sci.* **2013**, *285*, 150–154. (In Chinese)
8. People's Daily Online. Renmin ribao shenghuo manbu: Nongcun bushi guoqi shipin qingxiao de (Rural village is not a expired food market). Available online: http://opinion.people.com.cn/n/2014/0418 c1003-24911122.html (accessed on 26 Febeuary 2019). (In Chinese).
9. Oriental Daily News. Shenzhou guancha wenti shipin gong nongcun chrngxisng you bie liang chong tian (Observation in China: Problematic food supply in rural village, distinctive difference of food problem, between urban and rural area). Available online: https://hk.on.cc/hk/bkn/cnt/commentary/20140209/bkn-20140209011401057-0209_00832_001.html (accessed on 26 February 2019). (In Chinese).
10. Ministry of Commerce of the People's Republic of China. 2008 Nian liutong lingyu shipin anquan diaocha baogao.Doc (2008 safety investigation report of food product flow in China). Available online: http: //doc.mbalib.com/view/f23fae622d72c5315bf7749cf74dc288.html (accessed on 26 February 2019). (In Chinese)
11. Lozano, R.; Naghavi, M.; Foreman, K.; Lim, S.; Shibuya, K.; Aboyans, V.; Abraham, J.; Adair, T.; Aggarwal, R.; Ahn, S.Y.; et al. Global and regional mortality from 235 causes of death for 20 age groups in 1990 and 2010: A systematic analysis for the Global Burden of Disease Study 2010. *Lancet* **2012**, *380*, 2095–2128. [CrossRef
12. Wei, Q.; Sun, J.; Huang, J.; Zhou, H.Y.; Ding, Y.M.; Tao, Y.C.; He, S.M.; Liu, Y.L.; Niu, J.Q. Prevalence of hypertension and associated risk factors in Dehui City of Jilin Province in China. *J. Hum. Hypertens.* **2015**, *29* 64–68. [CrossRef]
13. Shao, S.; Hua, Y.; Yang, Y.; Liu, X.; Fan, J.; Zhang, A.; Xiang, J.; Li, M.; Yan, L.L. Salt reduction in china: A state-of-the-art review. *Risk Manag. Healthc. Policy* **2017**, *10*, 17–28. [CrossRef] [PubMed]
14. Chinese National Knowledge Infrastructure. Zhongguo jingji yu shehui fazhan tongji shujuku: Diaocha diqu jumin manxingbing huan bing lu (%) (Survey of chronic disease prevalence (%) among residents in various regions). Available online: http://tongji.cnki.net/kns55/Navi/result.aspx?id=N2015110062&file=N2015110062000236&floor=1 (accessed on 11 March 2019). (In Chinese).

15. Wang, Z.; Chen, Z.; Zhang, L.; Wang, X.; Hao, G.; Zhang, Z.; Shao, L.; Tian, Y.; Dong, Y.; Zheng, C.; et al. Status of hypertension in China: Results from the China hypertension survey, 2012–2015. *Circulation* **2018**. [CrossRef]
16. Hipgrave, D.B.; Chang, S.; Li, X.; Wu, Y. Salt and sodium intake in China. *J. Am. Med. Assoc.* **2016**, *315*, 703–705. [CrossRef] [PubMed]
17. Mente, A.; O'Donnell, M.; Rangarajan, S.; McQueen, M.; Dagenais, G.; Wielgosz, A.; Lear, S.; Ah, S.T.L.; Wei, L.; Diaz, R.; et al. Urinary sodium excretion, blood pressure, cardiovascular disease, and mortality: A community-level prospective epidemiological cohort study. *Lancet* **2018**, *392*, 496–506. [CrossRef]
18. Wong, J.; Sun, W.; Wells, G.; Li, Z.; Li, T.; Wu, J.; Zhang, Y.; Liu, Y.; Li, L.; Yu, Y.; et al. Differences in prevalence of hypertension and associated risk factors in urban and rural residents of the Northeastern region of the people's republic of China: A cross-sectional study. *PLoS ONE* **2018**, *13*, e0195340. [CrossRef]
19. Wang, Q.; Xu, L.; Sun, L.; Li, J.; Qin, W.; Ding, G.; Zhang, J.; Zhu, J.; Xie, S.; Yu, Z.; et al. Rural-urban difference in blood pressure measurement frequency among elderly with hypertension: A cross-sectional study in Shandong, China. *J. Health Popul. Nutr.* **2018**, *37*, 25. [CrossRef]
20. Li, J.; Shi, L.; Li, S.; Xu, L.; Qin, W.; Wang, H. Urban-rural disparities in hypertension prevalence, detection, and medication use among Chinese Adults from 1993 to 2011. *Int. J. Equity Health* **2017**, *16*, 50. [CrossRef]
21. Yuan, F.; Qian, D.; Huang, C.; Tian, M.; Xiang, Y.; He, Z.; Feng, Z. Analysis of awareness of health knowledge among rural residents in Western China. *BMC Public Health* **2015**, *15*, 55. [CrossRef]
22. Chan, E.Y.Y.; Huang, Z.; Lam, H.C.Y.; Wong, C.K.P.; Zou, Q. Health Vulnerability Index for Disaster Risk Reduction: Application in Belt and Road Initiative (BRI) Region. *Int. J. Environ. Res. Public Health* **2019**, *16*, 380. [CrossRef]
23. Chan, E.Y.Y.; Man, A.Y.T.; Lam, H.C.Y. Scientific evidence on natural disasters and health emergency and disaster risk management in Asian rural-based area. *Br. Med. Bull.* **2019**, *129*, 91. [CrossRef]
24. Chan, E.Y.Y.; Ho, J.Y.; Huang, Z.; Kim, J.H.; Lam, H.C.Y.; Chung, P.P.W.; Wong, C.K.P.; Liu, S.; Chow, S.; Man, A.Y.T.; et al. Long-Term and Immediate Impacts of Health Emergency and Disaster Risk Management (Health-EDRM) Education Interventions in a Rural Chinese Earthquake-Prone Transitional Village. *Int. J. Disaster Risk Sci.* **2018**, *9*, 319–330. [CrossRef]
25. Pickering, C.J.; O'Sullivan, T.L.; Morris, A.; Mark, C.; McQuirk, D.; Chan, E.Y.; Guy, E.; Chan, G.K.; Reddin, K.; Throp, R.; et al. The Promotion of "Grab Bags" as a Disaster Risk Reduction Strategy. *PLoS Curr.* **2018**, *10*.
26. Jiang, G.; Shi, J. Kun Ge Hua Yin Xi (phonetic System of Kunge). *J. Chongqing Univ. Technol.* **2015**, *29*, 302.
27. Jiang, G.; Shi, J. Kun Ge Ren Yu Yan Shi Yung Xian Zhuang Diao Cha (A Field Investigation of Language Use of the Kunge Ethnic Group). *J. China West Norm. Univ. Pilos. Soc. Sci.* **2013**, *1*, 80–85. (In Chinese)
28. The World Bank. The International Poverty Line Has Just Been Raised to $1.90 a Day, but Global Poverty Is Basically Unchanged. How Is That Even Possible? Available online: http://blogs.worldbank.org/developmenttalk/international-poverty-line-has-just-been-raised-190-day-global-poverty-basically-unchanged-how-even (accessed on 26 February 2019).
29. Howard, G.; Bogh, C.; Prüss, A.; Goldstein, G.; Shaw, R.; Morgan, J.; Teuton, J. *Healthy Villages: A Guide for Communities and Community Health Workers*; World health organization: Geneva, Switzerland, 2002.
30. Ge, K. The transition of Chinese dietary guidelines and the food guide pagoda. *Asia Pac. J. Clin. Nutr.* **2011**, *20*, 439–446.
31. China Country Commercial Guide. China—Labeling/Marking Requirements. Available online: https://www.export.gov/article?id=China-Labeling-Marking-Requirements (accessed on 11 April 2019).
32. National Bureau of Statistics of China. Yunnan sheng 2010 nian di liu ci quanguo renkou pucha zhuyao shuju gongbao (Main statistics report of Yunnan province of the Sixth National Population Census). Available online: http://www.stats.gov.cn/tjsj/tjgb/rkpcgb/dfrkpcgb/201202/t20120228_30408.html (accessed on 26 February 2019). (In Chinese)
33. Jain, S.; Gomathi, R.; Kar, S. Consumer awareness and status of food labeling in selected supermarkets of Puducherry: An exploratory study. *Int. J. Adv. Med. Health Res.* **2018**, *5*, 36.
34. Chen, L.; Zong, Y.; Wei, T.; Sheng, X.; Shen, W.; Li, J.; Niu, Z.; Zhou, H.; Zhang, Y.; Yuan, Y.; et al. Prevalence, awareness, medication, control, and risk factors associated with hypertension in Yi ethnic group aged 50 years and over in rural China: The Yunnan minority eye study. *BMC Public Health* **2015**, *15*, 383. [CrossRef]

35. Liu, A.; Niyongira, R. Chinese consumers food purchasing behaviors and awareness of food safety. *Food Control* **2017**, *79*, 185–191. [CrossRef]
36. Yim, L.P.; Li, Y.; Tong, W.; Lu, W.; Hu, Z.F.; Huang, P. Zhongguo chengxiang jumin anquan ren zhi nengli he jijiu zijiu nengli fenxi (Safety cognitive ability and first aid capacity in emergency event among urban and rural residents in China). *China J. Public Health* **2015**, *31*, 842–845. (In Chinses)
37. Chan, E.Y.Y.; Shaw, R. *Public Health and Disasters: Health Emergency and Disaster Risk Management in Asia*; Springer: Singapore, 2019; in press.

9

Infection Spread and High-Resolution Detection of Close Contact Behaviors

Nan Zhang [1], Boni Su [2], Pak-To Chan [1], Te Miao [1], Peihua Wang [1] and Yuguo Li [1,*]

[1] Department of Mechanical Engineering, The University of Hong Kong, Pokfulam Road, Hong Kong 999077, China; zhangnan@hku.hk (N.Z.); ptjchan@connect.hku.hk (P.-T.C.); miaote@connect.hku.hk (T.M.); phwang@connect.hku.hk (P.W.)

[2] China Electric Power Planning & Engineering Institute, Beijing 100120, China; bnsu@eppei.com

[*] Correspondence: liyg@hku.hk

Abstract: Knowledge of human behaviors is important for improving indoor-environment design, building-energy efficiency, and productivity, and for studies of infection spread. However, such data are lacking. In this study, we designed a device for detecting and recording, second by second, the 3D indoor positioning and head and body motions of each graduate student in an office. From more than 400 person hours of data. Students spent 92.2%, 4.1%, 2.9%, and 0.8% of their time in their own office cubicles, other office cubicles, aisles, and areas near public facilities, respectively. They spent 9.7% of time in close contact, and each student averagely had 4.0 close contacts/h. Students spent long time on close contact in the office which may lead to high infection risk. The average interpersonal distance during close contact was 0.81 m. When sitting, students preferred small relative face orientation angle. Pairs of standing students preferred a face-to-face orientation during close contact which means this pattern had a lower infection risk via close contact. Probability of close contact decreased exponentially with the increasing distance between two students' cubicles. Data on human behaviour during close contact is helpful for infection risk analysis and infection control and prevention.

Keywords: infection spread and control; infection risk; human behavior; close contact; sensor-based; indoor environment; indoor positioning; head and body motion; open-plan office

1. Introduction

Indoor human behaviors directly impact on indoor thermal comfort [1], energy efficiency [2], office design [3], and exposure to pollutants (e.g., infectious microbes) [4]. Indoor human behaviors in and between different environments also directly impact on the infection risk [5]. Close contacts are believed to facilitate the spread of many viral respiratory diseases such as influenza [6], SARS [7], MERS [8], and even Ebola [9].

Infection risk via close contact is influenced by interpersonal distance, respiratory activities, and movement of body parts. Interpersonal distance directly affects the risk of virus exposure due to inhalation and deposition, the so-called short-range airborne and large droplet routes, respectively [10]. A threshold distance of close contact less than 1.5 m to 2 m is generally accepted as risky [11–13]. Human respiratory activities such as breathing, talking, and coughing can generate droplets of different numbers and sizes [14–18]. Infectious pathogens are shed and exhaled by the infected during these respiratory activities, and transported by the exhaled air streams, while inhalation of fine droplets and exposure to large droplets are also affected by the inspiratory air streams and body/head/arm movement [19]. Relative face orientation (e.g., face-to-face, face-to-side) and posture are important factors in determining the cross-infection, especially over short distance [20]. Exposure of face-to-back close contact is much smaller than it of face-to-face pattern [21,22]. Posture also important in droplet deposition, for example, droplets deposited on trousers on the thighs of a sitting person should be more than on a standing person.

Very little data exist on indoor close contact behaviors, especially data combining all of the factors mentioned above. Some human behaviors are difficult to accurately monitor with high temporal resolution [11,19]. Electronic sensors such as radiofrequency identification devices (RFIDs) are the most commonly used to collect human contact data. These devices, however, can only detect close contact by taking readings of interpersonal distance every 20 s, and only one-on-one close contact can be detected [23,24]. A temporal resolution of 20 s is not sufficient, as the median value duration of a close contact is 17 s [11]. Moreover, human respiratory activities and movement of body parts (e.g., head and body) cannot be detected by this means. Body movements impact the air flows in a room. To collect close contact data with high temporal resolution, video recordings have been used, which can be processed second-by-second [11,19]. This approach is subject to human error on the part of the video analysts, and also time-consuming.

Office are the most common form of workplace for the most of employees, with open-plan designs widely used [25,26]. In this study, we monitored and analyzed indoor human behaviors in a graduate student office using automatic devices installed on the hats and clothes of the participants. These devices overcome nearly all of the shortcomings mentioned above and automatically collect high-resolution data on indoor human behaviors. The data monitored included the indoor position, head and body motion, and posture of each individual which are important for infectious disease transmission. We collected more than 1,440,000 s of data for 49 students across two days. This study supported data of indoor human behaviors on close contact. From indoor positioning distribution, we can know that which part in the office has higher infection risk. Combining individual inhalation and exhalation patterns with head's and body's motion during close contact, high-precision quantitative risk assessment on infection spread and control could be conducted.

2. Materials and Methods

The experiments were conducted in two close-by Chinese graduate student offices on two consecutive Saturdays. The choice of two nearly identical offices was due to the need of minimising microbial interference, as the experiment also contained another part on surface microbial monitoring, which is not reported in this paper.

2.1. Room Setting

Each room was designed for a maximum of 30 students, i.e., containing 30 cubicles (Figure 1). There were 26 students (13 male and 13 female) in Room 1 on the first experiment day (day 1), and 23 students (12 male and 11 female) in Room 2 on the second experiment day (day 2). A total of 32 students participated in the experiment, and 17 of them in both experiments. Among 32 participants, 27 students were those who worked in the institute and five students were invited by some students who were in the institute. In addition, three pairs of students were romantically involved. We selected these students because they were familiar with the experimental environment, which should minimize any bias caused by environment. The length (12.2 m) and height (2.73 m) of both rooms were the same, and the layouts of the cubicles in the two rooms were symmetrical, see Figure 1.

Each room had a water dispenser and a group of lockers. Only Room 2 had a printer. Each room was divided into six cubicle regions (marked by dotted lines in Figure 1), and students in the same cubicle region were more likely to communicate with each other. All of the students were monitored by 22 video cameras (1080P) from 8:30 a.m. to 9:30 p.m. The indoor temperature during the experimental days, which controlled by central air conditionings, was between 26 and 27 degrees. There were 27 fluorescent tubes on the ceiling of the office to keep the luminance, therefore, combing with the high-resolution cameras, most human behaviors can be captured. Each camera monitored one or two office cubicles, except for two with a global view, one camera for the door, and one camera for the water dispenser.

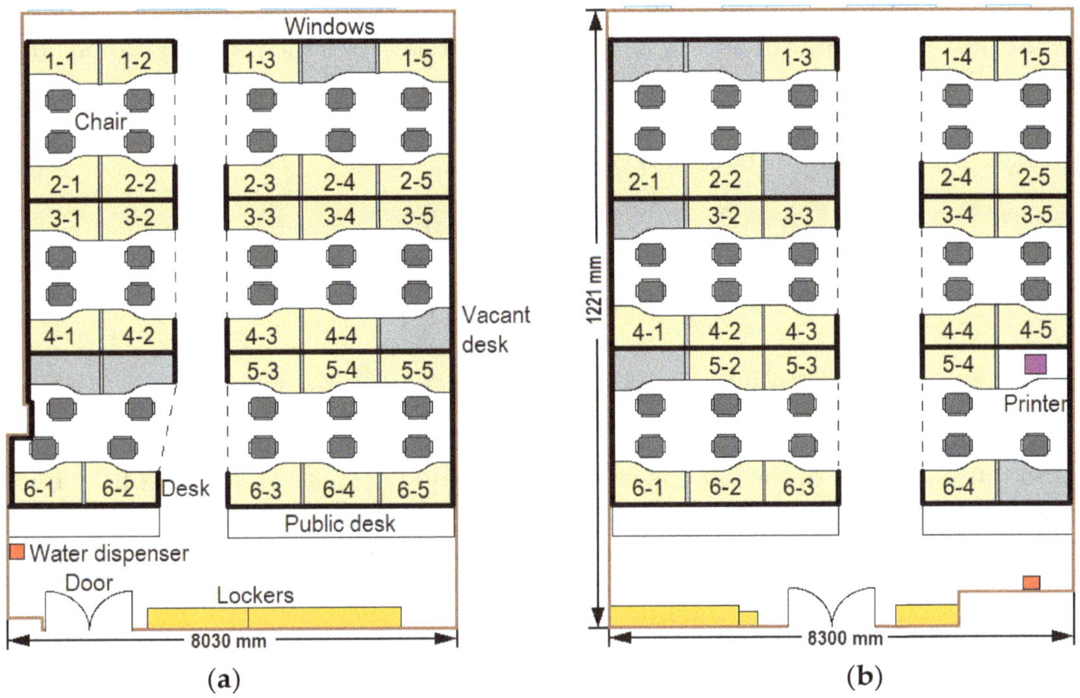

Figure 1. Room settings: (**a**) Room 1; (**b**) Room 2.

2.2. Detection Devices

The sensors we developed are shown in Figure 2a. The sensors for indoor positioning and head motion were installed on the participants' hats, and those for body motion were installed on the chest of a tight shirt. An ultrawide band (UWB) radio real-time location system (RTLS) was applied to obtain the indoor positions of all participants [27,28]. The distance resolution of UWB is within 0.1 m when there is no obstruction. To ensure continuous data transmission, the UWB tag was installed on the top of each hat, and four UWB anchors were installed on the office ceiling. An inertial measurement unit (IMU), which can measure and record the position and motion of the head and body (i.e., rotation), was also installed on the top of each hat and the front of each tight shirt. A microphone was installed on the collar band of the shirt to determine when the participants were talking. To protect privacy, only the sound level was recorded. Adjustable bands on the hat and around the head were used to avoid relative movement between the hat and head. Tight clothing was worn to avoid relative movement between the shirt and body. All of the data recorded during the experiment were saved in a chip. The weight of a device on hats and shirts was 73 g, and the weight of hat with fixed accessories was 159 g. Therefore, each student worn a hat of 232 g on the head and worn a device of 73 g on the shirt. Light weight brings a much smaller impact on human behaviors.

Rotations were recorded in the form of quaternions. To obtain the absolute (relative to the ground) rotation of the head and body, all of the participants underwent calibration after wearing and before taking off the hat and the shirt. During the calibration, the participant stood still and faced the same wall while keeping his/her head and body upright for 10 s. For any IMU (head or body), the quaternions during the calibrations before and after the experiment were denoted as q_{start} and q_{end}, respectively. If the difference between q_{start} and q_{end} was greater than a threshold value (equivalent to 10° rotation), it was probable that the participant had moved the hat or shirt during the experiment, and the data were discarded. Data were also regarded as invalid if the fluctuation of rotation between 10-s calibrations was more than 5°. To eliminate drift errors for all sensors, the quaternions were adjusted from all valid raw data based on spherical linear quaternion interpolation (Equation (1)):

$$q = q_{raw} q_{start}^{-1} \left(q_{start} q_{end}^{-1} \right)^{(t - t_{start})/(t_{end} - t_{start})}, \tag{1}$$

where t is time, t_{start} and t_{end} are the time of the calibrations before and after the experiment. The steering vectors ($\vec{x_h}$, $\vec{y_h}$, $\vec{z_h}$ for head and $\vec{x_b}$, $\vec{y_b}$, $\vec{z_b}$ for body, relative to the ground) can be obtained from the quaternions (Figure 2b). Usually, the horizontal rotation of the head relative to the body direction is more important. The relative steering vectors of head to body ($\vec{x_{hb}}$, $\vec{y_{hb}}$, and $\vec{z_{hb}}$) can be calculated using coordinate transformation (Equation (2)):

$$\left[\vec{x_{hb}}\ \vec{y_{hb}}\ \vec{z_{hb}}\right] = \begin{bmatrix} x_{\vec{x_b}} & y_{\vec{x_b}} & 0 \\ x_{\vec{y_b}} & y_{\vec{y_b}} & 0 \\ 0 & 0 & 1 \end{bmatrix} \left[\vec{y_h}\ \vec{y_h}\ \vec{z_h}\right], \tag{2}$$

where $x_{\vec{x_b}}$ and $y_{\vec{x_b}}$ are the components of $\vec{x_b}$ the in x and y directions and $x_{\vec{y_b}}$ and $y_{\vec{y_b}}$ are the components of $\vec{y_b}$ in the x and y directions, respectively. Here, the roll and pitch of the head are relative to the ground; only the yaw of the head is relative to the body. There is no yaw of the body because no relevant reference point on the waist was monitored. Therefore, data on three head motions (yaw, pitch, and roll) and two body motions (pitch and roll) were collected.

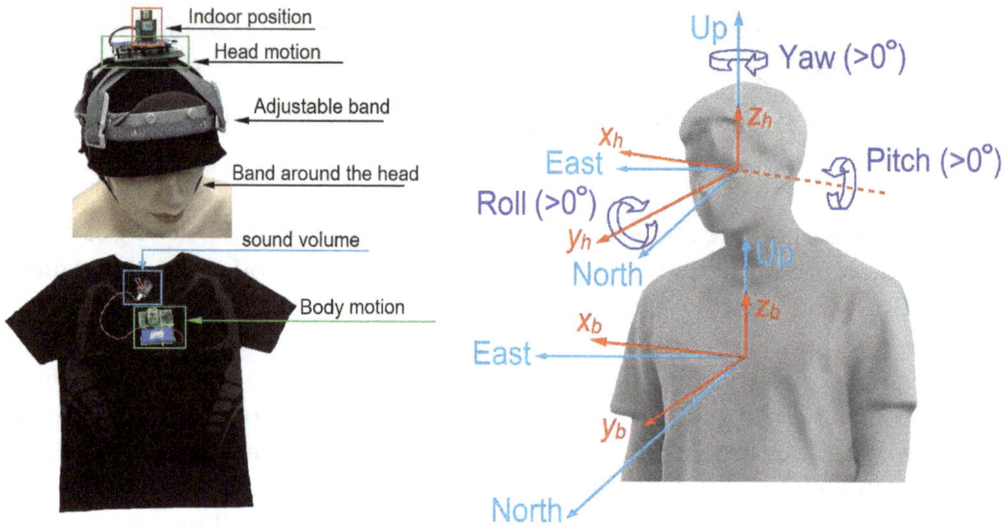

(a) (b)

Figure 2. Device design and motions of head and body. (**a**) Device for indoor positioning, and head and body motion detection; (**b**) current and base vectors for head and body.

All of the sensors were calibrated prior to the experiments. We first installed the IMUs on a large plate, and performed specific rotations with different angles (e.g., 45°, 90°, 135°, 180°) in three directions. The IMU was regarded as well-calibrated when the difference between all measured values and real values was less than 2°. The UWB sensors were also calibrated in the experimental rooms before the experiments. We chose five indoor points at which to perform calibration to reduce the error of indoor positioning to no more than 10 cm.

2.3. Close Contact Behavior

As motions relevant to the inhalation/exhalation flows, we considered individual head and upper body motions, human respiratory activities (e.g., coughing, sneezing, and speaking), and the features of relative position (e.g., interpersonal distance and relative face orientation) of two people. The definitions of head and body motions can be found in Zhang et al. [11].

Close contact was defined as any full or partial face-to-face interaction within 2 m [23,29–31]. A face-to-face interaction can occur with or without conversation, including when two individuals read a book or watch a computer screen together. An event was not counted as close contact if the distance between the two students was shorter than 2 m but there was no interaction between them; for example, if two students used their own computers in their own cubicles. If any close contact lasted for more than 1 s, it was counted as a single close contact. If the two students were separated (more than 2 m apart or with no interaction) by more than 1 s, the individual students' close contact behavior (e.g., with another student at that distance) was counted separately. In this study, interpersonal distance was defined as the distance between the sensors on the two participants other than those on their faces. In addition to interpersonal distance, the relative face orientation angle of the two participants was also obtained. This is the angle between the normal of the two students and ranges from 0° to 180° [11].

2.4. Data Processing

During the two experimental days, 1,440,492 s of human behavior data were collected. The first author processed all video episodes second by second, recording all visible close contacts between each pair of students in the office. The collected data include posture (standing, sitting, and squatting), whether two students were in close contact, the identities of those in close contact, and the start and end time of each episode of close contact. The indoor position and head and body motions were monitored by sensors. The indoor position data on *day 1* were unfortunately missed, which means that all of the valid indoor position data were from *day 2*. Out of the 23 participants, 21 had indoor position data during *day 2*, and in total 717,168 s of indoor position data were collected. Among these data, 10,827 s (1.5%) was lost or disrupted, and linear interpolation was used to approximate these data. To maintain the accuracy of all recorded data on head and body motions, we discarded the data for which the difference between two calibrations was more than 10° or the fluctuation during each calibration was more than 5°. After data filtering, 541,200 s of data on head and body motions were valid. Moreover, a total of 1,250,392 s of valid data on sound levels were recorded by the microphones over the two days. All of the results reported below are based on these valid data.

3. Results

3.1. General Human Behavior Data

While indoors, the students spent 5.3% of their time standing, 94.6% sitting, and only 0.1% squatting. We divided the office into functional areas, i.e., occupied office cubicles, vacant office cubicles, aisle, and areas near public facilities (Figure 3a). Figure 3b shows the distribution of indoor positions during *day 2*, where red indicates the highest coverage rate (≥40 times per 25 cm^2). Occupied office cubicles had the highest coverage rate, mainly due to occupation by their owner (Figure 3b). The students spent on average 92.2% of their time staying in their own cubicles. For the remaining 7.8% of the time, the students occupied other places. The results show that they spent most of the latter time in the aisle close to the doorway, the area close to the door, and areas close to the printer and the water dispenser (Figure 3c). Some students had a particularly close relationship with certain others or even a romantic relationship (e.g., boy-/girlfriend), and their office cubicles had a higher probability of being occupied by others. Most vacant office cubicles had a very low occupied percentage. In general, when outside their own cubicle, the students spent 47.9%, 4.5%, 37.4%, and 10.2% of their time in occupied office cubicles, vacant office cubicles, the aisle, and areas near public facilities.

Based on 541,200 valid data of head and body motions, we obtained the general characteristics of these motions for the overall group of students. Figure 4a illustrates the head and body motions. The circle shows the probability distribution of face orientation in the form of a projected half sphere; the reader can imagine that the eyes are located at the center of the sphere. This half sphere is divided into 1296 sectors, each of them 5° × 5°. The top, bottom, left, and right correspond to the participant raising, lowering, left-turning, and right-turning the head by 90°. The center indicates that the student is looking almost exactly forward.

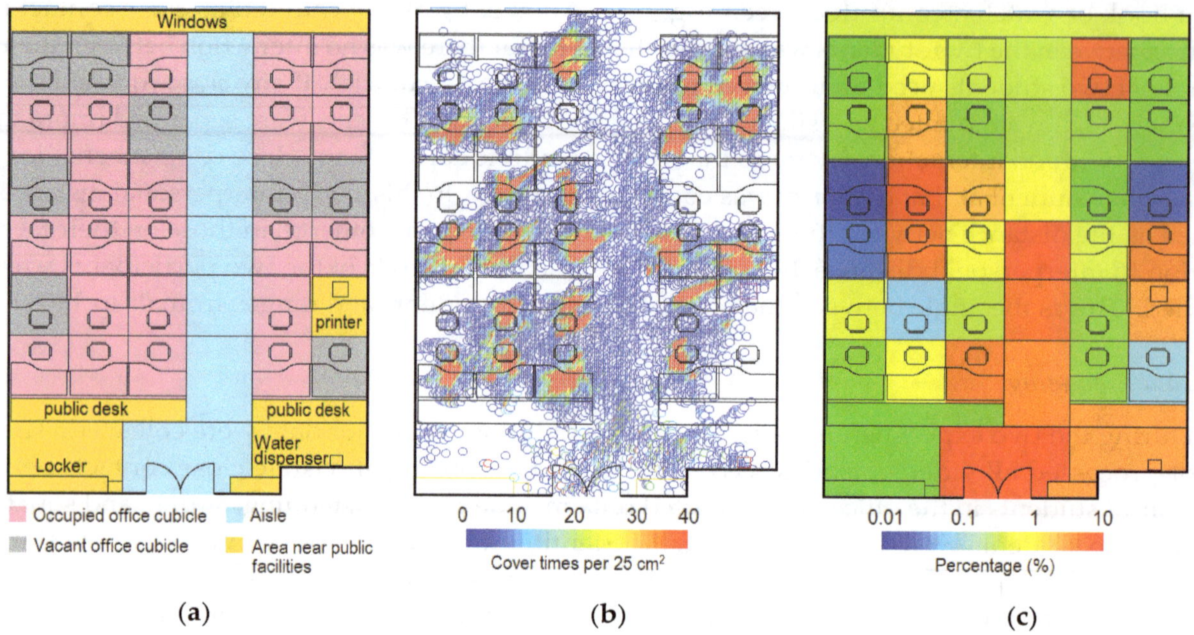

Figure 3. Indoor positioning in Room 2 (*day 2*). (**a**) Functional area; (**b**) Distribution of indoor positions; (**c**) Distribution of indoor positions by functional area during the time spent in other places (i.e., students outside their own cubicles). (Indoor positioning data for students 3-4 and 3-5 were lost).

This provides an intuitive visualization of the students' preferred head motions. In the office, the students preferred to look towards the red and orange grids in the circle (i.e., lower their head), and had a very low probability of raising their head (blue grids). To characterize the head motions, we considered the movement of the head in three directions independently. In the horizontal direction, the average degree of yaw was 4.1°, which means that the students on average slightly turned their head to the right by 4.1°.

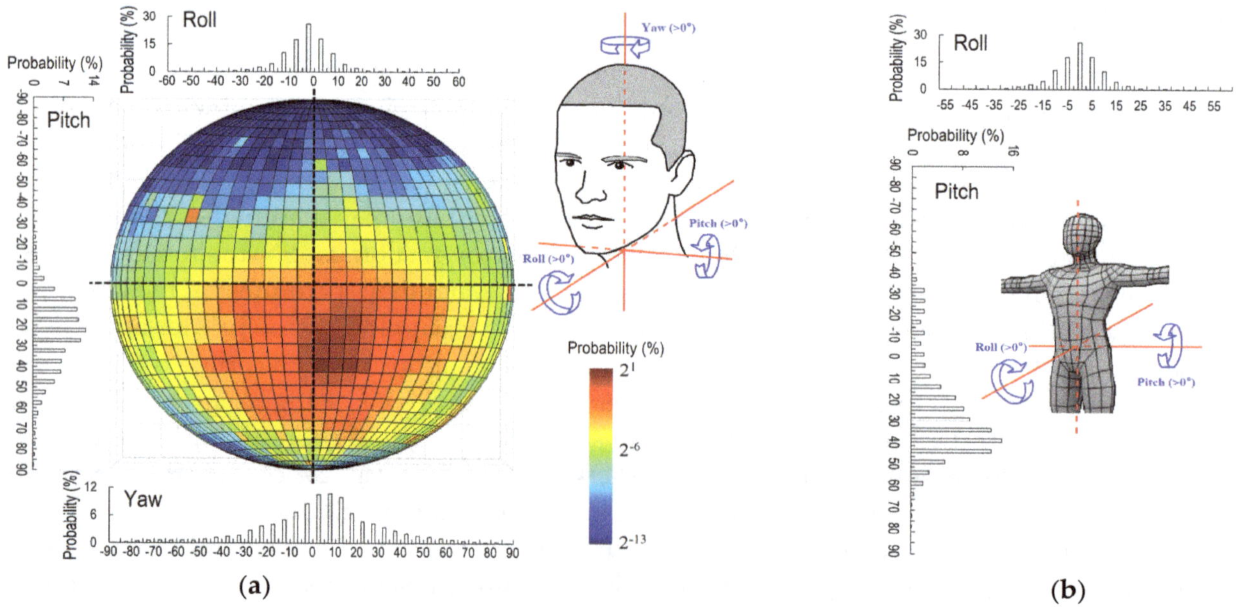

Figure 4. Indoor human behavior in terms of head and body motion. (**a**) Head motion; (**b**) Body motion. (Yaw of head is relative to the body; pitch and roll of head and all body motions are relative to the ground).

The students had almost equal probability of turning their head left and right, i.e., the probability distribution of yaw was symmetric. The average degree of pitch was 23.0°, which means that the students preferred to lower their head by 23.0° on average. Indeed, the head was lowered during 93.5% of indoor time. The students on average tilted (rolled) the head 2.8° to the left. The probability distributions of left and right tilts were almost the same. The students spent 86.1% and 97.4% of time tilting their head within 15° and 30°, respectively.

Figure 4b shows the body motions during indoor time. The students on average lowered their bodies (pitch) by 23.2°, and spent 85.6% of indoor time bending their bodies forward. The average degree of body roll was 3.7°, which means that the students on average slightly tilted their bodies to the right. The probability distribution of roll was almost symmetric. The students spent 86.7% and 98.2% of time tilting their bodies within 15° and 30°, respectively.

Three postures were considered in this study: standing, sitting, and squatting. Here we only analyzed head and body motions during standing and sitting because the students spent very little time squatting (0.1%). Figure 5 lists the probability distributions of head and body motions in three directions for all students during indoor time. The rolling of the head and body showed little difference between standing and sitting postures, and the participants had only a slightly higher probability of bending their head during sitting than during standing. However, the characteristics of yaw and pitch of the head, and pitch of the body, differed by posture. The average angles of head yaw during standing and sitting were −3.0° and 4.5°, respectively. The students on average lowered their heads by 30.9° and 24.1° while standing and sitting, respectively. The pitch of the body was strongly linked to posture. The average angles of pitch of the body during standing and sitting were 21.2° and 24.7°, respectively. However, the students had a higher probability of keeping their body bent forward at a large angle during standing ($\beta_b > 60°$ during 8.1% of the time) than during sitting ($\beta_b > 60°$ during 0.7% of the time). The most common forward-bending angle of the body during standing was between 10° and 15°, while that during sitting was 35° to 40°.

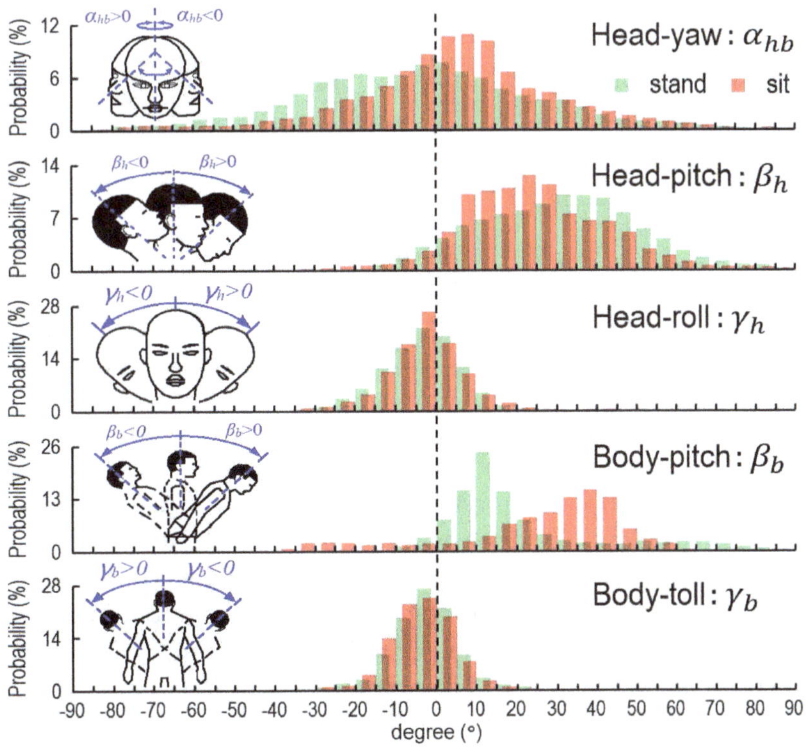

Figure 5. Probability distribution of head and body motions by posture.

3.2. Indoor Behavior During Close Contact

The students spent more than 9.7% of their time in close contact and each student had on average 4.0 close contact episodes per hour. The probability distribution of close contact fitted a log-normal distribution (Figure 6). The average and median durations of close contact were 54.5 and

15 s, respectively. Close contacts with duration between 8 and 16 s had the highest frequency. The durations of 38.2%, 68.8%, and 82.8% of close contacts were no more than 10, 30, and 60 s, respectively. From the microphone data, at least one student was speaking during 68.6% of the time during close contact. One-on-one close contacts accounted for more than 90% of close contact time, while 7.8%, 1.5%, and 0.6% of close contact time involved three, four, and five students simultaneously. Six-student conversations only accounted for 0.06% of close contact time.

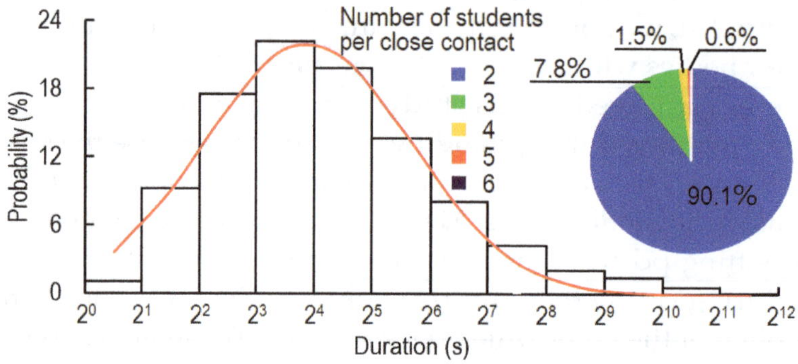

Figure 6. Probability distribution of duration per close contact.

During close contact, 22.9%, 76.3%, and 0.8% of students stood, sat, and squatted, respectively (Table 1). During 59.6% of the close contact time, both students were sitting. The pattern of one standing and one sitting was adopted during 33.5% of the close contact time. The students almost never chatted with each other while one stood and one squatted (0.1% of close contact time).

Table 1. Probability distribution of individual postures and posture pattern of students during close contact.

Description	Posture	Percentage
Individual posture	Sitting	76.3%
	Standing	22.9%
	Squatting	0.8%
Posture pattern	Sitting-sitting	59.6%
	Sitting-standing	33.5%
	Standing-standing	5.6%
	Sitting-squatting	1.2%
	Others	0.1%

Figure 7 shows the characteristics of close contact. As can be seen, 68.2% of the close contacts were between students in the same region, and most were between adjacent students. Only 13.2% of the close contacts were between students in remote regions (Figure 7a). Influenced by the circulation of people, students near the aisle and the door had a higher probability of being contacted (Figure 7b). From Figure 7c, the greater the distance between the office cubicles of two students was, the lower was the probability of a close contact. The average cubicle distance between two students for close contact was 1.25 areas (for the area distribution refer to Figure 3a), and 77.2% of close contacts occurred between two students with a cubicle distance of no more than three areas. The student who had the closest contacts had 50.5 episodes per hour (Figure 7d). On average each student had 4.0 close contact episodes per hour, and no one had zero close contacts during either day. During the two days, 12.2% (total pairs of contact: 141; possible pairs of contact: $1156 = 26 \times 25 + 23 \times 22$) of all possible pairs of students had close contact. Each pair of students had close contact on average 11.3 times per day, and the pair with the highest frequency of close contacts had 100 episodes per day (Figure 7e). As shown in Figure 7f, 22.4%, 40.8%, 59.2%, and 85.7% of the students spent no more than 1%, 5%, 10%, and 20% of their time in close contacts, respectively. The most sociable student spent 34% of her indoor time in close contact. The average and median ratios of close contact time to total indoor time were 9.7% and 6.4%, respectively. During the two days, the students had close contacts with an average of 8.4 and 4.2 students, respectively. The most sociable student had close contacts with 10 and 20 students during *day 1* and *day 2*, respectively (Figure 7g).

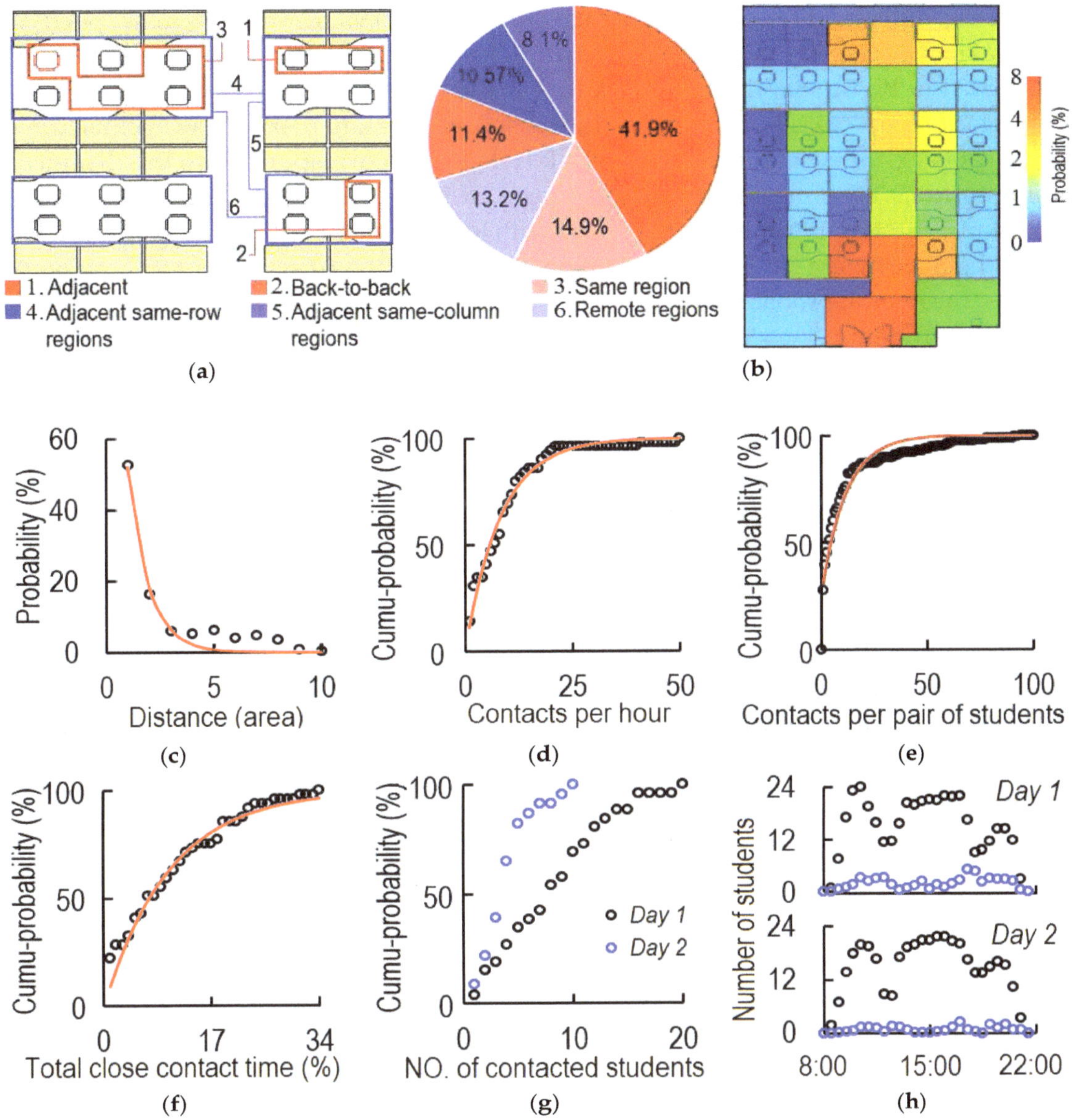

Figure 7. Characteristics of close contact. (**a**) Probability distribution by relative position of students' office cubicles (same region means two students are in the same region but not adjacent or back to back; percentage shows the episodes of close contact occurred in different relative positions); (**b**) Probability of area occupancy by area during close contact between remote students (students in different regions). The colour bar shows the ln values; (**c**) Probability distribution by distance between work cubicles of two students (distance is calculated as number of functional areas between cubicles of the two students, as illustrated in Figure 3a. For example, distance = 1 for adjacent or back-to-back office cubicles, and distance = 5 between *cubicles 2-2* and *3-2* (see Figures 1b and 3a)); (**d**) Cumulative probability distribution by frequency of close contact (episodes/hour); (**e**) Cumulative probability distribution by total episodes of close contact per day between each pair of participants (episodes/day); (**f**) Cumulative probability distribution by ratio of close contact time to total indoor time (%); (**g**) Cumulative probability distribution by number of contacted students per day; and (**h**) Distribution of number of students who stayed in the room and had close contact during *day 1* and *day 2* (black and blue points are total number of indoor students and total number of students in close contact, respectively).

From Figure 7h, the times of day with the most students in the office were between 9:30 and 11:30 and between 13:00 and 17:30. The peak frequency of close contact was between 11:00 and 12:30 and after 16:00.

Figure 8 shows the interpersonal distance by posture and gender. The average interpersonal distance during close contact was 0.81 m. The average interpersonal distances between sitting-sitting, standing-standing, and standing-sitting students were 0.74 m, 0.93 m, and 0.88 m, respectively. There were three peaks of interpersonal distance during close contact between two students who were sitting. As shown in Figure 8a, the first peak (0.1–0.3 m) was caused by pairs of participants with a very close relationship (e.g., boy-/girlfriend), the second peak (0.6–0.7 m) was caused by pairs of students who sat back-to-back, and the third peak (1.1–1.2 m) corresponded to the distance between two adjacent students. The probability distributions of interpersonal distance for sitting-standing students and standing-standing students accorded with log-normal distributions, and the most frequent interpersonal distances were 0.5 and 0.7 m, respectively. As 60% of close contact was between two sitting students, the overall probability distribution of interpersonal distance (black line) was similar to that of two sitting students.

From Figure 8b, 21.4%, 22.8%, 38.1%, and 17.7% of close contacts were between two male students (M-M), two female students (F-F), a male and a female student (non-couple) (M-F_NC), and couples (M-F_C). The contact rates (ratios of actual relationships with close contact to total possible relationships) for M-M, M-F, and F-F were 15.7%, 25.9%, and 10.3%, respectively. The average episodes of close contact per day between each pair of M-M, M-F_NC, M-F_C, and F-F who had contact with each other were 6.9, 8.2, 70.5, and 12.1, respectively. The average durations per close contact between each pair of M-M, M-F_NC, M-F_C, and F-F were 68.3, 48.7, 53.6, and 58.5 s, respectively. The average interpersonal distances during close contact between these four groups were 0.88 m, 0.70 m, 0.96 m, and 0.71 m, respectively. There was no interpersonal distance shorter than 0.2 m during close contact between two male students. Two female students preferred close contact at a short distance (0.1–0.4 m). Students of different genders (non-couple) had two peaks of interpersonal distance, which were related to their seating position. Couples had a normal distribution of interpersonal distance, and preferred distances between 0.4 and 0.6 m.

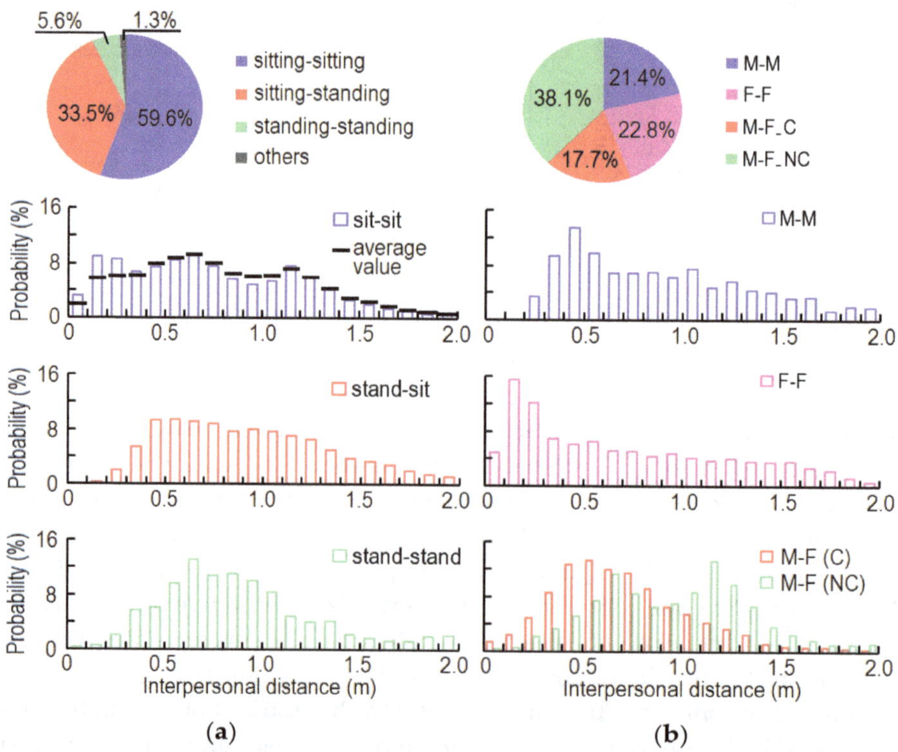

Figure 8. Probability distribution of interpersonal distance by: (**a**) Posture; (**b**) Gender.

There were three major posture patterns during close contacts in the office: sitting-sitting (both students sitting), standing-standing (both students standing), and sitting-standing (one student sitting, the other standing). The head and body motions of students and relative face orientation angles between students under different patterns of posture during close contact are shown in Figure 9. When two students were both standing or sitting, they preferred to look slightly downward. The average pitch angles of the head under sitting-sitting and standing-standing were 14.7° and 20.1°, respectively (Figure 9a,b). The average pitch angles of the body under these two conditions were 24.3° and 17.8°, respectively. However, under the sitting-standing condition (Figure 9c), the eye direction of the standing student was much lower than that of the sitting student.

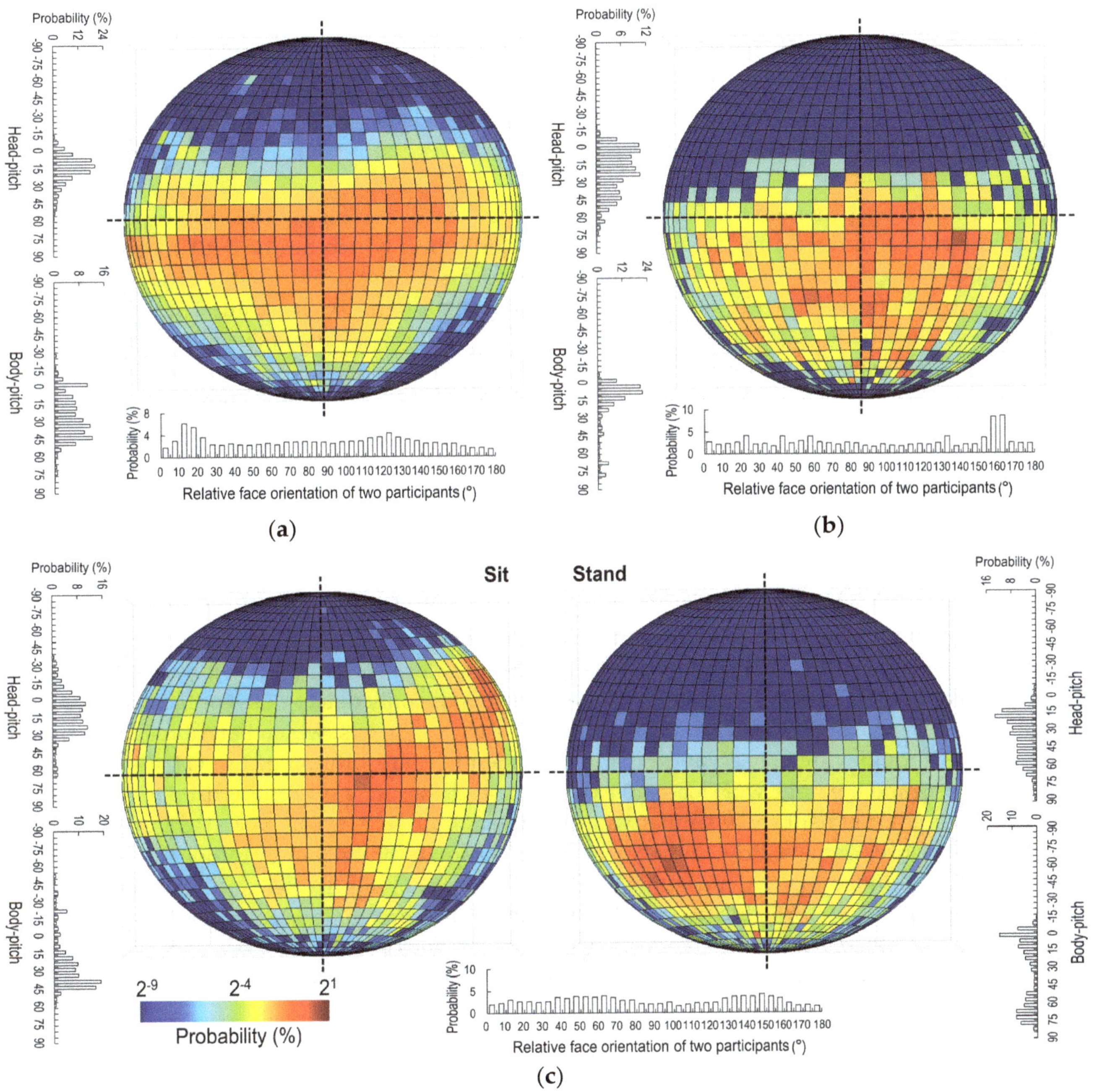

Figure 9. Head and body motions during close contact by posture of the two students: (**a**) Sitting-sitting; (**b**) Standing-standing; (**c**) Sitting-standing. (The circle shows the face orientation of the student; see Figure 4a).

The average pitch angles of the head of the sitting and the standing students in a sitting-standing pattern were 11.3° and 34.0°, respectively, and the average pitch angles of the body were 22.2° and 33.9°, respectively. The relatively low probability of looking downward for the sitting student implies that the standing student was usually located at the side of the sitting student rather than face-to-face. Standing students had a very high probability of facing downward.

Two sitting students had a high probability of only a slight relative angle of face orientation (5° to 25°) during close contact, which means that they usually faced in similar directions. Two standing students preferred face-to-face close contact with a relative face orientation angle between 150° and 170°. There was no obvious preference regarding relative face orientation angle under the sitting-standing pattern.

4. Discussion

4.1. Automatically Collected Indoor Human Behavior

In this study, we provided the first comprehensive dataset combining the indoor position, head and body motions, and posture of students at the same time which are helpful for infection risk assessment via close contact route. Indoor human behavior is strongly dependent on the type of indoor environment. In a hospital ward, patients usually lie in their beds, while health care workers walk between rooms and beds [32]. In an aircraft cabin or a cruise ship, passengers usually sit in their seats, while crew members walk through the aisle to provide service and food [33–35]. Both passengers in an aircraft cabin or a cruise ship and students in an office spend most of their time in their own seats or in aisles. Children in nurseries have been found to spend more time standing than sitting during indoor free-play time [36]. In a primary school, pupils have been found to spend 2.1 times more time sitting than standing during school hours [37]. However, in this study of a graduate student office, the students spent 94.6% of their time sitting. Therefore, people may tend to prefer sitting with increasing age, although the type of environment is also highly influential.

Close contact is an important activity in daily life, and also plays a critical role in infectious disease transmission. The duration of close contacts directly determines the exposure to viruses. Many researchers have reported the distribution of the duration of close contact (Figure 10) in different types of indoor environment. However, RFIDs or wireless sensors can only detect close contacts at intervals of 20 s [24,31,38–41], an insufficient temporal resolution for close contacts, which have a median duration of only 17 s. Although video observations can reach a temporal resolution of 1 s [11], the subjectivity of video analysts and the huge workload are two major shortcomings. As summarised in Figure 10, all types of indoor environment show similar values of the cumulative probability distribution (CDF) of the duration of close contacts. Brief close contacts (<20 s) are dominant, and prolonged close contacts (>300 s) are rare. Conferences and museums have a higher rate of long close contacts, while in hospitals and congress buildings shorter close contacts are more common. In a video observation study of a graduate student office, the average and median duration of close contact were 53.8 s and 17 s [11], respectively. Our study, meanwhile, found the average and median duration to be 54.5 s and 15 s, respectively.

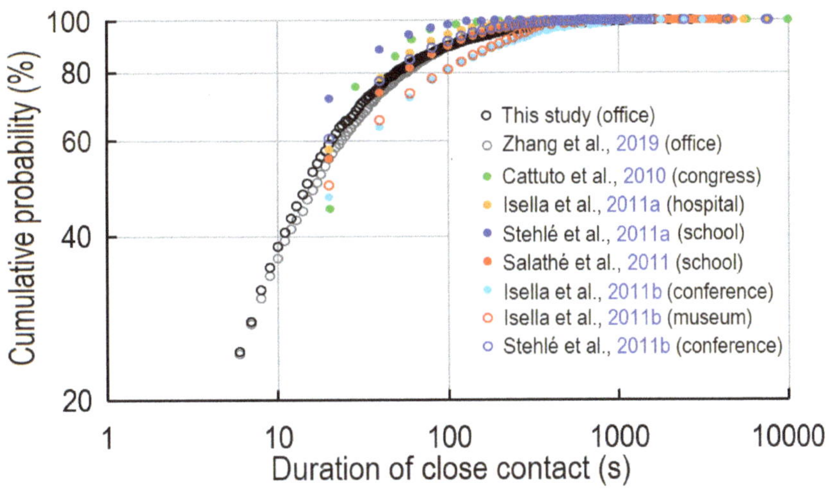

Figure 10. Cumulative probability distribution (CDF) of duration per close contact.

4.2. Close Contact Behavior

We collected and analyzed three types of data during close contact: indoor position, head and body motion/movement, and posture. These three factors are important to infectious disease transmission. Indoor position can help calculating the interpersonal distance of people during close contact. The infection risk decreases sharply with the increase of the interpersonal distance [12,20,42,43]. Posture, and head and body movement influence the body plume during close contact. For example, short-range exposure can be affected strongly by body plumes [44]. Frequent movement of the head and body during conversation can change not only the orientations of the exhaled/inhaled airflows, but also the patterns of body convective flows and the thermal plume. The exhaled airflows of two people also interact with and affect each other [12]. Various gestures involving small movements of the hands, palms, legs, eyebrows and other small-scale facial features may not significantly affect the body plume or exhaled flows [45,46]. Posture also important in droplet deposition. For example, more droplets may deposit on thighs of a sitting person if he/she talks with an infected. People have high probability to touch their thighs and legs with the frequency of more than 30 times per hour [19]. It may lead to a high infection risk because people also have high touch frequency on mucous membranes [47]. Relative face orientation is a critical factor for exposure during close contact, and it could be calculated by body and head motion. Previous studies found that the exposure during face-to-face close contact is the most, followed by face-to-side pattern, while face-to-back pattern had the lowest exposure [21,22].

As no such data on indoor human behavior in an office had previously been published, we mainly compared the sensor-collected data from this study with those of our previous experiment based on video observation [11] (Table 2). As head and body motions cannot easily be recorded using observation methods, the accuracy is difficult to guarantee. This may be the cause of the disagreements between the results in Table 2. In addition, in our previous experiment, all participants were students whose cubicles were in the studied office. In this study, however, some students were from the next room and some were invited into the office under study by students who worked there. Therefore, the various relationship networks may have caused the difference in the characteristics of close contact and of indoor human behaviors during close contact.

Table 2. Comparison of indoor human behaviors during close contact in a graduate student office between the previous observation study and the present sensor-based study.

Parameter.	Description	OB [1]	SB [2]	Parameter	Description	OB [1]	SB [2]
Individual posture	Sitting	59.5%	76.3%	Average ID [3]		0.67 m	0.81 m
	Standing	40.4%	22.9%	ID by gender	M-M	0.66 m	0.88 m
	Squatting	0.1%	0.8%		F-F	0.55 m	0.70 m
Posture pattern of two students	Sit-sit	34.3%	59.6%		M-F (NC)	0.79 m	0.96 m
	Sit-stand	46.2%	33.5%		M-F (C)	0.58 m	0.71 m
	Stand-stand	18.3%	5.6%	ID by posture	Sit-sit	0.59 m	0.74 m
	Others	1.2%	1.3%		Sit-stand	0.72 m	0.88 m
Number of students per close contact	2	87.5%	90.1%		Stand-stand	0.70 m	0.93 m
	3	11.1%	7.8%	Head/body motion	Head (yaw)	0.9°	2.3°
	4	1.2%	1.5%		Head (pitch)	10.3°	17.9°
	5	0.1%	0.6%		Body (pitch)	10.6°	25.3°
	≥6	<0.1%	<0.1%		Body (bend)	0.1°	3.7°

[1] Observation study: all data obtained through observation of video tapes by video analysts.11 [2] Sensor-based study (this study): all data obtained by sensor detection. [3] ID: interpersonal distance.

Our previous experiment showed that students spent 9.9% of their time in close contact interactions, while in this study that percentage was 9.7% ± 8.8%. The probability distributions of the students' posture during close contact differed between the two experiments, although sitting was always the most common posture, followed by standing. Almost none of the students had close contact when squatting. Sitting-sitting and sitting-standing were the most common posture patterns during close contact. In this study, the sitting-sitting pattern was much more dominant than in the previous experiment because all students chose their office cubicles before the experiment. Students with the closest relationships sat next to each other, and could chat without standing up or walking. During both experiments, one-on-one close contact accounted for almost 90% of all close contacts. The number of participants per close contacts depends on the type of indoor environment. For example, more people will participate in a close contact in a group discussion, while one-on-one close contact is very highly probable in a doctor's consulting room.

Preferred interpersonal distances differ by culture, ethnicity, relationship, personal habits, age, gender, and ambient environment [48]. Closer interpersonal distance means higher virus inhalation which increases infection risk via close contact route [42]. The average personal distances for acquaintances and intimately close persons in China are 83.6 and 57.6 cm, respectively [49]. However, there is no clear definition of interpersonal distance. Our previous study defined the interpersonal distance as that between two mouths, while this study defined it as the distance between two sensors worn on the top of the head. The previous study showed the average interpersonal distance in the office to be 0.67 m. In this study, the average interpersonal distance (0.81 m) was larger because of the different definitions of this parameter. Both experiments found the same effect of gender on interpersonal distance: two female students adopted the shortest distance while students of different genders (non-couples) were farthest apart. As an office is a public area, intimate couples do not interact at such close distance as they would otherwise. Posture also influences the interpersonal distance. Both experiments showed that two sitting students had the shortest interpersonal distance. In this study, more than 50% of close contacts were between adjacent or back-to-back students, and the probability distribution of interpersonal distance was strongly influenced by their cubicle positions. A compact indoor design would lead to shorter interpersonal distance during close contact.

The circulation of people around the office strongly influenced the probability of close contacts. Students at long distances apart had low probability of contact with each other. Therefore, a linear office cubicle design would lead to a lower close contact frequency compared with a matrix design because of longer average distance. People are generally disinclined to make close contact with someone a long distance away if there is no critical information to communicate. In this study, most close contacts were between students sitting in the same region because students with good relationships had chosen to sit together. Most students in this office were acquaintances, and had high probability of a brief close contact when encountering each other. Therefore, the students near the aisles, especially those near the door, had a high close-contact frequency with remote students (Figure 7b) as a result of office circulation. There was no close contact between 88% of the possible pairs of students (connection rate = 12%). In general, this value is strongly related to the level of intimacy between people indoors. For example, the connection rate tends to be very high in a home, but low in public environments such as conference rooms and aircraft cabins. This may explain why homes have a higher infection risk than other environments during an infectious outbreak [29].

This sensor-based study recorded higher pitch values of the head and body, which showed that students preferred to lower their head and lean their body forward. When sitting, they were usually looking at a computer monitor (mostly laptop computers) or reading a book from a desk, and therefore both the torso and head leaned forward. Over the long term, such a sitting posture may lead to a high prevalence of kyphosis among students [50]. Research has also showed that tilting the head forward by 15° places about 27 pounds of force on the neck [51]. This increases to 40 pounds at 30°, 49 pounds at 45°, and 60 pounds at 60° [51]. The damage caused by untreated 'text neck' can be of similar severity to occupational overuse syndrome or repetitive stress/strain injury. The office management team could be encouraged to educate their workers and provide ergonomic office equipment such as laptop stands to promote proper posture.

In simulations of infectious disease transmission via the close contact route, face to face is the most common orientation assumed, and all heads are assumed to be at the same height [12,20]. However, in our analysis, the students spent relatively little of their close contact time in a face-to-face position. Staring at the same screen, reading the same paper, or chatting without making eye contact were also common. Before this study, no data had been published on the percentage of time spent speaking during close contact. We found that students in close contact on average spent 68.6% of their time speaking. Studies have shown that talking for 5 min can generate the same number of droplet nuclei as a cough, i.e., some 3000 droplet nuclei [10], and speaking usually involves prolonged exhalation [52]. Our data may provide a reference for the simulation of infectious disease transmission via speaking during close contact. Moreover, combined with indoor surface touching behaviors [19], a comprehensive simulation of infection spread in an office considering the long-range airborne, fomite, and close contact routes could be performed [29]. The results would provide support for infection risk analysis on a large scale such as a city [5,53].

4.3. Limitations

This study has several limitations. The presence of the cameras might have had a psychological impact on the students' behaviors. The experimental hats and shirts showed slight relative movement when the participants moved their heads and bodies. Although we discarded some data with very large fluctuations, some error remained (resolution: 5°). Still, this error was much smaller than that of observation methods. Another limitation is that the interpersonal distance was defined as the distance between two sensors installed on the top of the experimental hats rather than between two mouths or noses. The interpersonal distances obtained in this study were longer than those between two mouths/noses, which are normally used to simulate close contact between two persons. Our experiment collected more than 1440,000 s of indoor data and more than 139,000 s of close contact data over 2 days. This data volume is large, but still insufficient to represent all indoor human behaviors in graduate student offices. Moreover, the close contact behaviors presents the characteristics in the office with around 25 students. Building type and total indoor population will influence the human behaviors.

5. Conclusions

Students spent long time on close contact (9.7%) in the office, which may explain the importance of the close contact route for many respiratory infections. The probability of close contact decreased exponentially with the increasing distance between two students' cubicles. Therefore, students who sit closer to the infected student, have much higher infection risk via close contact route than students who sit further. Comparing with pairs of sitting students, pairs of standing students had lower infection risk via close contact route because they did not prefer a face-to-face talk. The fact that standing students much preferred lower their head and body than sitting students may lead to a shorter distance of exhalation jet than we thought.

Author Contributions: Conceptualization, N.Z., Y.L. and P.W.; methodology, N.Z., B.S. AND P.W.; software, B.S.; formal analysis, N.Z. and P.-T.C.; investigation, N.Z., P.-T.C., T.M., B.S. and P.W.; resources, N.Z.; data curation, N.Z. and Y.L.; writing—original draft preparation, N.Z.; writing—review and editing, N.Z., Y.L., P.-T.C., T.M., B.S. and P.W.; visualization, B.S. and P.-T.C.; supervision, Y.L.; project administration, Y.L.; funding acquisition, Y.L. All authors have read and agreed to the published version of the manuscript.

References

1. Li, D.; Menassa, C.C.; Kamat, V.R. Non-intrusive interpretation of human thermal comfort through analysis of facial infrared thermography. *Energy Build.* **2018**, *176*, 246–261. [CrossRef]
2. Bornemann, B.; Sohre, A.; Burger, P. Future governance of individual energy consumption behavior change—A framework for reflexive designs. *Energy Res. Soc. Sci.* **2018**, *35*, 140–151. [CrossRef]
3. Bodin Danielsson, C.; Theorell, T. Office employees' perception of workspace contribution: A gender and office design perspective. *Environ. Behav.* **2019**, *51*, 995–1026. [CrossRef]
4. Waits, A.; Emelyanova, A.; Oksanen, A.; Abass, K.; Rautio, A. Human infectious diseases and the changing climate in the Arctic. *Environ. Int.* **2018**, *121*, 703–713. [CrossRef] [PubMed]
5. Zhang, N.; Huang, H.; Su, B.; Ma, X.; Li, Y. A human behavior integrated hierarchical model of airborne disease transmission in a large city. *Build. Environ.* **2018**, *127*, 211–220. [CrossRef]
6. Turgeon, N.; Hamelin, M.È.; Verreault, D.; Lévesque, A.; Rhéaume, C.; Carbonneau, J.; Checkmahomed, L.; Girard, M.; Boivin, G.; Duchaine, C. Design and validation with influenza A virus of an aerosol transmission chamber for ferrets. *Int. J. Environ. Res. Public Health* **2019**, *16*, 609. [CrossRef]
7. Lee, K.M.; Jung, K. Factors influencing the response to infectious diseases: Focusing on the case of SARS and MERS in South Korea. *Int. J. Environ. Res. Public Health* **2019**, *16*, 1432. [CrossRef]
8. Weber, D.J.; Rutala, W.A.; Fischer, W.A.; Kanamori, H.; Sickbert-Bennett, E.E. Emerging infectious diseases: Focus on infection control issues for novel coronaviruses (Severe Acute Respiratory Syndrome-CoV and Middle East Respiratory Syndrome-CoV), hemorrhagic fever viruses (Lassa and Ebola), and highly pathogenic avian influenza viruses, A (H5N1) and A (H7N9). *Am. J. Infect. Control* **2016**, *44*, e91–e100.
9. Umar, A.A.; Sheshi, M.A.; Abubakar, A.A. Knowledge and practice of Ebola virus disease preventive measures among health workers in a tertiary hospital in Northern Nigeria. *Arch. Med. Surg.* **2018**, *3*, 1–5. [CrossRef]
10. Xie, X.; Li, Y.; Chwang, A.T.; Ho, P.L.; Seto, W.H. How far droplets can move in indoor environments—Revisiting the Wells evaporation-falling curve. *Indoor Air* **2007**, *17*, 211–225. [CrossRef]
11. Zhang, N.; Tang, J.W.; Li, Y. Human behavior during close contact in a graduate student office. *Indoor Air* **2019**, *29*, 577–590. [CrossRef] [PubMed]
12. Liu, L.; Li, Y.; Nielsen, P.V.; Jensen, R.L. Short-range airborne transmission of expiratory droplets between two people. *Indoor Air* **2017**, *27*, 452–462. [CrossRef] [PubMed]
13. Wei, J.; Li, Y. Enhanced spread of expiratory droplets by turbulence in a cough jet. *Build. Environ.* **2015**, *93*, 86–96. [CrossRef]
14. Duguid, J.P. The size and the duration of air-carriage of respiratory droplets and droplet-nuclei. *Epidemiol. Infect.* **1946**, *44*, 471–479. [CrossRef]
15. Loudon, R.G.; Roberts, R.M. Relation between the airborne diameters of respiratory droplets and the diameter of the stains left after recovery. *Nature* **1967** *213*, 95–96. [CrossRef]

16. Chao, C.Y.H.; Wan, M.P.; Morawska, L.; Johnson, G.R.; Ristovski, Z.D.; Hargreaves, M.; Mengersen, K.; Corbett, S.; Li, Y.; Xie, X.; et al. Characterization of expiration air jets and droplet size distributions immediately at the mouth opening. *J. Aerosol Sci.* **2009**, *40*, 122–133. [CrossRef]
17. Fabian, P.; McDevitt, J.J.; DeHaan, W.H.; Fang, R.O.P.; Cowling, B.J.; Chan, K.H. Influenza virus in human exhaled breath: An observational study. *PLoS ONE* **2008**, *3*, e2691. [CrossRef]
18. Xie, X.; Li, Y.; Sun, H.; Liu, L. Exhaled droplets due to talking and coughing. *J. R. Soc. Interface* **2009**, *6*, S703. [CrossRef]
19. Zhang, N.; Li, Y.; Huang, H. Surface touch and its network growth in a graduate student office. *Indoor Air* **2018**, *28*, 963–972. [CrossRef]
20. Ai, Z.T.; Melikov, A.K. Airborne spread of expiratory droplet nuclei between the occupants of indoor environments: A review. *Indoor Air* **2018**, *28*, 500–524. [CrossRef]
21. Pantelic, J.; Tham, K.W.; Licina, D. Effectiveness of a personalized ventilation system in reducing personal exposure against directly released simulated cough droplets. *Indoor Air* **2015**, *25*, 683–693. [CrossRef] [PubMed]
22. Olmedo, I.; Nielsen, P.V.; Ruiz de Adana, M.; Jensen, R.L.; Grzelecki, P. Distribution of exhaled contaminants and personal exposure in a room using three different air distribution strategies. *Indoor Air* **2012**, *22*, 64–76. [CrossRef] [PubMed]
23. Cattuto, C.; Van den Broeck, W.; Barrat, A.; Colizza, V.; Pinton, J.F.; Vespignani, A. Dynamics of person-to-person interactions from distributed RFID sensor networks. *PLoS ONE* **2010**, *5*, e11596. [CrossRef] [PubMed]
24. Vanhems, P.; Barrat, A.; Cattuto, C.; Pinton, J.F.; Khanafer, N.; Régis, C.; Kim, B.-A.; Comte, B.; Voirin, N. Estimating potential infection transmission routes in hospital wards using wearable proximity sensors. *PLoS ONE* **2013**, *8*, e73970. [CrossRef]
25. Di Blasio, S.; Shtrepi, L.; Puglisi, G.E.; Astolfi, A. A cross-sectional survey on the impact of irrelevant speech noise on annoyance, mental health and well-being, performance and occupants' behavior in shared and open-plan offices. *Int. J. Environ. Res. Public Health* **2019**, *16*, 280. [CrossRef]
26. Davis, M.C.; Leach, D.J.; Clegg, C.W. Breaking out of open-plan: Extending social interference theory through an evaluation of contemporary offices. *Environ. Behav.* **2019**. [CrossRef]
27. Martinez-Millana, A.; Lizondo, A.; Gatta, R.; Vera, S.; Salcedo, V.T.; Fernandez-Llatas, C. Process mining dashboard in operating rooms: Analysis of staff expectations with analytic hierarchy process. *Int. J. Environ. Res. Public Health* **2019**, *16*, 199. [CrossRef]
28. Alarifi, A.; Al-Salman, A.; Alsaleh, M.; Alnafessah, A.; Al-Hadhrami, S.; Al-Ammar, M.A.; Al-Khalifa, H. Ultra wideband indoor positioning technologies: Analysis and recent advances. *Sensors* **2016**, *16*, 707. [CrossRef]
29. Zhang, N.; Li, Y. Transmission of influenza A in a student office based on realistic person-to-person contact and surface touch behavior. *Int. J. Environ. Res. Public Health* **2018**, *15*, 1699. [CrossRef]
30. Hornbeck, T.; Naylor, D.; Segre, A.M.; Thomas, G.; Herman, T.; Polgreen, P.M. Using sensor networks to study the effect of peripatetic healthcare workers on the spread of hospital-associated infections. *J. Infect. Dis.* **2012**, *206*, 1549–1557. [CrossRef]
31. Isella, L.; Romano, M.; Barrat, A.; Cattuto, C.; Colizza, V.; Van den Broeck, W.; Gesualdo, F.; Pandolfi, E.; Ravà, L.; Rizzo, C.; et al. Close encounters in a pediatric ward: Measuring face-to-face proximity and mixing patterns with wearable sensors. *PLoS ONE* **2011**, *6*, e17144. [CrossRef] [PubMed]
32. Hang, J.; Li, Y.; Jin, R. The influence of human walking on the flow and airborne transmission in a six-bed isolation room: Tracer gas simulation. *Build. Environ.* **2014**, *77*, 119–134. [CrossRef]
33. Lei, H.; Li, Y.; Xiao, S.; Lin, C.H.; Norris, S.L.; Wei, D.; Hu, Z.; Ji, S.; Norris, S.L. Routes of transmission of influenza A H1N1, SARS CoV, and norovirus in air cabin: Comparative analyzes. *Indoor Air* **2018**, *28*, 394–403. [CrossRef] [PubMed]
34. Xiao, S.; Li, Y.; Lei, H.; Lin, C.H.; Norris, S.L.; Yang, X.; Zhao, P. Characterizing dynamic transmission of contaminants on a surface touch network. *Build. Environ.* **2018**, *129*, 107–116. [CrossRef]
35. Zhang, N.; Miao, R.; Huang, H.; Chan, E.Y.Y. Contact infection of infectious disease onboard a cruise ship. *Sci. Rep.* **2016**, *6*, 38790. [CrossRef]
36. Fees, B.S.; Fischer, E.; Haar, S.; Crowe, L.K. Toddler activity intensity during indoor free-play: Stand and watch. *J. Nutr. Educ. Behav.* **2015** *47*, 170–175. [CrossRef]

37. Aminian, S.; Hinckson, E.A.; Stewart, T. Modifying the classroom environment to increase standing and reduce sitting. *Build. Res. Informat.* **2015**, *43*, 631–645. [CrossRef]
38. Isella, L.; Stehlé, J.; Barrat, A.; Cattuto, C.; Pinton, J.F.; Van den Broeck, W. What's in a crowd? Analysis of face-to-face behavioral networks. *J. Theor. Biol.* **2011**, *271*, 166–180. [CrossRef]
39. Salathé, M.; Kazandjieva, M.; Lee, J.W.; Levis, P.; Feldman, M.W.; Jones, J.H. A high-resolution human contact network for infectious disease transmission. *Proc. Natl. Acad. Sci. USA* **2010**, *107*, 22020–22025. [CrossRef]
40. Stehlé, J.; Voirin, N.; Barrat, A.; Cattuto, C.; Isella, L.; Pinton, J.F.; Quaggiotto, M.; Broeck, W.V.D.; Regis, C.; Lina, B.; et al. High-resolution measurements of face-to-face contact patterns in a primary school. *PLoS ONE* **2011**, *6*, e23176. [CrossRef]
41. Stehlé, J.; Voirin, N.; Barrat, A.; Cattuto, C.; Colizza, V.; Isella, L.; Régis, C.; Pinton, J.-F.; Khanafer, N.; Broeck, W.V.D.; et al. Simulation of an SEIR infectious disease model on the dynamic contact network of conference attendees. *BMC Med.* **2011**, *9*, 87. [CrossRef] [PubMed]
42. Villafruela, J.M.; Olmedo, I.; San José, J.F. Influence of human breathing modes on airborne cross infection risk. *Build. Environ.* **2016**, *106*, 340–351. [CrossRef]
43. Olmedo, I.; Nielsen, P.V.; Ruiz de Adana, M.; Jensen, R.L. The risk of airborne cross-infection in a room with vertical low-velocity ventilation. *Indoor Air* **2013**, *23*, 62–73. [CrossRef] [PubMed]
44. Murakami, S.; Kato, S.; Zeng, J. Combined simulation of airflow, radiation and moisture transport for heat release from a human body. *Build. Environ.* **2000**, *35*, 489–500. [CrossRef]
45. Pease, A. *Body Language: How to Read others' Thoughts by Their Gestures*; Sheldon Press: London, UK, 1988.
46. Rim, D.; Novoselac, A. Transport of particulate and gaseous pollutants in the vicinity of a human body. *Build. Environ.* **2009**, *44*, 1840–1849. [CrossRef]
47. Nicas, M.; Best, D. A study quantifying the hand-to-face contact rate and its potential application to predicting respiratory tract infection. *J. Occup. Environ. Hyg.* **2008**, *5*, 347–352. [CrossRef]
48. Heshka, S.; Nelson, Y. Interpersonal speaking distance as a function of age, sex, and relationship. *Sociometry* **1972**, *35*, 491–498. [CrossRef]
49. Sorokowska, A.; Sorokowski, P.; Hilpert, P.; Cantarero, K.; Frackowiak, T.; Ahmadi, K. Preferred interpersonal distances: A global comparison. *J. Cross Cult. Psychol.* **2017**, *48*, 577–592. [CrossRef]
50. Mirbagheri, S.S.; Rahmani-Rasa, A.; Farmani, F.; Amini, P.; Nikoo, M.R. Evaluating kyphosis and lordosis in students by using a flexible ruler and their relationship with severity and frequency of thoracic and lumbar pain. *Asian Spine J.* **2015**, *9*, 416. [CrossRef]
51. Neupane, S.; Ali, U.; Mathew, A. Text neck syndrome-systematic review. *Imp. J. Interdiscip. Res.* **2017**, *3*, 141–148.
52. McFarland, D.H. Respiratory markers of conversational interaction. *J. Speech Lang. Hear. Res.* **2001**, *44*, 128–143. [CrossRef]
53. Zhang, N.; Huang, H.; Duarte, M.; Zhang, J. Dynamic population flow based risk analysis of infectious disease propagation in a metropolis. *Environ. Int.* **2016**, *94*, 369–379. [CrossRef] [PubMed]

10

Health Consequences of an Armed Conflict in Zamboanga, Philippines Using a Syndromic Surveillance Database

Miguel Antonio Salazar [1,2,*], Ronald Law [3,4] and Volker Winkler [1,*]

1 Institute of Global Health, University of Heidelberg, Im Neuenheimer Feld 324, 69120 Heidelberg, Germany
2 Graduate School, Angeles University Foundation, Angeles City, Pampanga 2009, Philippines
3 Department of Health, Health Emergency Management Bureau, Sta. Cruz, Manila 1003, Philippines; rplaw@doh.gov.ph
4 College of Public Health, University of the Philippines, Manila 1000, Philippines
* Correspondence: mike.salazar@uni-heidelberg.de (M.A.S.); v.winkler@uni-heidelberg.de (V.W.)

Abstract: The Zamboanga armed conflict was a 19-day long encounter in the Philippines in 2013 that displaced 119,000 people from their homes. This study describes the health consequences of this complex emergency in different age groups, time periods, and health facilities using data from Surveillance in Post Extreme Emergencies and Disasters (SPEED). This is a descriptive study of the SPEED database spanning 196 days of observation post-disaster and 1065 SPEED reports from 49 health facilities. Evacuation centers and village health centers, both primary care facilities, had the highest number of consults. Common infections and noncommunicable diseases were the most common reasons for consultations, namely, acute respiratory infections, fever, watery diarrhea, skin disease, and hypertension. Infections can be associated with environmental conditions in displaced populations, while hypertension has a high prevalence in the country and implies long-term care. Conflict-related injuries and deaths were not frequently observed due to the volatile situation that influenced health-seeking behavior as well as possible reporting gaps. In conclusion, in complex emergencies, as in natural disasters, wherein early alert and warning for potential outbreaks is crucial, SPEED can assist decision makers on response and recovery interventions. Linkages between SPEED and other surveillance and reporting systems need to be explored.

Keywords: disasters; armed conflict; complex emergencies; syndromic surveillance

---

1. Introduction

On September 9, 2013, in the city of Zamboanga, Philippines, a gun battle ensued between the Philippine Armed Forces and the Moro National Liberation Front (MNLF). The MNLF engaged government forces in five villages, or barangays, the country's smallest governance division. The hostilities ended 19 days after the start of the encounter. During the course and in the aftermath of the military skirmish, 118,819 individuals were affected and evacuated from their homes [1]. Six months after the encounter, only half of the affected population were able to return to their homes. The conflict compromised the nutrition and hygiene of the 20,000 internally displaced people in the two largest evacuation sites [2]. The Zamboanga armed conflict may be considered a complex emergency, as it fits the definition of a humanitarian event due to armed conflict, political destabilization, food supply shortages, displacement of populations, and health systems disruption [3].

Conflict and the resulting displacement of affected residents leads to health consequences. Traditionally, communicable diseases have been the focus of disaster management and refugee health [4,5]. Displaced populations are particularly susceptible to communicable diseases because of risk factors such as cramped housing, environmental damage, economic difficulty, lack of hygiene and clean water supply, inadequate nutrition, and lack of basic health services. Diarrhea and acute respiratory infections are the two most common causes of morbidity and mortality in displaced populations [5]. Measles, on the other hand, is a highly deadly disease in situations where shelter is poorly planned, people live in close proximity to each other, and immunization rates are low [4–7].

Furthermore, noncommunicable diseases (NCDs) have been seen to have a significant burden on health services post-disaster regardless of whether the event is due to natural hazards or conflict [5,8,9]. NCDs, due to prolonged treatment and the need for coordinated long-term care, pose a challenge during disaster response and recovery because of the resulting disrupted and unresponsive health system [8]. NCD treatment may either be neglected or inadequate in a disaster setting if response is poorly planned and NCDs are not considered a priority [9].

Complex emergencies are situations where livelihood and life are threatened by war, civil disturbance, and migration of people in the midst of political instability and security threats, all of which make emergency response difficult [10]. The types of injuries observed from complex emergencies may be different from disasters due to natural hazards such as typhoons and earthquakes. Violent trauma comprises one of the major direct health impacts in armed conflicts. Its effects may vary from the type and location of the conflict. In complex emergencies in Eastern Europe, violent trauma contributed to the majority of direct morbidity and mortality; however, its significance in complex emergencies in Asia and Africa was typically less due to the predominance of infectious diseases [3]. Natural hazards due to typhoons and earthquakes cause more deaths from injuries, which may be due to drowning and crush injuries, respectively [11–13]. For morbidity, minor injuries such as bruises, cuts, and burns played a more significant role compared to fractures in natural hazards in the Philippines in 2013 [14,15].

Surveillance for Post Extreme Emergencies and Disasters (SPEED) is a syndromic surveillance system deployed specifically after disasters and emergencies and is a joint project of the Philippine Department of Health (DOH) and the World Health Organization established in 2011 [16,17]. Disease surveillance and early warning systems have the ability to inform decision makers on possible disaster risks [18]. Multi-hazard early warning systems are integral parts of understanding disaster risk—one of the priorities under the Sendai Framework for Disaster Risk Reduction 2015–2030 [19]. Health Emergency and Disaster Risk Management (H-EDRM) is a concept that covers the intersection between disaster risk reduction management and health. It is suggested that research in this field should include needs assessments, monitoring, and evaluation and reporting systems that can measure health indicators in all phases of disasters: mitigation, preparedness, response, and recovery [20]. SPEED is an example of a reporting system in H-EDRM focused on disaster response and recovery.

Previous studies in the Philippines have looked into the health effects of natural hazards using SPEED. In the aftermath of the natural hazards in the Philippines in 2013, namely a flood, typhoon, and an earthquake, SPEED data showed that infectious diseases still dominated in morbidity; however, NCDs had a substantial burden to the health systems of the affected populations [14,15,21]. Although SPEED was also deployed in the Zamboanga armed conflict, the health effects of this complex emergency have yet to be studied using SPEED data. This study aims to describe the health consequences of the Zamboanga armed conflict on consultations for communicable diseases, injuries, and NCDs in different age groups, time periods, and health facility types using data from SPEED and their health system implications.

2. Materials and Methods

This study analyzed the SPEED database specifically for the Zamboanga armed conflict in 2013. SPEED was activated in Zamboanga City from 11 September 2013 to 24 March 2014, thereby beginning two days after the onset of the Zamboanga siege and spanning 196 days in total. The SPEED reports are comprised of all disease consultations for a particular day fitting the case definitions regardless of attribution to the disaster for a specific health facility, which includes village health centers, evacuation centers, hospitals, and community health centers. SPEED reports can be submitted to the system on a daily basis either manually, via Short-Messaging System (SMS), or through the internet by the designated public health nurse or data encoder [17].

Similar to previous studies done for SPEED, the 21 disease entities were divided into three groups: communicable diseases, NCDs, and injuries [14,15]. Communicable diseases included in SPEED are acute bloody diarrhea, acute flaccid paralysis, acute hemorrhagic fever, acute jaundice syndrome, acute respiratory infection (ARI), acute watery diarrhea, animal bites, conjunctivitis, fever, fever with other symptoms (FOS), suspected leptospirosis, skin disease, suspected measles, suspected meningitis, and tetanus. Fractures and wounds (including bruises and burns) make up the injury group, while noncommunicable diseases are comprised of acute asthmatic attack, acute malnutrition, high blood pressure, and known diabetes mellitus. Descriptions for each of the 21 syndromes have been mentioned by Salazar et al. in 2016 and in the SPEED Operations Manual [14,17].

The database is composed of reports with disease or syndrome counts for a particular health facility per day. There were two observed age groups: individuals under the age of five and those aged five and older. Rates were established with the denominator as either the population of the village or municipality, depending on the health facility type. Village health centers and evacuation centers used the village population, while hospitals and community health centers used the city population. The 2010 Philippine census data for villages was used for the denominator for village health center and evacuation center rates, while municipality census data was used for hospital and community health center rates. Rates were presented as per 10,000 population, similar to other studies conducted on SPEED [14,15,22].

Similar to the analysis of SPEED for typhoon Haiyan, the Bohol earthquake, and the Luzon flood in the Philippines, two time periods, less than or equal to two months and greater than two months post-disaster, were compared in this study. These time periods corresponded to disaster response and recovery, respectively [14]. To compare rates for the two disaster time periods, Poisson regression was used [23]. Consultation rates for health facility types and the mean difference between age groups (under five and five and older) were presented as mean rates with 95% confidence intervals. To illustrate total daily consultation rates among the four health facility types across the observed time period, models for each of the health facility types were derived using the multivariable fractional polynomial method [24]. Day zero for this study was pegged at the onset of the conflict.

This is a descriptive study of the SPEED database managed by the Health Emergency Management Bureau (HEMB) of the DOH. SPEED uses aggregated and anonymized data from health facilities and evacuation centers affected by emergencies and disasters. The SPEED data for the Zamboanga armed conflict was requested from the director of HEMB and the authors had exclusive access to the data.

3. Results

3.1. Health Facilities

There were 1065 SPEED reports during the Zamboanga armed conflict within a 196-day period of observation post-disaster. The first SPEED report was transmitted on the second day of the armed conflict. There was a decrease in the number of SPEED reports after the first day of reporting; however, the most notable drop happened around the 60th to 80th day, where the number of reports thereafter plateaued (see Figure 1).

Among the 49 reporting health facilities, 21 were evacuation centers, 15 were village health centers, nine were hospitals, and four were community health centers. Evacuation centers (448) had the most reports, followed by village health centers (297), hospitals (266), and community health centers (54). Comparing the total rates of consultations seen per day for the four facilities, evacuation centers (32.3 per 10,000 population) were on top, with village health centers (24.8 per 10,000 population), hospitals (0.3 per 10,000 population), and community health centers (0.2 per 10,000 population) following suit. For all health facility types, there were more daily consultations in the response period than during the recovery period (see Table 1).

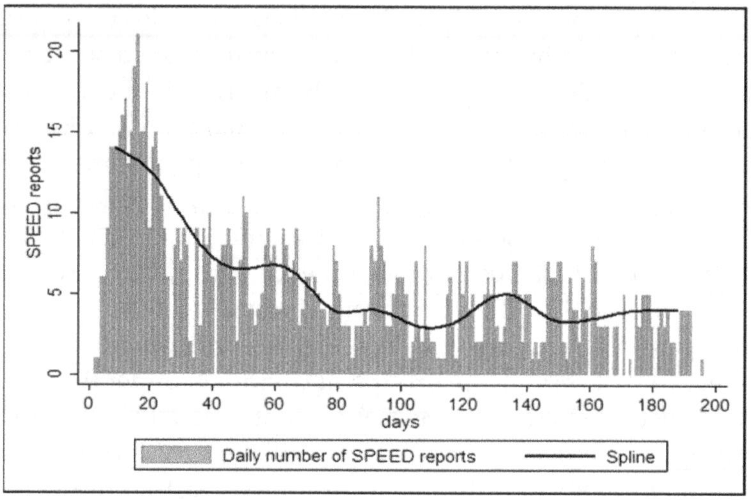

Figure 1. Bar graph of daily number of Surveillance in Post Extreme Emergencies and Disasters (SPEED) reports with spline.

Table 1. Total consultation rates per 10,000 individuals for health facility types comparing time post-disaster.

Health Facility Type	Mean Number of Consultations per Day (95% Confidence Intervals) (*n*)	≤2 Months (Response) (*n*)	>2 Months (Recovery) (*n*)	Difference between ≤2 Months and >2 Months (*p*-value)
Evacuation center	32.3 (27.9–36.7) (n = 448)	34.3 (n = 373)	22.4 (n = 75)	11.9 (<0.01)
Village health center	28.5 (24.5–32.5) (n = 297)	65.5 (n = 70)	17.1 (n = 227)	48.4 (<0.01)
Hospital	0.3 (0.2–0.3) (n = 266)	0.5 (n = 68)	0.2 (n = 198)	0.3 (<0.01)
Community health center	0.2 (0.1–0.2) (n = 54)	0.4 (n = 13)	0.1 (n = 41)	0.3 (0.03)
Regardless of facility type	21.6 (19.3–23.9) (n = 1065)	33.2 (n = 524)	10.3 (n = 541)	22.9 (<0.01)

Modeled rates for hospitals and community health centers showed little variability. Evacuation centers and village health centers differed considerably in their modeled rates. For village health centers, there was an exponential decrease in the total daily consultation rates, while evacuation centers had a delayed peak with a less profound decline (see Figure 2).

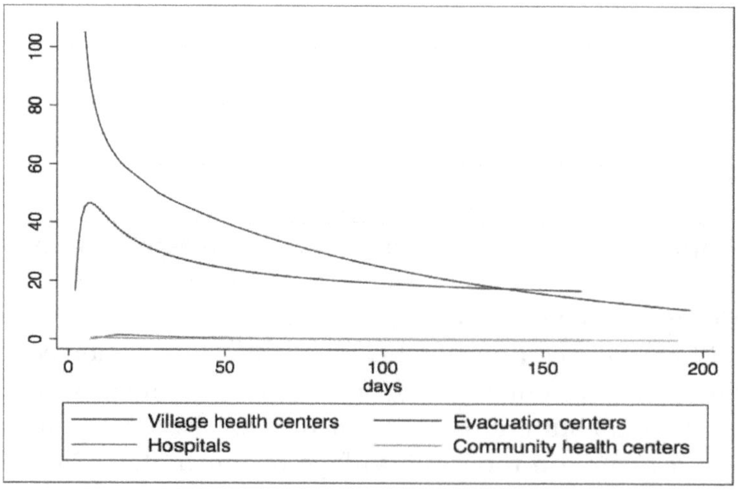

Figure 2. Poisson regressions for daily total consultations per 10,000 individuals across time for different health facility types.

There was a notable difference between the time periods, within two months (response) and after two months (recovery), regardless of health facility type. There were similar numbers of SPEED reports for both the response (524) and recovery (541) periods. When disaggregated by health facility type, evacuation centers had more reports in the response period. The other three health facility types had more SPEED reports during the recovery period. Similar to the visualized models, village health centers had the highest difference between the rates of the two time periods. The disaster response period had significantly higher rates for all four health facilities when comparing total consultation rates (see Table 1).

3.2. Syndrome Rates

Communicable diseases such as acute respiratory infections (11.3 per 10,000 population), fever (3.5), acute watery diarrhea (2.3), and skin disease (1.7) had the highest syndrome rates among all 21 syndromes. Hypertension was the only disease entity that had a syndrome rate ≥1 per 10,000 population and was not communicable in nature (see Table 2). Injuries such as fractures and wounds had daily rates below 1 per 10,000 individuals, but there were more cases of wounds (1982) than of fractures (154) in terms of absolute number of cases.

Table 2. Top syndrome rates per 10,000 individuals separated by time post-disaster and by age.

Syndrome	Total n = 1065	≤2 Months (Response) n = 524	>2 Months (Recovery) n = 541	Difference between ≤2 Months and >2 Months (p-value)	<5 Years of Age	≥5 Years of Age	Difference between <5 Years and ≥5 Years (95% Confidence Interval)
				Communicable diseases			
Acute respiratory infection (ARI)	11.3	18.0	4.8	13.2 (<0.01)	41.8	7.2	34.7 (30.7–38.6)
Fever	3.5	4.9	2.2	2.7 (<0.01)	14.0	2.1	11.8 (10.1–13.6)
Acute watery diarrhea	2.3	3.8	0.9	2.9 (<0.01)	8.5	1.5	7.0 (5.9–8.1)
Skin disease	1.7	2.4	1	1.4 (<0.01)	5.7	1.2	4.5 (3.7–5.3)
Fever with other symptoms (FOS)	0.3	<0.1	0.1	0.5 (<0.01)	0.3	0.3	<0.1 (−0.1–0.2)
Communicable disease total	19.4	29.9	9.3	20.6 (<0.01)	71.1	12.5	58.6 (52.0–65.2)
				Injuries			
Open wounds and bruises/burns	0.7	0.9	0.4	0.4 (<0.01)	0.9	0.6	0.3 (0.1–0.5)
Injury total	0.7	0.9	0.4	0.4 (<0.01)	0.9	0.6	0.3 (0.1–0.5)
				Non-communicable diseases (NCDs)			
High blood pressure	1.0	1.8	0.3	1.4 (<0.01)	<0.1	1.2	1.2 (1.0–1.4)
Acute asthmatic attack	0.4	0.6	0.2	0.4 (<0.01)	1.1	0.3	0.8 (0.6–1.0)
NCD total	1.5	2.4	0.6	1.8 (<0.01)	1.4	1.5	0.1 (−0.3–0.5)

The majority of the disease entities had higher rates in the disaster response period compared to the recovery period. Comparing the two disaster phases, among the 21 diseases, 13 had p-values less than 0.05. For communicable diseases, these were ARI, fever, acute watery diarrhea, skin disease, FOS, conjunctivitis, suspected measles, acute bloody diarrhea, and animal bites. ARI, fever, acute watery diarrhea, skin disease, acute bloody diarrhea, and animal bites had higher rates for the disaster response period compared to the recovery period. FOS, suspected measles, and acute bloody diarrhea, on the other hand, had higher rates for the disaster recovery period. The other four were wounds, bruises, and burns for injuries and high blood pressure, acute asthmatic attack, and diabetes for NCDs (See Table 2). Acute flaccid paralysis had no consults for the whole period of observation.

All the disease entities for communicable diseases had higher rates for the under-five age group, except for FOS, tetanus, and suspected meningitis. High blood pressure, diabetes mellitus, and fractures were the other diseases with higher rates for those five years and older. Of these six syndromes, the communicable diseases, FOS, tetanus, and suspected meningitis had 95% confidence intervals crossing zero.

3.3. Syndromes of Outbreak Potential

The DOH has a list of diseases of epidemic potential that are classified as either an immediately notifiable or a weekly notifiable disease or syndrome [25]. Among the diseases and syndromes in SPEED, acute flaccid paralysis, tetanus, animal bites (proxy for rabies), and suspected measles warrant immediate notification based on the directives of the DOH. Notifiable diseases for weekly reporting included in SPEED are the following: acute bloody diarrhea, suspected meningitis, acute watery diarrhea (which could be cholera), suspected leptospirosis, and FOS (which could be either typhoid or malaria) [25,26]. For the whole observation period, looking at the actual number of cases, there was no consult for acute flaccid paralysis, 12 for tetanus, 235 for animal bites, 60 for suspected measles, 60 for acute bloody diarrhea, 4 for suspected meningitis, 4781 for acute watery diarrhea, 31 for suspected leptospirosis, and 794 for FOS.

When visualized across time, the top immediately notifiable and weekly notifiable diseases were seen to have differing characteristics. Again, looking at the actual number of cases per day, there were more reported cases of acute watery diarrhea and FOS, which are weekly notifiable diseases, compared to animal bites and suspected measles, which are immediately notifiable diseases. Suspected measles had spikes in both the response and recovery periods, while animal bite cases had a peak in the end of the disaster response period (around the 2-month mark) and decreased thereafter. Acute watery diarrhea consistently had a higher number of cases during the disaster response period, while there were variable peaks for FOS across the observed time period (see Figure 3).

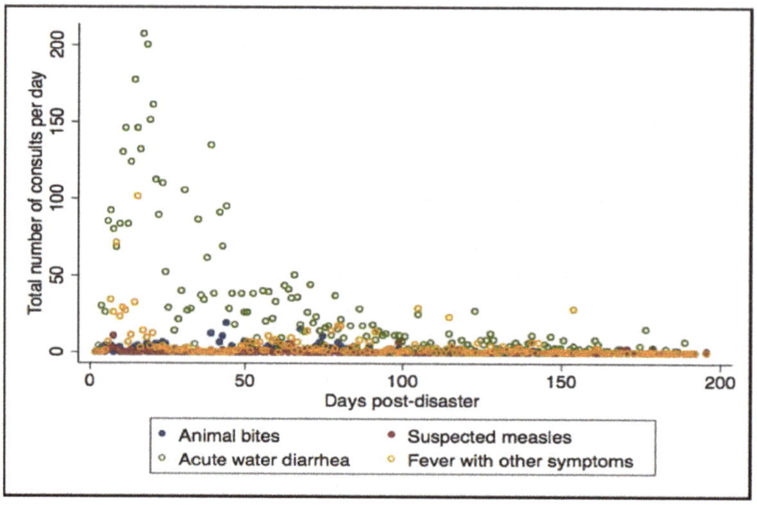

Figure 3. Total daily consultations of the most common immediately notifiable syndromes (animal bites and suspected measles) and the most common weekly notifiable syndromes (acute watery diarrhea and fever with other symptoms) across time among all reporting health facilities.

4. Discussion

4.1. Common Syndromes

In complex emergencies, communicable diseases are the usual primary care conditions [5,27]. The Zamboanga armed conflict was no exception. The top five syndromes observed can be managed in primary care settings. Similarly, in disasters in the same year (Bohol earthquake, typhoon Haiyan, and the Luzon flood), acute respiratory infections were also the most common followed by fever, acute water diarrhea, and skin disease. NCDs were also part of the top six syndromes in the form of hypertension [14,15]. However, compared to the disasters ensuing from natural hazards, wounds did not figure prominently in the disease burden in this armed conflict [14].

The top communicable disease in the Zamboanga armed conflict, ARI, reflected the yearly morbidity profile of the Zamboanga peninsula [28]. This was not the case for fever, acute watery diarrhea, and skin disease, which garnered the succeeding top numbers of consultations during the response and recovery periods post-disaster. However, the three syndromes can be associated to the environmental conditions experienced by the displaced individuals in the aftermath of the conflict, namely loss of shelter, decreased food security, and compromised access to water, sanitation, and hygiene [5,10]. The conflict displaced 80,757 individuals who were placed in 60 evacuation centers while 38,062 displaced people went to the homes of their families or relatives [1]. Those living in evacuation centers were faced with difficulties in accessing food, clean water, sanitation, and proper shelter [29]. All top four disease syndromes are communicable in nature and may be attributed to conditions in evacuation areas or temporary homes where basic services are sub-optimally provided [5,30].

NCDs represented by hypertension, the fifth most common syndrome seen in this study, are included in the top morbidities in the Zamboanga region and the Philippines in general [28]. Hypertension had been previously studied in disasters in the Philippines. In Typhoon Haiyan, hypertension was also the most common NCD and the third most common among the 21 syndromes of SPEED [15,21]. In another study done after Haiyan, hypertension was included in the top three diagnoses for adults seeking consult from mobile medical teams in 40 villages in the provinces of Samar and Leyte [31]. In 2013, hypertension was the third most common cause of morbidity in the general Philippine population, while in the Zamboanga Peninsula, the region of Zamboanga City, it was the second highest [28]. As the population is moving towards increased food availability and having sedentary work environments during normal times, people already have an increased risk of having NCDs [32]. When displaced populations who are exposed to protracted emergencies or a prolonged rehabilitation process such as in Zamboanga [29] are given packaged food with low nutritional value, have limited space for free movement, and have decreased physical activity, vulnerability to NCDs is further magnified.

Compared to other studies looking at natural hazards also using the SPEED database, the Zamboanga armed conflict had lower rates for injuries, namely wounds and fractures. In typhoon Haiyan and the Bohol earthquake, injuries resulted in rates of 1.4 and 1.2 consultations per 10,000 population, respectively. The Zamboanga armed conflict witnessed 0.7 consultations per 10,000 for injuries. The injuries seen in the typhoon and the earthquake were mostly minor in nature [14]. These injuries could be attributed to the magnitude and force of the disaster, where the affected population sustained direct injuries because of fallen structures and debris as a result of the earthquake or flying and floating debris brought about by typhoons and floods. Susceptibility to injuries is inversely related to the capacity for physical protection [33,34]. In contrast, the injuries in conflict can be attributed to gunshots or other forms of violence; however, it is hypothesized that not all people displaced by the conflict actually dealt with hazards such as gunshots, bombings, or grenades, or if they did, SPEED was not able to capture it. The consultations seen in SPEED reflected this disparity, where minor injuries were not as common in the conflict compared to natural hazards. However, these rates may also be underestimated because not all people who are injured will seek medical care or will be brought to health facilities because of several factors unique in the context of complex emergencies [35].

4.2. Mortality

Deaths related to violence are usually the perceived hallmark of conflicts. In Eastern Europe, trauma-related deaths predominated in the conflict in Bosnia-Herzegovina. In Asia and Africa, on the other hand, deaths due to infectious diseases and those related to malnutrition predominated [3]. In total, there were 13 deaths reported in SPEED across the observed time period ranging from day 2 to day 196. There were five deaths within the response period and eight deaths in the recovery period. There were 11 deaths reported from hospitals, while there was one death each for village health centers and community health centers. Fever was the cause of the most number of deaths among disease syndromes, with six deaths, followed by four for leptospirosis, two for hypertension, and one for wounds. The deaths reflected in SPEED, mostly communicable in nature, do not give a comprehensive picture of deaths that occurred as a consequence of the conflict.

There were differences in the deaths reported through SPEED to that of the DOH's official mortality tally. According to the DOH, there were 268 deaths due to gunshot wounds in the Zamboanga armed conflict; however, these were not reflected in SPEED [36]. As these deaths were direct effects of the 19-day long conflict and may not have been treated in a health facility, these records could not be captured by SPEED, a health facility-dependent reporting system. In addition, as health facilities did not report daily, there were deaths that could have been missed on days in which the health facility did not send a SPEED report. Nevertheless, the reporting of deaths in the SPEED database should be further scrutinized. A time series analysis on the different systems of certifying and registering deaths after disasters, whether natural or human-induced, is suggested. Also, a delineation between direct and indirect causes of deaths will be essential. These would give a more complete picture of the impact of complex emergencies and natural disasters on mortality, such as the causes of deaths and the temporality or the relation to time post-disaster.

4.3. Health Facility Type

Evacuation centers had the highest number of consults per health facility per day regardless of time period post-disaster. However, during the response period to the Zamboanga armed conflict, there were more consults during the first two months post-disaster in village health centers. This may be the time when the situation had stabilized. It also shows the importance of evacuation centers as points for delivery of basic health services to the displaced population. It is hypothesized that the affected population was familiar with the village health centers, the frontline primary health care facilities, and their services, thus they sought health care in these facilities. However, as the population moved to temporary shelters, health services were delivered in the evacuation centers, explaining the large number of consultations reported from evacuation centers.

There were more SPEED reports and a higher number of consultations coming from village health centers and evacuation centers in the Zamboanga armed conflict compared to typhoon Haiyan, where SPEED was also used. In typhoon Haiyan, village health centers had the most consultations on average; however, village health centers comprised only a minority of the SPEED reports and had the highest variability. Furthermore, the distribution of consultations for health facilities across time were not discussed in publications on Haiyan using SPEED [15]. This study, on the other hand, gives a visualization of the consultations for evacuations centers and village health centers across time, showing the difference between disaster response and recovery. Reports from village health centers and evacuation centers also made up the majority of SPEED reports for this particular disaster. This study demonstrates the importance of evacuation centers and village health centers as health facilities being utilized by the displaced population to gain access to basic health services during response and recovery.

The magnitude of the disaster could have played a role in the predominance of reports from village health centers in the Zamboanga armed conflict, which was isolated to one city, compared to typhoon Haiyan, where nine regions of the Philippines were affected. The importance of community health centers in typhoon Haiyan could have reflected the need to optimize aid, since these were the main health facilities and seats of health governance of the municipalities affected [15]. Since the health system disruption of the conflict was less than typhoon Haiyan and localized within one city, relief efforts could have been distributed more to village health centers and evacuation centers.

4.4. Policy and Health System Implications

As part of its mandate of informing the decisions of health policy makers and providing them with early warning systems to detect possible outbreaks of conditions expected in disasters and emergencies [17], SPEED's performance during the Zamboanga armed conflict showed that it was able to detect possible measles and cholera outbreaks. Episodes of animal bites were also recorded, which could have prompted public health measures to control stray dogs and other animals in the city. However, syndromic surveillance was shown to have limited capacity in investigating conditions that are not part of the case definitions. As disease entities are not specific and are not confirmed in the laboratory, these reported cases must be investigated further.

Event-based surveillance can feed from the real-time, location-specific reports from SPEED and lead surveillance teams to areas with unusual increases in syndrome consultations. As event-based surveillance entails rapid detection and assessment of public health events and emergencies, the team can further examine and respond to possible outbreaks identified from SPEED [37].

For SPEED to be fully utilized by public health decision makers and H-EDRM researchers, the system has to be integrated with other surveillance systems already used by the DOH. The suggestions by Foldy in 2004 to improve outcomes of surveillance systems adapted to SPEED are the following: (1) the SPEED database should be available to be mined, (2) the results from SPEED should have user-friendly visual displays or a SPEED dashboard, (3) there should be capacity for diverse technical inputs to understand complex data, (4) surveillance should be linked to response, and (5) there should be institutional capacity to confirm the diagnosis, both clinical and laboratory [38]. This entails coordination among different bureaus within the DOH. SPEED is under the Health Emergency Management Bureau, while the other surveillance systems are under the Epidemiology Bureau of the DOH. Moreover, it was observed that health facilities were not consistent in sending daily SPEED reports. The gaps in the reporting in SPEED, whether in terms of morbidity and mortality, shows the need for further validation through different data sources within and outside government to get the best picture of the complex emergency or disaster. It is also prudent to assess the reporting system for deaths post-disasters in health facilities and investigate the process of certification and reporting. These can provide information on the mechanisms of death, classification, and possible public health interventions.

Since disasters from natural hazards and complex emergencies amplify health systems' weaknesses and needs [10,14], other health services should be monitored aside from infectious diseases, non-communicable diseases, and injuries. Mental health services during and after conflicts are essential during disaster response and recovery. In a humanitarian setting, mental health conditions could be preexisting, trauma-induced, or triggered by failures in basic services during response and recovery [39,40]. On the other hand, women still needed to access maternal health services during the on-going conflict in Zamboanga. Consultations for antenatal, delivery, and postnatal care were seen in evacuation centers and in health facilities [41]. Aside from emergency obstetric care, the minimum initial service package in humanitarian emergencies also includes other interventions under reproductive health, such as those for sexual violence, contraception, and HIV [42]. When it was first developed in 2011, SPEED did not include syndromes or diseases pertaining to mental health or maternal health. The inclusion of mental health and reproductive health in SPEED can be further studied by the DOH to be able to capture important concerns that can guide provision of more specific health services.

4.5. Limitations

The SPEED database is dependent on the use of the health workforce who may be preoccupied and overworked during times of emergencies and disasters. The use of the system and its activation is dependent on the decisions of either the local chief executive, health officer, or the DOH. This in turn affects the allocated human resources and logistics deployed to support SPEED's operational requirement [17]. The required continued monitoring and governance by health officials coupled with other external stressors in disaster response and recovery could have led to the inconsistencies in the reporting of health facilities in the aftermath of the complex emergency.

The data quality of SPEED needs to be further evaluated even though SPEED results are initially validated by HEMB [14]. As a secondary data source without confirmed diagnoses, results from SPEED can only be used for descriptive studies and not for confirming the need for declaring outbreaks [17]. Furthermore, as SPEED is housed in HEMB and isolated from other disease surveillance systems, coordination among DOH bureaus needs to be improved in order to have an integrated disease surveillance and response system both in disasters and in normal times.

5. Conclusions

The SPEED data for the Zamboanga armed conflict showed that primary care conditions such as common infections and NCDs were the most prevalent reasons for consultations. Evacuation centers had the highest rates and the highest number of SPEED reports, thus highlighting the importance of the health facilities nearest to the population affected. Common infectious diseases, such as ARI, fever, watery diarrhea, and skin disease, may be associated with environmental conditions of displaced populations in contexts wherein essential health services are lacking or inadequate. Hypertension, on the other hand, is a common condition needing chronic and long-term care. These forms of considerations validate the emphasis that must be placed on primary health care in the immediate aftermath of disasters, whether natural or human-induced. Lastly, SPEED was able to assist decision makers on identifying possible outbreaks, which were averted; however, it did not pick up a high number of injuries and deaths due to violence expected from complex emergencies. SPEED is also in isolation from other reporting systems. It is suggested that linkages between SPEED and other surveillance systems, such as event-based surveillance and indicator-based surveillance and other reporting systems used especially for trauma and deaths, be strengthened to better illustrate the public health impacts of complex emergencies. Coordination within the DOH needs to be improved in order to have a truly integrated disease surveillance system.

Author Contributions: The authors of this manuscript were involved in the conception and design of the study or have contributed to the acquisition, analysis, or interpretation of the data of the study. They took part in its critical revision. They have agreed to be accountable for all aspects of the work. M.A.S. wrote the manuscript, conceptualized the study, interpreted the results, and collated the responses and comments from other authors. R.L. was vital in the acquisition of data and was part of the analysis of the results and the revision of the manuscript. V.W. contributed to the writing of the manuscript, conceptualization of the study, and the analysis of the results.

Acknowledgments: The authors would like to thank the leadership and staff of the Health Emergency Management Bureau of the Department of Health for their technical support and guidance in the completion of this study. The views stated in this article are those of the authors and do not necessarily reflect the official policy or position of the Health Emergency Management Bureau or the Philippine Department of Health.

References

1. National Disaster Risk Reduction and Management Council. *Final Report Re Armed Conflict in Zamboanga City and Basilan Province*; National Disaster Risk Reduction and Management Council: Quezon City, Philippines, 2013.
2. United Nations Office for the Coordination of Humanitarian Affairs. *Philippines: Zamboanga Action Plan 2014 (Revision)*; United Nations Office for the Coordination of Humanitarian Affairs: Makati, Philippines, 2014; Volume 30.
3. Brennan, R.J.; Nandy, R. Complex Humanitarian Emergencies: A Major Global Health Challenge. *Emerg. Med.* **2001**, *13*, 147–156. [CrossRef]
4. Médecins, S.F. *Refugee Health: An Approach to Emergency Situations*; Médecins Sans Frontières: Geneva, Switzerland, 1997.
5. Connolly, M.A.; Gayer, M.; Ryan, M.J.; Salama, P.; Spiegel, P.; Heymann, D.L. Communicable Diseases in Complex Emergencies: Impact and Challenges. *Lancet* **2004**, *364*, 1974–1983. [CrossRef]
6. Lam, E.; McCarthy, A.; Brennan, M. Vaccine-Preventable Diseases in Humanitarian Emergencies among Refugee and Internally-Displaced Populations. *Hum. Vaccin. Immunother.* **2015**, *11*, 2627–2636. [CrossRef] [PubMed]
7. Kouadio, I.K.; Kamigaki, T.; Oshitani, H. Measles Outbreaks in Displaced Populations: A Review of Transmission, Morbidity and Mortality Associated Factors. *BMC Int. Health Hum. Rights* **2010**, *10*, 5. [CrossRef] [PubMed]
8. Slama, S.; Kim, H.J.; Roglic, G.; Boulle, P.; Hering, H.; Varghese, C.; Rasheed, S.; Tonelli, M. Care of Non-Communicable Diseases in Emergencies. *Lancet* **2016**, *389*, 326–330. [CrossRef]
9. Demaio, A.; Jamieson, J.; Horn, R. Non-Communicable Diseases in Emergencies: A Call to Action. *PLoS Curr.* **2013**, *5*. [CrossRef] [PubMed]
10. Wisner, B.; Adams, J. *Environmental Health in Emergencies and Disasters*; World Health Organization: Geneva, Switzerland, 2002.

11. Centers for Disease Control and Prevention (U.S.). Deaths Associated with Hurricane Sandy—October–November 2012. *Morb. Mortal. Wkly. Rep.* **2013**, *62*, 393–397.
12. Ochi, S.; Murray, V.; Hodgson, S. The Great East Japan Earthquake Disaster: A Compilation of Published Literature on Health Needs and Relief Activities, March 2011–September 2012. *PLoS Curr.* **2013**, *5*. [CrossRef] [PubMed]
13. Ching, P.K.; de los Reyes, V.C.; Sucaldito, M.N.; Tayag, E. An Assessment of Disaster-Related Mortality Post-Haiyan in Tacloban City. *West Pacific Surveill. Response J.* **2015**, *6* (Suppl. 1), 34–38. [CrossRef]
14. Salazar, M.A.; Pesigan, A.M.; Law, R.; Winkler, V. Post-Disaster Health Impact of Natural Hazards in the Philippines in 2013. *Glob. Health Action* **2016**, *9*, 31320. [CrossRef] [PubMed]
15. Salazar, M.A.; Law, R.; Pesigan, A.; Winkler, V. Health Consequences of Typhoon Haiyan in the Eastern Visayas Region Using a Syndromic Surveillance Database. *PLoS Curr.* **2017**, *9*. [CrossRef]
16. Banwell, N.; Montoya, J.; Opeña, M.; IJsselmuiden, C.; Law, R.; Rutherford, S.; Chu, C.; Murray, V.; Balboa, G.J. Developing the Philippines as a Global Hub for Disaster Risk Reduction—A Health Research Initiative as Presented at the 10th Philippine National Health Research System Week Celebration. *PLoS Curr.* **2016**, *8*. [CrossRef] [PubMed]
17. Health Emergency Management Bureau. *Surveillance in Post Extreme Emergencies and Disasters Operations Manual for Managers*; Department of Health Philippines: Manila, Philippines, 2011.
18. Aitsi-Selmi, A.; Murray, V.; Wannous, C.; Dickinson, C.; Johnston, D.; Kawasaki, A.; Stevance, A.S.; Yeung, T. Reflections on a Science and Technology Agenda for 21st Century Disaster Risk Reduction: Based on the Scientific Content of the 2016 UNISDR Science and Technology Conference on the Implementation of the Sendai Framework for Disaster Risk Reduction 2015–2020. *Int. J. Disaster Risk Sci.* **2016**, *7*, 1–29.
19. UNISDR (United Nations International Strategy for Disaster Reduction). *Sendai Framework for Disaster Risk Reduction 2015–2030*; UNISDR: Geneva, Switzerland, 2015.
20. Lo, S.T.T.; Chan, E.Y.Y.; Chan, G.K.W.; Murray, V.; Abrahams, J.; Ardalan, A.; Kayano, R.; Yau, J.C.W. Health Emergency and Disaster Risk Management (Health-EDRM): Developing the Research Field within the Sendai Framework Paradigm. *Int. J. Disaster Risk Sci.* **2017**, *8*, 145–149. [CrossRef]
21. Martinez, R.E.; Quintana, R.; Go, J.J.; Marquez, M.A.; Kim, J.K.; Villones, M.S.; Salazar, M.A. Surveillance for and Issues Relating to Noncommunicable Diseases Post-Haiyan in Region 8. *West Pacific Surveill. Response J.* **2015**, *6* (Suppl. 1), 21–24. [CrossRef] [PubMed]
22. National Statistics Office. The 2010 Census of Population and Housing Reveals the Philippine Population at 92.34 Million. Available online: https://psa.gov.ph/content/2010-census-population-and-housing-reveals-philippine-population-9234-million (accessed on 30 November 2015).
23. Hutchinson, M.K.; Holtman, M.C. Analysis of Count Data Using Poisson Regression. *Res. Nurs. Health* **2005**, *28*, 408–418. [CrossRef] [PubMed]
24. Zhang, Z. Multivariable Fractional Polynomial Method for Regression Model. *Ann. Transl. Med.* **2016**, *4*, 174. [CrossRef] [PubMed]
25. Department of Health Philippines. *Adopting the 2008 Revised List of Notifiable Diseases, Syndromes, Health-Related Events and Conditions, AO 2008–0009*; Department of Health Philippines: Manila, Philippines, 2008.
26. Health Emergency Management Bureau. *Manual of Treatment Protocols of Common Communicable Diseases and Other Ailments During Emergencies and Disasters*, 2nd ed.; Banatin, C., Dominguez, N., Eds.; Department of Health Philippines: Manila, Philippines, 2013.
27. Gayer, M.; Legros, D.; Formenty, P.; Connolly, M.A. Conflict and Emerging Infectious Diseases. *Emerg. Infect. Dis.* **2007**, *13*, 1625–1631. [CrossRef] [PubMed]
28. Epidemiology Bureau. *The 2013 Philippine Health Statistics*; Asuncion, I., Benegas-Segarra, A., Timbang, T., Sinson, F., Rebanal, L., Eds.; Department of Health Philippines: Manila, Philippines, 2013.
29. Asian Institute of Journalism and Communication. *Zamboanga Learning Review on Post-Conflict Community Engagement*; Asian Institute of Journalism and Communication: Manila, Philippines, 2015.
30. Elfaituri, S.S. Skin Diseases among Internally Displaced Tawerghans Living in Camps in Benghazi, Libya. *Int. J. Dermatol.* **2016**, *55*, 1000–1004. [CrossRef] [PubMed]
31. Mobula, L.M.; Fisher, M.L.; Wood, T.; Plyler, W. Prevalence of Hypertension among Patients Attending Mobile Medical Clinics in the Philippines after Typhoon Haiyan. *PLoS Curr.* **2016**, *8*. [CrossRef] [PubMed]
32. WHO Regional Office for Europe. *Gaining Health: The European Strategy for the Prevention and Control of Noncommunicable Diseases*; WHO Regional Office for Europe: Copenhagen, Denmark, 2006.

33. Doocy, S.; Daniels, A.; Packer, C.; Dick, A.; Kirsch, T.D. The Human Impact of Earthquakes: A Historical Review of Events 1980–2009 and Systematic Literature Review. *PLoS Curr.* **2016**, *28*, 237–244. [CrossRef] [PubMed]
34. Doocy, S.; Dick, A.; Daniels, A.; Kirsch, T.D.; Hopkins, J. The Human Impact of Tropical Cyclones: A Historical Review of Events 1980-2009 and Systematic Literature Review Citation Abstract Authors. *PLoS Curr.* **2013**, *1* 1–25.
35. Murray, C.J.L.; King, G.; Lopez, A.D.; Tomijima, N.; Krug, E.G. Armed Conflict as a Public Health Problem. *BMJ* **2002**, *324*, 346–349. [CrossRef] [PubMed]
36. Health Emergency Management Bureau. *Final Report: Armed Conflict in Zamboanga City*; Health Emergency Management Bureau: Manila, Philippines, 2014.
37. WHO Regional Office for the Western Pacific. *A Guide to Establishing Event-Based Surveillance*; WHO Western Pacific Regional Office: Manila, Philippines, 2008.
38. Foldy, S.L. Linking Better Surveillance to Better Outcomes. *Morb. Mortal. Wkly. Rep.* **2004**, *53*, 12–17.
39. World Health Organization; United Nations High Commissioner for Refugees. *MhGAP Humanitarian Intervention Guide (MhGAP-HIG): Clinical Management of Mental, Neurological and Substance Use Conditions in Humanitarian Emergencies*; WHO: Geneva, Switzerland, 2015.
40. Health Emergency Management Bureau. *Pocket Emergency Tool*, 4th ed.; Department of Health Philippines: Manila, Philippines, 2012.
41. United Nations Office for the Coordination of Humanitarian Affairs. *Philippines: Zamoanga and Basilan Emgerency Situtaion Report No. 8*; UN OCHA: Manila, Philippines, 2013.
42. Women's Refugee Commission. *Minimum Initial Service Package (MISP) for Reproductive Health in Crisis Situations: A Distance Learning Module*, 3rd ed.; Women's Refugee Commission: New York, NY, USA, 2011.

11

Nurses' Readiness for Emergencies and Public Health Challenges

Mohammed Ali Salem Sultan [1,2,*], Amir Khorram-Manesh [3,4], Eric Carlström [2,5], Jarle Løwe Sørensen [5], Hadi Jaber Al Sulayyim [6] and Fabian Taube [4,7]

1 Model of Care, Directorate of Health Affairs, Najran 66255, Saudi Arabia
2 Institute of Health and Care Sciences, Sahlgrenska Academy, Gothenburg University, 413 46 Göteborg, Sweden; eric.carlstrom@gu.se
3 Institute of Clinical Sciences, Sahlgrenska Academy, Gothenburg University, 413 90 Göteborg, Sweden; amir.khorram-manesh@surgery.gu.se
4 Department of Research and Development, Swedish Armed Forces Centre for Defence Medicine, 426 76 Göteborg, Sweden; fabian.taube@amm.gu.se
5 USN School of Business, Campus Vestfold, University of South-Eastern Norway, 3603 Kongsberg, Norway; jarle.sorensen@usn.no
6 Department of Infection and Prevention and Control, Directorate of Health Affairs, Najran 66255, Saudi Arabia; hadialsleem@hotmail.com
7 Institute of Medicine, Sahlgrenska Academy, Gothenburg University, 41345 Göteborg, Sweden
* Correspondence: mohammed.sultan@gu.se

Abstract: This study was aimed at assessing the readiness of 200 emergency nurses in the southern part of Saudi Arabia in the management of public health emergencies, major incidents, and disasters by using quantitative research through a self-reporting validated questionnaire containing 10 different dimensions. All registered nurses working in emergency departments who were willing to participate, of all ages and gender groups, were included. Nurses who were not present during the study period because of vacation or maternity leave, nurses at the managerial level, and nursing aides were excluded. The participating nurses reported good knowledge in almost all investigated aspects of the theoretical dimensions of emergency management. However, they revealed perceived weaknesses in practical dimensions of emergency management and difficulties in assessing their own efforts. There was a significant correlation between qualification and the dimensions of emergency preparedness, epidemiology and surveillance, isolation and quarantine and critical resources, which indicates a need for strengthening their practical contribution as well as their theoretical knowledge. Educational initiatives combining theoretical and practical aspects of emergency management may provide an opportunity to examine nurses' knowledge, skills, and abilities continuously in an environment with no harm to patients.

Keywords: disaster; emergency; healthcare; nurse; readiness; preparedness; public health

1. Introduction

The increasing incidences of public health emergencies and disasters necessitate global awareness, multiagency collaboration, and emergency system readiness to respond [1]. Major incidents and disasters (MIDs) might be inevitable, but they can be mitigated by performing an appropriate risk and vulnerability assessment (RVA) as the foundation for creating a disaster response plan [2]. Risks and vulnerabilities causing a public health emergency or an MID may vary in different countries; however, the current coronavirus 2019 (COVID-19) pandemic has clearly demonstrated how a local outbreak can influence the spread of a disease and how it can result in lessons learned for global benefits. A response plan targets all possible risks, not only to enable countries to act based on their resources but also to share knowledge and compare their outcome to improve their response. Global threats can be man-made or natural (e.g., terrorism, pandemics and disasters). Vulnerabilities are the weaknesses that can be exploited by threats, and they can be dimensions which are either missing, such as strategic leadership, or of poor quality, such as the lack of proper education [3]. Although all parts of a healthcare system should be ready to manage an MID, hospital preparedness is particularly important since hospitals should serve not only the affected people but also other emergency or elective cases in need of help simultaneously. Therefore, a well-prepared hospital needs an RVA-based response plan and should facilitate educational initiatives to build up a pool of well-educated and skilled staff [4].

Because of their numbers and distribution, nurses are the largest group in the healthcare domain who face MIDs, and their knowledge and level of preparedness play a crucial role in the pre-, peri-, and post-MID periods [5]. In previous studies, about 80% of Philippine nurses were found to be neither fully prepared nor knowledgeable about disaster preparedness and response, and they lacked an awareness of existing management protocols [6]. Furthermore, 65.4% of Pakistani nurses had theoretical knowledge related to disaster plans, drills, and preparedness but very little practical knowledge about MID management [7]. Finally, in Egypt and China, the majority of nurses had unsatisfactory levels of information and knowledge about disaster management and needed to join specific training programmes [8,9]. These studies reveal the importance of theoretical and practical dimensions in nurses' preparedness.

The Kingdom of Saudi Arabia (KSA) engages nearly 80% of the Arabian Peninsula, and its desert area accommodates the largest continuous sand desert in the world [10]. The KSA is a disaster-prone country with varying grades of emergencies. It has one of the world's highest mortality rates in motor vehicle crashes [11]. Terrorist incidents such as bombings have resulted in periodic internal instability as well as shifts in regional and international political dynamics [12]. Mass gatherings (Ramadan and Hajj) are two special events on the Islamic calendar that contribute to overcrowding during prayer performance and other rituals, resulting in numerous incidents [13]. Finally, many cities experience building collapses regularly as a result of mass gatherings, insufficient building safety, and a lack of control by the authorities, leading to injuries and deaths [14]. Natural disasters, such as flooding, earthquakes, and drought, occur frequently in the KSA. Floods are the most frequently experienced natural event because of unplanned urban development and improper drainage or the low ground of some high-populated areas, such as Jeddah and Mecca, which are surrounded by mountains and are easily affected by rainfall, resulting in flooding [15]. These threats make a good case for the KSA's preparedness in MIDs to be studied. One recent study from the KSA on emergency nurses' disaster preparedness showed that 28% of the nurses had inadequate knowledge [16]. The number of participants, however, was small (n = 72). Other studies such as the one from Australia have also confirmed these results, showing nurses' confusion about their role in MID management and their shortcomings in basic knowledge regarding standard disaster terminology and types of disasters [17]. Altogether, these studies highlight a knowledge gap in the overall preparedness of the nurses to deal with disasters.

2. Aim

This study aims to assess the theoretical and practical MID readiness of emergency nurses in the southern KSA, where MIDs frequently occur and well-educated, multinational nurses are employed to increase its response capacity.

3. Materials and Methods

3.1. Study Design

This study employed a descriptive quantitative design using a validated questionnaire to assess the knowledge and awareness among licensed nursing staff of preparedness to respond to emergencies and specific healthcare scenarios.

3.2. *Questionnaire*

This study used the Emergency Preparedness Information Questionnaire (EPIQ) to assess the disaster preparedness of nurses [18]. EPIQ contains a variety of topical areas, of which two are relevant for the present study, i.e., (1) the 10 specific competency dimensions related to preparedness in the case of large-scale emergency events and (2) self-assessed familiarity across these competency areas. EPIQ is the only reliable and validated tool in the literature that evaluates nurses' perceived familiarity of emergency preparedness and disaster response core competencies. It uses familiarity as an important measure of the acquisition of new information. Wisniewski et al. developed EPIQ by performing an extensive search in the literature, combined with nurses' perceptions of perceived familiarity with these capabilities. They also sought to determine preferred education methods and demographics for future educational endeavours. EPIQ has been validated by psychometric testing and used in several studies aiming to measure levels of disaster preparedness and provides a comprehensive analysis of the topic of study since it covers broad areas [19,20]. It works to individually assess all areas of healthcare and delves into in-depth information relevant to the research. Additionally, it is simple to read and interpret and provides a user-friendly interface.

EPIQ consists of 51 items divided into two parts: the first six questions relate to demographic and individual information. Secondly, 45 knowledge-based questions are distributed among the 10 emergency preparedness competency dimensions, which are (1) Emergency Preparedness Terms and Activities, (2) Incident Command System (ICS) and own role within it, (3) Ethical Issues in Triage, (4) Epidemiology and Surveillance, (5) Isolation/Quarantine, (6) Decontamination, (7) Communication/Connectivity, (8) Psychological Issues, (9) Special Populations, and (10) Accessing Critical Resources (Appendix A).

3.3. *Setting*

The research was conducted at the Ministry of Health's (MOH) hospitals (n = 10) in the Najran region, located in the southern part of the KSA.

3.4. *Population and Sample*

All nurses at the 10 hospitals included in the study were informed about the study by the nursing office director at each hospital. The participants were randomly included from the list of nurses working in each emergency department (ED), thus avoiding the bias of choosing a specific group. They were ensured that their participation was voluntary, they could withdraw from the study whenever they decided to, and the obtained data were handled confidentially. They received basic information about the study and its goals, and informed consent was obtained from each participant. A power analysis with a standardised statistical power of 0.80 and medium effect size of 0.5 premediated the appropriate sample size to 200 nurses. The self-completion questionnaire was presented to the participants through the SurveyMonkey website.

3.5. *Data Collection and Processing*

Collected data were stored at the hospitals' research centres. Nurses answered the questionnaires on a specific research day to prevent response influence. The respondents were asked to provide correct information. The information provided was subject only to research, and the researcher could not disclose the respondents' identities at any time, no matter the circumstances. The included participants were registered nurses working in EDs who were willing to participate, in all age and gender groups. Nurses who were not present during the study period because of vacation or maternity leave, nurses at the managerial level, and nursing aides were excluded.

All data concerning the 10 emergency preparedness competency dimensions were analysed by the authors. The primary investigator was responsible for collecting data and categorising them for further analysis by the teammate. Each dimension consisted of a number of questions, in which participants could indicate their familiarity with a topic based on a five-point Likert scale (see results).

3.6. Ethical Approval

For this study, an ethical committee certificate of approval was obtained from the Institutional Review Board at the General Directorate of Health Affairs in the Najran region (IRB Log Number 2020-27 E—Date of approval: 1 July 2020).

3.7. Statistics

The homogeneity of the items in the subscales of the EPIQ was analysed by calculating Cronbach's alpha using Statistical Package for the Social Sciences (SPSS) software version 20. Cronbach's alpha was 0.98, which shows high internal consistency and, according to Brace, Kemp and Snelgar [21], is considered satisfactory. Other results are descriptively presented in actual numbers and percentages. A Kolmogorov–Smirnov test was used to explore normality. As a result of skewness in the data, Spearman's rho was used to test co-variation. Means were compared using the Mann–Whitney U and Kruskal–Wallis tests. Statistical significance was recognised at $p < 0.05$, and all tests were two-tailed.

4. Results

Of the 200 nurses who answered the questionnaire, 181 (90.5%) were female and 19 (9.5%) were male. A majority of the respondents (45.5%) were 22–30 years old. About 39% of the nurses were 31–40 years old, while the remaining 15.5% were 40 years old or older. About 93.5% of the nurses had a Bachelor of Science in Nursing (BSN), 6% had a Master of Science in Nursing (MSN), and 0.5% had a Doctor of Philosophy (PhD) in Nursing. Most of the practicing nurses, especially those in EDs within MOH hospitals, possessed undergraduate qualifications from MOH-certified education and training institutions. About 12% of the nurses had more than 16 years of experience within EDs, 20% had 11–15 years of experience, and 34% had 6–10 years of experience, while the remaining 34% had 1–5 years of experience.

The remaining results of the study were categorised into the following 10 dimensions, which denote the extent to which nurses are aware of disaster risks and preparedness. Each dimension consisted of several questions, in which nurses were asked to indicate their familiarity with a topic based on a five-point Likert scale as follows: very familiar (5), somewhat familiar (4), familiar to neutral (3), somewhat unfamiliar (2), and not familiar (1). The positive threshold was 'familiar to neutral' to 'very familiar'.

Table 1 shows that most of the participants had good knowledge (familiar to very familiar) in most items of these dimensions: signs and symptoms (different biological agents: 49.5%, and better for Anthrax: 75%), modes of transmission (56.5%), antidote and adverse reaction (66% and 69.5%, respectively). However, participants seemed to be uncertain about their practical capabilities, skills, and evaluations of their own actions, including necessary first aid interventions such as ventilation and oxygen administration during a public health emergency (32% and 39.5%, respectively).

Table 1. Description of 200 nurses' responses regarding familiarity with Emergency Preparedness Terms and Activities.

Items	Very Familiar	Somewhat Familiar	Familiar to Neutral	Somewhat Unfamiliar	Not Familiar	Total
1. Signs/symptoms of exposure to different biological agents	11 (5.5%)	16 (8%)	72 (36%)	82 (41%)	19 (9.5%)	100%
2. Signs/symptoms of Anthrax inhalation	26 (13%)	56 (28%)	68 (34%)	42 (21%)	8 (4%)	100%
3. Modes of transmission for different types of biological agents (anthrax, smallpox, etc.)	12 (6%)	24 (12%)	77 (38.5%)	71 (35.5%)	16 (8%)	100%
4. Match antidote and prophylactic medications to specific biological/chemical agents	9 (4.5%)	35 (17.5%)	88 (44%)	55 (27.5%)	13 (6.5%)	100%
5. Possible adverse reactions to smallpox vaccination	16 (8%)	37 (18.5%)	86 (43%)	44 (22%)	17 (8.5%)	100%
6. Basic first aid in a large-scale emergency event (including oxygen administration and ventilation)	6 (6%)	4 (2%)	48 (24%)	84 (42%)	58 (29%)	100%
7. How to evaluate the effectiveness of your own actions during a large-scale emergency	4 (2%)	11 (5.5%)	64 (32%)	92 (46%)	29 (14.5%)	100%

Table 2 shows that a majority of the nurses surveyed had good knowledge regarding what they needed to do during a large-scale emergency. They also appeared to have good knowledge about the emergency operations plan (EOP), Incident Command System (ICS), physical locations of all entities, the importance of medical decision-making, etc.

Table 2. Description of nurses' responses regarding their familiarity with the Incident Command System (ICS) and their role (n = 200).

Items	Very Familiar	Somewhat Familiar	Familiar to Neutral	Somewhat Unfamiliar	Not Familiar	Total
1. The content of emergency operations plan (EOP) in your agency/organisation	25 (12.5%)	84 (42%)	72 (36%)	15 (7.5%)	4 (2%)	100%
2. To which functional group in the Incident Command System (ICS) you would be assigned during a large-scale emergency event	23 (11.5%)	62 (31%)	84 (42%)	24 (12%)	7 (3.5%)	100%
3. The physical location to which you would report if a large-scale emergency event occurred	27 (13.5%)	78 (39%)	76 (38%)	14 (7%)	5 (2.5%)	100%
4. Assess and respond to site safety issues for self, co-workers and affected people during a large-scale emergency event	25 (12.5%)	77 (38.5%)	80 (40%)	13 (6.5%)	5 (2.5%)	100%
5. The strategic rationale used to develop the ICS response/action plan	13 (6.5%)	68 (34%)	89 (44.5%)	25 (12.5%)	5 (2.5%)	100%
6. Your agency's preparedness for responding to a large-scale emergency event	22 (11%)	81 (40.5%)	73 (36.5%)	18 (9%)	6 (3%)	100%
7. Differences between decision-making processes in the Incident Command System for a large-scale emergency event and non-emergency situations	24 (12%)	76 (38%)	82 (41%)	14 (7%)	4 (2%)	100%
8. Tasks which should NOT be delegated to volunteers in a large-scale emergency event	22 (11%)	65 (32.5%)	86 (43%)	21 (10.5%)	6 (3%)	100%

Table 3 shows nurses' approaches to the assessment of affected people's health following a crisis and their familiarity with ethical issues in MIDs, such as during triage. Overall, they claimed that they had good knowledge and understanding of these issues.

Table 3. Description of nurses' responses regarding their familiarity with Ethical Issues in Triage (N = 200).

Items	Very Familiar	Somewhat Familiar	Familiar to Neutral	Somewhat Unfamiliar	Not Familiar	Total
1. How to perform a rapid physical assessment of a victim of a large-scale emergency event	28 (14%)	78 (39%)	77 (38.5%)	13 (6.5%)	4 (2%)	100%
2. How to perform a rapid mental health assessment of a victim of a large-scale emergency event	25 (12.5%)	64 (32%)	86 (43%)	20 (10%)	5 (2.5%)	100%
3. How to assist with triage in a large-scale emergency event	32 (16%)	73 (36.5%)	72 (36%)	18 (9%)	5 (2.5%)	100%
4. General issues related to the proper handling of the dead during a large-scale emergency event (ethical, legal, cultural, and safety)	29 (14.5%)	65 (32.5%)	84 (42%)	19 (9.5%)	3 (1.5%)	100%

Table 4 shows nurses' knowledge in mitigating the further outbreak of a disease. Overall, most of the nurses claimed that they had good knowledge in handling the administrative measures needed in chemical, biological, radiological, and nuclear (CBRN) surveillance.

Table 4. Description of nurses' responses regarding their familiarity with Epidemiology and Surveillance (N = 200).

Items	Very Familiar	Somewhat Familiar	Familiar to Neutral	Somewhat Unfamiliar	Not Familiar	Total
1. History and assessment surveillance data for creating a high index of suspicion that a patient has been exposed to a biological agent	20 (10%)	62 (31%)	92 (46%)	21 (10.5%)	5 (2.5%)	100%
2. When to report an unusual set of symptoms to an epidemiologist	19 (9.5%)	80 (40%)	74 (37%)	23 (11.5%)	4 (2%)	100%
3. Diseases that are immediately reportable to state health departments	26 (13%)	86 (43%)	72 (36%)	13 (6.5%)	3 (1.5%)	100%
4. Ability to identify the exacerbation of an underlying disease as a result of exposure to a chemical or biological agent or to radiation	20 (10%)	67 (33.5%)	95 (47.5%)	14 (7%)	4 (2%)	100%

In Table 5, nurses evaluated their knowledge of isolation and quarantine issues. Most of the surveyed nurses seemed to have good knowledge in these areas.

Table 5. Description of nurses' responses regarding their familiarity with Isolation/Quarantine (N = 200).

Items	Very Familiar	Somewhat Familiar	Familiar to Neutral	Somewhat Unfamiliar	Not Familiar	Total
1. Isolation procedures for people exposed to biological or chemical agents	33 (16.5%)	80 (40%)	66 (33%)	17 (8.5%)	4 (2%)	100%
2. Your facility's/community's quarantine process	36 (18%)	90 (45%)	60 (30%)	10 (5%)	4 (2%)	100%

Table 6 shows that most of the nurses had good knowledge of the decontamination process in their hospitals, including the use of personal protective equipment (PPE).

Table 6. Description of nurses' responses regarding their familiarity with Decontamination (N = 200).

Items	Very Familiar	Somewhat Familiar	Familiar to Neutral	Somewhat Unfamiliar	Not Familiar	Total
1. Selection of the appropriate personal protective equipment when caring for patients exposed to chemical, biological, radiological, and nuclear (CBRN) agents	63 (31.5%)	95 (47.5%)	35 (17.5%)	4 (2%)	3 (1.5%)	100%
2. The decontamination procedures stated in your facility's emergency operations plan	36 (18%)	89 (44.5%)	61 (30.5%)	10 (5%)	4 (2%)	100%
3. The impact on the environment from a large-scale emergency event	24 (12%)	82 (41%)	72 (36%)	18 (9%)	4 (2%)	100%

Table 7 addresses the communication aspect of emergency response. A majority of the nurses had good knowledge of communication and information sharing during an emergency and of the need for debriefing and communication devices.

Table 7. Description of nurses' responses regarding their familiarity with Communication/Connectivity (N = 200).

Items	Very Familiar	Somewhat Familiar	Familiar to Neutral	Somewhat Unfamiliar	Not Familiar	Total
1. The procedure used to document provision of care in a large-scale emergency event	21 (10.5%)	77 (38.5%)	79 (39.5%)	19 (9.5%)	4 (2%)	100%
2. Chain of custody during a large-scale emergency event	15 (7.5%)	63 (31.5%)	92 (46%)	26 (13%)	4 (2%)	100%
3. Procedure for communicating critical patient information to those transporting patients	24 (12%)	86 (43%)	74 (37%)	11 (5.5%)	5 (2.5%)	100%
4. Effectively present information about degree of risk to various audiences	23 (11.5%)	60 (30%)	95 (47.5%)	17 (8.5%)	5 (2.5%)	100%
5. Identify the different abilities of key partners in your emergency operations plan (EOP)	18 (9%)	65 (32.5%)	88 (44%)	24 (12%)	5 (2.5%)	100%
6. Appropriate debriefing activities during a large-scale emergency event	19 (9.5%)	53 (26.5%)	102 (52%)	19 (9.5%)	7 (3.5%)	100%
7. Use of all types of communication devices (phone, fax, email, personal digital assistant (PDAs), etc.)	31 (15.5%)	64 (32%)	88 (44%)	13 (6.5%)	4 (2%)	100%

Table 8 shows that a majority of the nurses had good knowledge of appropriate and necessary psychological support during MIDs, claimed that they could provide health counselling/education in issues related to chemical, biological, radiological, nuclear, and explosive (CBRNE) agents, and could communicate with, identify, and evaluate youth and adults with post-traumatic stress disorder (PTSD).

Table 8. Description of nurses' responses regarding their familiarity with Psychological Issues (N = 200).

Items	Very Familiar	Somewhat Familiar	Familiar to Neutral	Somewhat Unfamiliar	Not Familiar	Total
1. Appropriate psychological support for all parties involved in a large-scale emergency event	23 (11.5%)	67 (33.5%)	88 (44%)	17 (8.5%)	5 (2.5%)	100%
2. Provide health counselling/education to patients regarding the long-term impact of chemical, biological, radiological, nuclear, and explosive (CBRNE) agents	31 (15.5%)	48 (24%)	89 (44.5%)	26 (13%)	6 (3%)	100%
3. Signs of post-traumatic stress in patients seen for routine health care following an event	21 (10.5%)	68 (34%)	86 (43%)	20 (10%)	5 (2.5%)	100%
4. How to evaluate a teenager to detect post-traumatic mental health problems	17 (8.5%)	59 (29.5%)	87 (43.5%)	28 (14%)	9 (4.5%)	100%

Table 9 shows nurses' knowledge in handling special populations affected by a disaster. A majority of nurses claimed to have good knowledge and understanding of the unique needs and expectations required for care of vulnerable groups.

Table 9. Description of nurses' responses regarding their familiarity with Special Populations (N = 200).

Items	Very Familiar	Somewhat Familiar	Familiar to Neutral	Somewhat Unfamiliar	Not Familiar	Total
1. Procedures for providing care to children/youth during a large-scale emergency event in cases in which prior consent from parent/legal guardian is possible	20 (10%)	61 (30.5%)	88 (44%)	27 (13.5%)	4 (2%)	100%
2. The appropriate care of sensitive/vulnerable patient groups during a large-scale emergency (i.e., aged, pregnant women, and the disabled)	18 (9%)	65 (32.5%)	87 (43.5%)	25 (12.5%)	5 (2.5%)	100%

Table 10 shows the ability of nurses to access critical resources during an MID. They seemed to have good knowledge and capabilities to perform necessary measures in all areas within this dimension.

Table 10. Description of nurses' familiarity responses rate of Accessing Critical Resources (N = 200).

Items	Very Familiar	Somewhat Familiar	Familiar to Neutral	Somewhat Unfamiliar	Not Familiar	Total
1. During an event, where to quickly access up-to-date resources for specific CBRNE incidents	17 (8.5%)	52 (26%)	90 (45%)	35 (17.5%)	6 (3%)	100%
2. Determine the appropriate agency to which reportable diseases are to be directed	18 (9%)	54 (27%)	91 (45.5%)	27 (13.5%)	10 (5%)	100%
3. The process for gaining access to the Strategic National Stockpile	11 (5.5%)	36 (18%)	86 (43%)	48 (24%)	19 (9.5%)	100%
4. Please provide an assessment of your overall familiarity with response activities/preparedness in the case of a large-scale emergency event	19 (9.5%)	63 (31.5%)	88 (44%)	25 (12.5%)	5 (2.5%)	100%

The results of normality, measured with the Kolmogorov–Smirnov test, indicated the data to be significantly skewed (sig. 0.00). As a result of the skewness and the fact that the data were ordinal and presented as ranks, a non-parametric test, Spearman's rho, was chosen to measure bivariate correlations. The variables of age, qualification, and experience were tested for the 10 studied dimensions of nurses' familiarity responses. Significant correlations were found in the correlations on qualification and dimensions of Emergency Preparedness (sig. 0.006), Epidemiology and Surveillance (sig. 0.008), Isolation and Quarantine (sig. 0.000) and Critical Resources (sig. 0.019). All significant correlations represented a small to moderate association (Critical Resources, 0.185–Isolation and Quarantine, 0.266) (Table 11).

Table 11. Ranks and statistics of nurses' responses regarding their familiarity with Emergency Preparedness Terms and Activities, Epidemiology and Surveillance, Isolation/Quarantine, and Accessing Critical Resources/Qualification (sign ≤ 0.05, N = 200).

		Emergency Preparedness	Qualification			Epidemiology and Surveillance	Qualification
Emergency preparedness	CC	1.0	0.195	Epidemiology & Surveillance	CC	1.0	0.188
	Sig.tt		0.006		Sig.tt		0.008
Qualification	CC	0.195	1.0	Qualification	CC	0.188	1.0
	Sig.tt	0.006			Sig.tt	0.008	
		Isolation/ Quarantine	Qualification			Critical Resources	Qualification
Isolation/ Quarantine	CC	1.0	0.266	Critical Resources	CC	1.0	0.185
	Sig.tt		0.000		Sig.tt		0.019
Qualification	CC	0.266	1.0	Qualification	CC	0.185	1.0
	Sig.tt	0.000			Sig.tt	0.019	

CC = Correlation Coefficient, Sig.tt = Significant two-tailed.

The psychological issues dimension was significant when correlated to age (sig. 0.029), qualification (sig. 0.026), and experience (sig. 0.027). The correlations represented a small association (0.154–0.158) (Table 12).

Table 12. Ranks and statistics of nurses' responses regarding their familiarity with Psychological Issues/Age, Qualification and Experience (sign ≤ 0.05, N = 200).

		Psychologi-Cal Issues	Age			Psychologi-Cal Issues	Qualification			Psychologi-Cal Issues	Experience
Psychological issues	CC	1.0	0.154	Psychological issues	CC	1.0	0.158	Psychological issues	CC	1.0	0.157
	Sig.tt		0.029		Sig.tt		0.026		Sig.tt		0.027
Age	CC	0.154	1.0	Qualification	CC	0.158	1.0	Experience	CC	0.157	1.0
	Sig.tt	0.029			Sig.tt	0.026			Sig.tt	0.027	
		Psychologi-Cal Issues	Age			Psychologi-Cal Issues	Qualification			Psychologi-Cal Issues	Experience
Psychological issues	CC	1.0	0.154	Psychological issues	CC	1.0	0.158	Psychological issues	CC	1.0	0.157
	Sig.tt		0.029		Sig.tt		0.026		Sig.tt		0.027
Age	CC	0.154	1.0	Qualification	CC	0.158	1.0	Experience	CC	0.157	1.0
	Sig.tt	0.029			Sig.tt	0.026			Sig.tt	0.027	

CC = Correlation Coefficient, Sig.tt = Significant two-tailed.

5. Discussions

In this paper, we assessed the readiness of emergency nurses in the southern region of the KSA in the management of public health emergencies, major incidents, and disasters. The reasons for such evaluation were the continuous exposure of the region to both man-made and natural disasters and the advanced educational backgrounds of the nursing staff.

The results of this study indicate a good preparedness in all theoretical dimensions of MID management, including emergency preparedness terms and activities, Incident Command Systems and their role in MID management, ethical issues in triage, epidemiology and surveillance, isolation and quarantine, decontamination, communication issues, psychological issues, management of special/vulnerable populations, and assessment of critical resources. However, the nurses appeared to be uncertain about their skills and practical performance and the evaluation of their own abilities. These results are opposite to what was reported earlier from the KSA [16] and thus confirm a good theoretical knowledge and a need for practical opportunities. Bearing in mind that 93.5% of nurses had a BSN, 6% had an MSN, and 0.5% had a PhD in nursing and that most of the practicing nurses (66%) had more than five years of experience, these results might be indicative of a need for further educational initiatives to improve the skills and practical performance of all nurses working in the management of MIDs [6–9].

The quantitative nature of this study and the collected data provide an understanding of the preparedness of nurses working at MOH hospitals in the southern region of the KSA and reveal both strengths and weaknesses that can be implementable and relevant in other regions and countries.

The current COVID-19 pandemic has demonstrated difficulties in MID management, such as resource scarcity and medical decision-making, which seem to be more complicated in practice than in theory [22]. The EPIQ questionnaire enabled the researchers to capture various dimensions of disaster preparedness and response in nursing environments [23]. However, the nurses' lack of confidence in their own skills and performance should be considered a critical shortcoming. Several studies have shown that healthcare workers who are confident in their own level of competence are more likely to react effectively in real crises than those who are not [24–28]. Nurses' theoretical knowledge, such as their ability to identify the signs and symptoms associated with highly infectious biological and chemical agents, is essential for enhancing disaster preparedness; however, this theoretical knowledge should be incorporated in practical performance to yield a robust preparedness. Proper education and training in an environment where nurses can act without hesitation, make mistakes with no harm to patients, and establish contact with necessary agencies without getting rejected will enable them to attain the required knowledge and skills to identify and report signs and symptoms that are unclear and to treat and intervene with necessary and evaluable measures [4,29–32]. Such performance and collaborative action will ensure their confidence in their response activities as key players in an MID.

Nurses' emergency preparedness is determined by their familiarity with their organisation's emergency operations plan (EOP), which allows them to follow the recommended procedures for crisis intervention from a healthcare perspective [33]. Nurses' knowledge of the ethical, legal, cultural, psychological, and safety dimensions of emergency response is critical for effective intervention and recovery [23,34]. Planning to address the needs of special populations is a strategic dimension of emergency response and recovery initiatives [17]. Effective communication during an emergency is essential for ensuring nurses' collaboration with other stakeholders involved in a crisis event. The epidemiology and surveillance aspects of disaster management require streamlined communication among various departments and agencies [17].

Most of the nurses in this study reported knowledge of and familiarity with all aforementioned dimensions. However, since MIDs are rare events, they have no chance to evaluate their theoretical and practical abilities in a real situation. Simulation exercises may offer a chance to examine these abilities in a safe environment with no harm to patients [4,35,36]. These exercises may also offer an opportunity to raise their awareness about pandemics, quarantine, isolation, the use of PPE, and other critical resources to foster recovery and minimise the spread of highly infectious diseases. A majority of nurses in this study understood the methods for isolation but lacked adequate knowledge concerning the community quarantine process and the impact it may have on the mental health of both affected people and workers. This finding supports earlier findings by McCarthy [23,37], which as part of building modern contemporary emergency nurses, argued the need for nurses to increase their understating of procedures performed and competency in practice. This shortcoming would be addressed in collaborative simulation exercises [4].

In this study, there was a significant correlation between qualification and the dimensions of emergency preparedness, epidemiology and surveillance, isolation and quarantine, and critical resources. These findings are in accordance with Gladston, who reported a significant correlation between nurses' perceptions and qualifications [38], and similar to studies showing statistically significant associations between the dimensions of psychological issues and age, qualification and experience [38–41].

6. Limitations

This study focussed on nursing staff working in emergency departments only and did not consider other nurses' roles and responses. The sample consisted overwhelmingly of women. The small number of male nurses was not a representative sample of the male population of nurses in the region. The non-parametric correlations provided some useful data possible to generalise to a broader population. However, when comparing means, the results were mainly non-significant. Repeated non-parametric tests on the data (Mann–Whitney U and Kruskal–Wallis Test) indicated the need for an extended study. Data for this study were collected in the Najran region only, which is one of 13 regions in Saudi Arabia, so there was a limitation to the ability to generalise the results to all parts of Saudi Arabia. Furthermore, this study focussed on nurses working in MOH hospitals, while nurses working in other agencies, such as Saudi Arabian Oil Company (ARAMCO) Medical Services, Security Forces hospitals, National Guard hospitals, and the Armed Forces Hospitals of Saudi Arabia were not included. Finally, self-reported surveys by nature have bias: response recall, the possibility that questions will be misinterpreted, and the possibility that respondents' perceived knowledge may not be what they actually know.

7. Conclusions

The aim of this study was to evaluate the theoretical and practical readiness of nurses in MID management. The results indicate that nurses working in Najran EDs in the southern part of the KSA have good theoretical knowledge but lack confidence in their practical performance. Several studies have shown the significance of self-confidence in healthcare workers' responses to real crises [24–28]. Since theoretical knowledge should go hand in hand with practical knowledge to achieve successful outcomes in MIDs, bolstering practical emergency preparedness exercises, for example, with scenario-based simulation exercises [4] may enhance nurses' readiness for crisis response.

Author Contributions: Conceptualization: M.A.S.S., A.K.-M.; Data curation: M.A.S.S., H.J.A.S.; Formal analysis: M.A.S.S., H.J.A.S., A.K.-M., E.C., J.L.S., and F.T.; Investigation: M.A.S.S.; Methodology: M.A.S.S., E.C., A.K.-M.; Project administration: M.A.S.S.; Resources: M.A.S.S.; Supervision: A.K.-M.; Validation: E.C., J.L.S. and F.T.; Writing—original draft: M.A.S.S.; Writing—review and editing: A.K.-M., E.C., J.L.S., and F.T. All authors have read and agreed to the published version of the manuscript.

Acknowledgments: All authors would like to thank James W. Peltier for providing us the questionnaire.

Appendix A Questionnaire

The questionnaire is divided into two parts. The first six questions related to demographic and individual information, while the remaining 45 knowledge-based questions are distributed in the 10 emergency preparedness competency dimensions.

Appendix A.1 PART I

Demographics

Kindly tick the box where necessary

1. State your age □ 22–30 years □ 31–40 years □ > 40 years

2. State your gender □ Male □ Female

3. What is your academic degree? □ BS □ MS □ PhD

4. What is your nursing experience? □ 1–5 years □ 6–10 □ 11–15 □ > 16

5. What is your experience in the ED? □ 1–5 □ 6–8□ > 9

6. What is your marital status? □ Single □ Married □ Divorced □ Widow/widower

Appendix A.2 PART II

Table A1. Emergency Preparedness Information Questionnaire (EPIQ).

S. No	Components	Not Familiar		Somewhat Unfamiliar		Familiar to Neutral		Somewhat Familiar		Very Familiar	
I	**Emergency Preparedness Terms and Activities**	**N**	%	**N**	%	**N**	%	**N**	%	**N**	%
1	Signs/symptoms of exposure to different biological agents										
2	Signs/symptoms of Anthrax inhalation										
3	Modes of transmission for different types of biological agents (anthrax, smallpox, etc.)										
4	Match antidote and prophylactic medications to specific biological/chemical agents										
5	Possible adverse reactions to smallpox vaccination										
6	Basic first aid in a large-scale emergency event (including oxygen administration and ventilation)										
7	How to evaluate the effectiveness of your own actions during a large-scale emergency										
II	**Incident Command System (ICS) and your role within it**	**N**	%	**N**	%	**N**	%	**N**	%	**N**	%
8	The content of emergency operations plan (EOP) in your agency/organisation										
9	To which functional group in the Incident Command System (ICS) you would be assigned during a large-scale emergency event										
10	The physical location to which you would report if a large-scale emergency event occurred										
11	Assess and respond to site safety issues for self, co-workers and affected people during a large-scale emergency event										
12	The strategic rationale used to develop the ICS response/action plan										
13	Your agency's preparedness for responding to a large-scale emergency event										
14	Differences between decision-making processes in the Incident Command System for a large-scale emergency event and non-emergency situations.										
15	Tasks which should NOT be delegated to volunteers in a large-scale emergency event										

Table A1. *Cont.*

S. No	Components	Not Familiar		Somewhat Unfamiliar		Familiar to Neutral		Somewhat Familiar		Very Familiar	
III	**Ethical Issues in Triage**	**N**	**%**	**N**	**%**	**N**	**%**	**N**	**%**	**N**	**%**
16	How to perform a rapid physical assessment of a victim of a large-scale emergency event										
17	How to perform a rapid mental health assessment of a victim of a large-scale emergency event										
18	How to assist with triage in a large-scale emergency event										
19	General issues related to the proper handling of the dead during a large-scale emergency event (ethical, legal, cultural and safety)										
IV	**Epidemiology and Surveillance**	**N**	**%**	**N**	**%**	**N**	**%**	**N**	**%**	**N**	**%**
20	History and assessment surveillance data for creating a high index of suspicion that a patient has been exposed to a biological agent										
21	When to report an unusual set of symptoms to an epidemiologist										
22	Diseases that are immediately reportable to state health departments										
23	Ability to identify the exacerbation of an underlying disease as a result of exposure to a chemical or biological agent or to radiation										
V	**Isolation/Quarantine**	**N**	**%**	**N**	**%**	**N**	**%**	**N**	**%**	**N**	**%**
24	Isolation procedures for people exposed to biological or chemical agents										
25	Your facility's/community's quarantine process										
VI	**Decontamination**	**N**	**%**	**N**	**%**	**N**	**%**	**N**	**%**	**N**	**%**
26	Selection of the appropriate personal protective equipment when caring for patients exposed to CBRN agents										
27	The decontamination procedures stated in your facility's emergency operations plan										
28	The impact on the environment from a large-scale emergency event										

Table A1. *Cont.*

S. No	Components	Not Familiar		Somewhat Unfamiliar		Familiar to Neutral		Somewhat Familiar		Very Familiar	
VII	**Communication/Connectivity**	**N**	%	**N**	%	**N**	%	**N**	%	**N**	%
29	The procedure used to document provision of care in a large-scale emergency event										
30	Chain of custody during a large-scale emergency event										
31	Procedure for communicating critical patient information to those transporting patients										
32	Effectively present information about degree of risk to various audiences										
33	Identify the different abilities of key partners in your emergency operations plan (EOP)										
34	Appropriate debriefing activities during a large-scale emergency event										
35	Use of all types of communication devices (phone, fax, email, personal digital assistant (PDAs), etc.)										
VIII	**Psychological Issues**	**N**	%	**N**	%	**N**	%	**N**	%	**N**	%
36	Appropriate psychological support for all parties involved in a large-scale emergency event										
37	Provide health counselling/education to patients regarding the long-term impact of CBRNE agents										
38	Signs of post-traumatic stress in patients seen for routine health care following an event										
39	How to evaluate a teenager to detect post-traumatic mental health problems										

Table A1. *Cont.*

S. No	Components	Not Familiar		Somewhat Unfamiliar		Familiar to Neutral		Somewhat Familiar		Very Familiar	
IX	**Special Populations**	**N**	%	**N**	%	**N**	%	**N**	%	**N**	%
40	Procedures for providing care to children/youth during a large-scale emergency event in cases in which prior consent from parent/legal guardian is possible										
41	The appropriate care of sensitive/vulnerable patient groups during a large-scale emergency (i.e., aged, pregnant women and the disabled)										
X	**Accessing Critical Resources**	**N**	%	**N**	%	**N**	%	**N**	%	**N**	%
42	During an event, where to quickly access up-to-date resources for specific CBRNE incidents										
43	Determine the appropriate agency to which reportable diseases are to be directed										
44	The process for gaining access to the Strategic National Stockpile										
45	Please provide an assessment of your overall familiarity with response activities/preparedness in the case of a large-scale emergency event										

References

1. Skliarov, S.; Kaptan, K.; Khorram-Manesh, A. Definition and General Principles of Disasters. In *Handbook of Disaster and Emergency Management*; Khorram-Manesh, A., Ed.; Kompendiet: Göteborg, Sweden, 2017; Chapter 1; pp. 17–22.
2. Khorram-Manesh, A.; Nyberg, L. Risk and Vulnerability Analysis. In *Handbook of Disaster and Emergency Management*; Khorram-Manesh, A., Ed.; Kompendiet: Göteborg, Sweden, 2017; Chapter 4, pp. 35–37.
3. Khorram-Manesh, A. Flexible surge capacity—Public health, public education, and disaster management. *Health Promot. Perspect.* **2020**, *10*, 175–179. [CrossRef] [PubMed]
4. Khorram-Manesh, A.; Berlin, J.; Carlström, E. Two Validated Ways of Improving the Ability of Decision-Making in Emergencies; Results from a Literature Review. *Bull. Emerg. Trauma* **2016**, *4*, 186–196. [PubMed]
5. Schultz, C.H.; Koenig, K.L.; Whiteside, M.; Murray, R. Development of National Standardized All-Hazard Disaster Core Competencies for Acute Care Physicians, Nurses, and EMS Professionals. *Ann. Emerg. Med.* **2012**, *59*, 196–208. [CrossRef] [PubMed]
6. Labrague, L.J.; Yboa, B.C.; McEnroe-Petitte, D.M.; Lobrino, L.R.; Brennan, M.G.B. Disaster Preparedness in Philippine Nurses. *J. Nurs. Sch.* **2016**, *48*, 98–105. [CrossRef] [PubMed]
7. Shabbir, R.; Afzal, M.; Sarwar, H.; Gilani, S.A.; Waqas, A. Nurses knowledge and practices regarding disasters management and emergency preparedness. *Saudi J. Med. Pharm. Sci.* **2017**, *3*, 464–476.
8. Khalil, N.S.; Atia, A.S.M.; Moustafa, M.F.; Soliman, H.T.T. Emergency nurses' knowledge and practice regarding preparedness of disaster management at a university hospital, Egypt. *Nurs. Healthc. Int. J.* **2019**, *3*, 1–12.
9. Xu, Y.; Zeng, X.; Yehua, X.; Xia, Z. Necessity for disaster-related nursing competency training of emergency nurses in China. *Int. J. Nurs. Sci.* **2016**, *3*, 198–201. [CrossRef]
10. Emil, M.; Sultan, M.; Sefry, S.; Ahmed, M.; AboAbdallah, M.; Chouinard, K.; Krawczyk, M. Reconstruction of the paleohydrological setting of the Rub Al Khali, Saudi Arabia. In Proceedings of the American Geophysical Union Fall Meeting Abstracts, San Francisco, CA, USA, 9–13 December 2013.
11. Hassan, H.M.; Al-Faleh, H. Exploring the risk factors associated with the size and severity of roadway crashes in Riyad. *J. Saf. Res.* **2013**, *47*, 67–74.
12. Alamri, Y.A. Emergency Management in Saudi Arabia: Past, Present and Future. In *Comparative Emergency Management: Understanding Disaster Policies, Organizations, and Initiatives from Around the World*; McEntire, D.A., Ed.; Federal Emergency Management Agency: Washington, DC, USA, 2010; p. 21.
13. Fadhlullah, S.Y.; Ismail, W. A Statistical Approach in Designing an RF-Based Human Crowd Density Estimation System. *Int. J. Distrib. Sens. Netw.* **2016**, *12*, 8351017. [CrossRef]
14. Rahman, J.; Thu, M.; Arshad, N.; Van Der Putten, M. Mass Gatherings and Public Health: Case Studies from the Hajj to Mecca. *Ann. Glob. Health* **2017**, *83*, 386–393. [CrossRef]
15. Global Facility for Disaster Reduction and Recovery GFDRR. 2020. Saudi Arabia. Available online: https://www.gfdrr.org/en/saudi-arabia (accessed on 11 April 2020).
16. AlShehri, B. Emergency nurses' preparedness for disaster in the Kingdom of Saudi Arabia. *J. Nurs. Educ. Pr.* **2017**, *7*, e013563. [CrossRef]
17. Hammad, K.; Arbon, P.; Gebbie, K.M. Emergency nurses and disaster response: An exploration of South Australian emergency nurses' knowledge and perceptions of their roles in disaster response. *Australas. Emerg. Nurs. J.* **2011**, *14*, 87–94. [CrossRef]
18. Wisniewski, R.; Dennik-Champion, G.; Peltier, J.W. Emergency Preparedness Competencies. *JONA J. Nurs. Adm.* **2004**, *34*, 475–480. [CrossRef] [PubMed]
19. Garbutt, S.J.; Peltier, J.W.; Fitzpatrick, J.J. Evaluation of an instrument to measure nurses' familiarity with emergency preparedness. *Mil. Med.* **2008**, *173*, 1073–1077. [CrossRef] [PubMed]
20. McKibbin, A.E.; Sekula, K.; Colbert, A.M.; Peltier, J.W. Assessing the Learning Needs of South Carolina Nurses by Exploring Their Perceived Knowledge of Emergency Preparedness: Evaluation of a Tool. *J. Contin. Educ. Nurs.* **2011**, *42*, 547–558. [CrossRef] [PubMed]
21. Brace, N.; Kemp, R.; Snelgar, R. *SPSS for Psychologists: A Guide to Data Analysis Using SPSS for Windows*, 3rd ed.; Lawrence Erlbaum Associates Publishers: New York, NY, USA, 2006.

22. Goniewicz, K.; Khorram-Manesh, A.; Hertelendy, A.J.; Goniewicz, M.; Naylor, K.; Burkle, F.M. Current Response and Management Decisions of the European Union to the COVID-19 Outbreak: A Review. *Sustainability* **2020**, *12*, 3838. [CrossRef]
23. McCarthy, G.; Cornally, N.; Mahoney, C.O.; White, G.; Weathers, E. Emergency nurses: Procedures performed and competence in practice. *Int. Emerg. Nurs.* **2013**, *21*, 50–57. [CrossRef]
24. Li, H.-Y.; Bi, R.-X.; Zhong, Q.-L. The development and psychometric testing of a Disaster Response Self-Efficacy Scale among undergraduate nursing students. *Nurse Educ. Today* **2017**, *59*, 16–20. [CrossRef]
25. Al Thobaity, A.; Williams, B.; Plummer, V. A new scale for disaster nursing core competencies: Development and psychometric testing. *Australas. Emerg. Nurs. J.* **2016**, *19*, 11–19. [CrossRef]
26. Lee, Y.; Lee, M.; Park, S. Development of the disaster nursing competency scale for nursing students. *J. Korean Soc. Disaster Inform.* **2013**, *9*, 511–520.
27. Valentine, M.A.; Nembhard, I.M.; Edmondson, A.C. Measuring teamwork in health care settings: A review of survey instruments. *Med. Care.* **2015**, *53*, e16–e30. [CrossRef] [PubMed]
28. Regan, S.; Laschinger, H.K.; Wong, C.A. The influence of empowerment, authentic leadership, and professional practice environments on nurses' perceived interprofessional collaboration. *J. Nurs Manag.* **2016**, *24*, E54–E61. [CrossRef] [PubMed]
29. Al Khalaileh, M.A.; Bond, E.; Alasad, J.A. Jordanian nurses' perceptions of their preparedness for disaster management. *Int. Emerg. Nurs.* **2012**, *20*, 14–23. [CrossRef]
30. Fung, O.W.M.; Loke, A.Y.; Lai, C.K.Y. Disaster preparedness among Hong Kong nurses. *J. Adv. Nurs.* **2008**, *62*, 698–703. [CrossRef]
31. Veenema, T.G.; Griffin, A.; Gable, A.R.; MacIntyre, L.; Simons, R.N.; Couig, M.P.; Walsh, J.J.; Lavin, M.C.C.; Dobalian, A.; Larson, E. Nurses as Leaders in Disaster Preparedness and Response-A Call to Action. *J. Nurs. Sch.* **2016**, *48*, 187–200. [CrossRef] [PubMed]
32. Alim, S.; Kawabata, M.; Nakazawa, M. Evaluation of disaster preparedness training and disaster drill for nursing students. *Nurse Educ. Today* **2015**, *35*, 25–31. [CrossRef]
33. Ireland, M.; Ea, E.; Kontzamanis, E.; Michel, C. Integrating Disaster Preparedness into a Community Health Nursing Course: One School's Experience. *Disaster Manag. Response* **2006**, *4*, 72–76. [CrossRef] [PubMed]
34. Ibrahim, F.A.A. Nurses Knowledge, Attitudes, Practices and Familiarity Regarding Disaster and Emergency Preparedness—Saudi Arabia. *Am. J. Nurs. Sci.* **2014**, *3*, 18–25. [CrossRef]
35. Chapman, K.; Arbon, P. Are nurses ready? Disaster preparedness in the acute setting. *Australas. Emerg. Nurs. J.* **2008**, *11*, 135–144. [CrossRef]
36. Weiner, E.; Irwin, M.; Trangenstein, P.; Gordon, J. Emergency preparedness curriculum in nursing schools in the United States. *Nurs. Educ. Perspect.* **2006**, *26*, 334–339.
37. Volkman, J.C.; Rebmann, T.; Hilley, S.; Alexander, S.; Russell, B.; Wagner, W. Infection prevention disaster preparedness planning for long-term care facilities. *Am. J. Infect. Control* **2012**, *40*, 206–210. [CrossRef] [PubMed]
38. Gladston, S.; Nayak, R. Disaster preparedness among nurses working in a paediatric acute care setting of a tertiary hospital, south India. *IOSR J. Nurs. Health Sci.* **2017**, *18*, 25–35.
39. Al-Hunaishi, W.; Hoe, V.C.; Chinna, K. Factors associated with healthcare workers willingness to participate in disasters: A cross-sectional study in Sana'a, Yemen. *BMJ Open* **2019**, *9*, e030547. [CrossRef]
40. Bella Magnaye, R.N.; Muñoz, M.S.; Muñoz, M.A.; Muñoz, R.G.; Muro, J.H. The role, preparedness and management of nurses during disasters. *Int. Sci. Res. J.* **2011**, *3*, 269–294.
41. Tzeng, W.-C.; Feng, H.-P.; Cheng, W.-T.; Lin, C.-H.; Chiang, L.-C.; Pai, L.; Lee, C.-L. Readiness of hospital nurses for disaster responses in Taiwan: A cross-sectional study. *Nurse Educ. Today* **2016**, *47*, 37–42. [CrossRef]

12

A Coronavirus (COVID-19) Triage Framework for (Sub)National Public–Private Partnership (PPP) Programs

David Baxter [1] **and Carter B. Casady** [2,*]

[1] Infrastructure Development/PPP Consultant and Steering Committee Member for the World Association of PPP Units & Professionals (WAPPP), Washington, DC 22312, USA; dbaxter@wappp.org
[2] Bartlett School of Construction and Project Management, University College London, London WC1E 7HB, UK
* Correspondence: c.casady@ucl.ac.uk

Abstract: Around the world, countries are struggling to address the immediate and long-term impacts of the novel coronavirus (COVID-19) pandemic on their (sub)national public–private partnership (PPP) programs. Burdened with the real possibility of widespread project failures and constrained budgets, governments are searching for ways to prioritize projects in need of relief and bolster post-pandemic recovery plans. To meet this need, this article conceptualizes a triage system for PPP programs based on five categories: (1) projects without a need for economic stimulus (blue); (2) projects experiencing minor economic/financial losses (green); (3) projects needing temporary/stop-gap support or restructuring (yellow); (4) projects unable to survive without significant economic relief (red); and (5) projects that cannot survive, even with government intervention (black). This research also stresses the importance of launching and sustaining a crisis command center to support PPP triage decisions and encourages PPP stakeholders to collectively craft win–win solutions for post-pandemic recovery efforts.

Keywords: coronavirus (COVID-19); public–private partnerships (PPPs) triage; crisis management; resilience

1. An Unprecedented Battle

The novel coronavirus (COVID-19) pandemic caught most public agencies at all levels of government off-guard, leaving them ill-equipped to address the immediate and long-term impacts on their (sub)national public–private partnership (PPP) programs. In the United States alone, procurements for several infrastructure PPP projects have already been delayed, put on hold, or cancelled altogether [1]. With uncertainty increasing around demand–risk transit and toll road projects, more project failures are anticipated. States are also projected to face a 30 percent drop in transportation-related revenues (e.g., gas tax) over the next 12–18 months. Combined with sharp declines in sales tax revenue, the fiscal position of state and local governments will continue to deteriorate through at least fiscal year (FY) 2021 [2] and "catch-up" funding mechanisms may be needed for state and local infrastructure development and recovery efforts [3].

Without flexible surge capacity "to scale up and down resources in a fast, smooth, and productive way" [4] (p. 1), many governments, banking organizations, and development institutions still do not fully understand the current strengths and weaknesses of their existing PPP programs. They are, therefore, looking for ways to assess the massive, sudden, and unprecedented impacts of the COVID-19 pandemic on PPP projects and (sub)national programs. More specifically, "a new model to exercise or simulate all phases of multiagency disaster management" is needed, "based on real scenarios, to find out strengths and weaknesses of [their PPP] organizations and to improve ... access to all resources" [4] (p. 4). This article thus offers a conceptual triage framework for PPP programs. Borrowing from medical and business triage procedures, we outline several triage heuristics for PPP practitioners. We begin by briefly describing the concept of medical triage. Next, we discuss how medical triage models have been adapted by the private sector into decision-making frameworks. Then, we use both medical and business triage approaches as a template for conceptualizing a PPP triage framework. After reflecting on additional considerations for PPP triage actions, we ultimately conclude by encouraging PPP stakeholders to collectively craft win–win solutions for post-pandemic recovery efforts.

2. Medical Triage

Medical triage involves identifying and sorting people most urgently in need of care. Adopted from battlefield medicine, triage procedures assess a patient's health status to determine their relative priority for treatment. In practice, triage is reserved for situations (e.g., wars, natural disasters, pandemics, etc.) when both supplies and staff are limited and care must be rationed [5]. In medical settings, injured or ill patients are typically categorized into various treatment groups based on need and urgency. These groupings generally use the following color scheme to identify priority levels:

1. Blue: patients not in need of urgent medical attention or hospitalization;
2. Green: patients with minor injuries or illnesses (i.e., "walking wounded");
3. Yellow: more serious cases whose lives are not yet threatened;
4. Red: those who will die without immediate treatment, and
5. Black: a fifth category reserved for the deceased, or those with no chance of survival [5,6].

With so many patients becoming critical ill simultaneously, many countries have found it impossible to meet the unprecedented healthcare demands of the COVID-19 pandemic [7]. This has forced doctors to make excruciating triage decisions on who to treat [8]. Although some scholars, such as Ouyang, Argon, and Ziya [9], have recently developed mathematical modeling and analysis techniques to improve intensive care unit (ICU) allocation decisions during periods of high patient demand, many of these triage decisions are often based on heuristics (e.g., age, comorbidities, etc.), which value "saving people with the greatest chance of short-term survival, followed by saving those who, thanks to a relative lack of coexisting conditions, have the greatest chance of long-term survival" [7] (p. 1875); see also [10]. When faced with such ethical dilemmas, many scenarios "will still feel morally untenable, particularly in the face of heightened prognostic uncertainty" and resource scarcity [7] (p. 1875). Nevertheless, rationing is often required in the direst circumstances. The COVID-19 pandemic is no exception. King and Kissoon [11] (p. 1794) stress that, "while research during pandemics is fraught with many obstacles, we must be courageous" and test triage models when the opportunity presents.

3. Business Triage

Over time, medical triage approaches have been adapted by the private sector into decision-making frameworks. These frameworks help businesses prioritize organizational goals and resource allocation. In global disasters like the COVID-19 pandemic, business enterprises must face "difficult decisions with regard to allocating limited resources between multiple 'mission-critical' functions" [12] (p. 21). In such times of crisis, business triage methodologies offer a simplified means of decision making based on objective, evidence-based criteria. Using similar categories employed by military and disaster–medical services—i.e., red (essential/critical), yellow (important/urgent), and green (optional/supportive)—these models identify tiers of service/operational criticality for the long-term health of a company. Crises force businesses to prioritize their essential/critical (red) expenses and relieve obvious "pain points" plaguing the organization. Once these "urgent care" needs are stabilized, other important (yellow) functions can be addressed, followed by auxiliary/supportive capabilities [13]. To determine relative organizational priorities, triage determinations will typically involve:

1. centralized decision making for consistency, speed, and decisiveness;
2. cataloging sources of funds (e.g., cash, lines of credit, equity infusions, etc.);
3. rapidly identifying economic scenarios;
4. modeling projected impacts;
5. defining non-negotiables (i.e., essential/critical functions);
6. drawing on available levers of leadership (expense reductions; hiring freezes, etc.);
7. determining immediate actions to take [14].

Accepted and understood throughout the organization, these triage procedures ultimately promote business continuity during rapidly evolving and unpredictable events. By identifying the sickest "patients" (i.e., processes) first and quickly stabilizing them, businesses can then prioritize other urgent operations that will need more planning and resources to fix [15].

4. Public–Private Partnership (PPP) Triage: A Conceptual Framework

Taken together, both medical and business triage processes offer a useful template for conceptualizing a PPP triage framework in the COVID-19 epoch. Because the likelihood of widespread PPP project failures is all but inevitable, governments will soon face the difficult and unenviable task of triaging PPP projects in their (sub)national programs so they can maximize project survival and kickstart national recovery efforts. Such a "mass-casualty event" will require rapid assessment of the "current health" of PPP projects to determine if they are in a terminal downward trajectory or show signs of resuscitation and recovery.

In this assessment process, government institutions (i.e., PPP units, ministries of finance, treasury units, and other line ministries) may find themselves in almost the same situation as hospital ICUs, facing critical shortages of funding, financing, and material resources to keep their projects functioning. Governments facing such constraints should thus develop "several triage heuristics policies that can potentially be used in practice" [9] (p. 592). For instance, a sophisticated and objective PPP triage system might begin by separating current PPP projects (and candidate projects) into the following categories (see Table 1).

Table 1. Public–Private Partnership (PPP) Triage Framework.

Triage Code	Criteria	Action or Priority
Blue	Project without a need for economic stimulus	Periodically (re)assess project key performance indicators (KPIs)
Green	Project experiencing minor financial/economic losses	Closely monitor project KPIs for early signs of project distress/default
Yellow	Project needs temporary/stop-gap support or restructuring	Explore contractual renegotiation procedures and other conciliation mechanisms
Red	Project will not survive without significant economic relief	Evaluate existing government guarantees and other opportunities for economic resuscitation
Black	Project cannot survive, even with government intervention	Prepare for contract termination and/or buyout procedures

To illustrate, take, for example, the LBJ-managed lanes in Texas. This PPP recorded a 20 percent traffic drop in March due to the COVID-19 pandemic. However, Ferrovial (the private concessionaire) still recorded growth in both revenues and EBITDA across its toll road division. This stronger-than-expected performance led Moody's to revise its outlook on the LBJ PPP from positive to stable and reaffirm its Baa3 rating despite uncertainty about the project's traffic and revenue recovery [16]. Because the liquidity of the PPP is also expected to remain strong, this project would likely be coded in the triage framework as "blue" and only need to be periodically (re)assessed.

A similar performance assessment could also be applied to airport PPPs affected by the COVID-19 pandemic. For instance, passenger numbers at Heathrow Airport have declined by 18.3 percent, and both revenues and EBITDA have fallen 12.7 percent and 22.4 percent, respectively. However, since Heathrow "has the necessary resources to continue operating for at least the next 12 months even in the absence of passengers[,] this PPP would be initially coded as "green" (i.e., experiencing minor financial/economic losses) but potentially reclassified as "yellow" if signs of project distress and/or potential default persist [16].

Finally, the COVID-19 pandemic is exacerbating problems plaguing transit projects like the $2 billion Purple Line light-rail PPP in Maryland. Already 976 days—more than $2\frac{1}{2}$ years—behind schedule and $755 million (i.e., 37 percent) over budget, Purple Line Transit Constructors (i.e., the joint-venture between Fluor, Lane Construction Corp. and Traylor Bros) is now threatening to walk away from the 36-year PPP. Efforts are currently underway to save this code "red" project, but a failed settlement could add up to a year to the project's schedule, cost millions more, and end in a protracted legal battle. If the parties are going to find a resolution, all will likely need to share in the sacrifice. However, this prospect comes at a particularly bad time for government budgets suffering from tax revenue losses due to the pandemic [17]. Without any relief or new significant funding from Maryland's Department of Transportation, this PPP may ultimately have to be re-triaged as "black" and prepared for contract termination.

Overall, governments (in conjunction with private sector counterparties, consultants, etc.) could begin using this conceptual PPP triage framework to label each "patient" (i.e., project) by sector or specific service offered, develop preliminary damage assessment records (see, e.g., FEMA [18]), identify project triage priorities for economic mitigation, track triage statuses, and identify additional risks associated with context-specific political, economic, and social factors. Categorizing desired outcomes/goals using such a PPP triage model would ultimately ensure limited resource allocation support and maintain national recovery goals.

5. Additional Considerations for PPP Triage Actions

Naturally, the utility of any PPP triage framework for decision making, goal prioritization, and resource allocation will depend on a country's institutional capacity and surrounding PPP-enabling environment [19,20]. Governments should thus consider launching and sustaining a crisis command center to effectively triage PPP projects [14]. Within this center, one of the first and most important tasks is to separate PPP specialists providing "care" for projects from those making triage decisions. A "triage officer", backed by a team with expertise in PPP preparation, procurement, and management, would make resource allocation decisions and communicate them within their PPP unit, ministry of finance, treasury unit, or other line ministry overseeing a country's (sub)national PPP program. Using revised and recalibrated Value for Money (VfM) assessments, Public Sector Comparators (PSCs), and other PPP screening tools, this triage team would provide economic and commercial rationales for triage decisions rather than quick fixes based on political headwinds. These decisions would then be reviewed regularly by a centralized (sub)national-level monitoring committee to ensure other factors, such as "People First PPP" considerations, project sustainability, and resilience, are given weight in decisions to rescue current PPP projects and reprioritize procurements for future PPPs [21]. Such oversight and governance will ensure countries do not mortgage their futures for ill-conceived, short-term recovery actions.

Finally, the triage framework should be reviewed regularly, as knowledge about the impacts of the pandemic evolves [7]. In this phase, governments may revisit commitments to Sustainable Development Goals (SDGs), see how the pandemic has affected them, and recalibrate national development strategies accordingly. Governments may also wish to (re)consider unsolicited proposals for stalled PPP program initiatives, (re)evaluate the resilience of PPPs to force majeure events, and develop short-, medium- and long-term solutions that strike a balance between investing in the future and reducing costs to survive [22,23]. Overall, post-pandemic recovery efforts should produce new PPP policy guidance and sector-specific models "that may respond, in a logical, consistent, and consultative way, to inevitable changes in policy and the market" [24] (p. 19).

6. Conclusions

Although the "point at which preparedness dissolves into panic will always be context-dependent ... the best outcome of this pandemic would be being accused of having overprepared" [7] (p. 1875). Governments will thus need to begin carrying out extensive and systematic triage assessments of their (sub)national PPPs in order to mitigate the impacts of the COVID-19 pandemic. This article offers an initial conceptualization of PPP triage processes, but hard and decisive decisions still need to be made on both current and planned PPP projects. If PPPs are going to be a central tool for national economic recovery efforts, "trust, shared vision and long-term commitments" are needed so "contracting parties [can] change their adversarial relationships to a more cooperative, team-based approach" [25] (p. 441); see also [26]. Through cooperation, openness, and innovation, PPP stakeholders can collectively craft win–win incentives that maximize opportunities in the face of shared risks [27].

Overall, "[d]ue to the complexity, intensity, and frequency of complex disasters, global leaders in healthcare, government, and business will need to pivot from siloed approaches of decision-making to embrace multidisciplinary and transdisciplinary levels of cooperation" [28] (p. 3838). Doing so will fundamentally change the way transportation, transit, school, and hospital PPPs are designed and operated. Although "a lot of projects have been able to continue, and some, such as hospitals and schools, have even been accelerated[,]" governments still need to provide relief to struggling projects to get them through this tough time [29]. After all, "[p]erfect is the enemy of good, especially during crises when prompt action is required" [14]. Moving forward, much more work still needs to be done to combat COVID-19 and prepare for the next pandemic. Let us not repeat the same mistakes. Instead, let us challenge the complacency of construction management research, "engage in more robust critique and analysis of construction systems, as they are realised in practice[,]" and develop sustainable, resilient, and future-proofed PPPs [30] (p. 1).

Author Contributions: The authors confirm contribution to the paper as follows: conceptualization (D.B. and C.B.C.); writing—original draft preparation (D.B.); writing—review and editing (C.B.C). All authors have read and agreed to the published version of the manuscript.

References

1. Inframation. *US P3 Market Summary|May 2020*; Inframation—An Acuris Company: New York, NY, USA, 2020.
2. American Association of State Highway and Transportation Officials (AASHTO). State DOTs Feeling the Budgetary Impact of COVID-19. 2020. Available online: https://aashtojournal.org/2020/04/24/state-dots-feeling-the-budgetary-impact-of-covid-19/ (accessed on 25 May 2020).
3. Casady, C.B.; Geddes, R.R. Asset Recycling for Social Infrastructure in the United States. *Public Works Manag. Policy* **2020**, *25*, 281–297. [CrossRef]
4. Khorram-Manesh, A. Flexible surge capacity–public health, public education, and disaster management. *Health Promot. Perspect.* **2020**, *10*, 1–5.
5. Harbaugh, K. The Next, Terrible Phase of This Crisis|After Cancellation Comes Triage. 2020. Available online: https://www.theatlantic.com/ideas/archive/2020/03/after-cancellation-comes-triage/608146/ (accessed on 25 May 2020).
6. Barfod, C.; Danker, J.; Forberg, J.; Lauritzen, M.M. The distribution of triage categories and the impact of emergency symptoms and signs on the triage level. *Scand. J. Trauma Resusc. Emerg. Med.* **2010**, *18*, 34. [CrossRef]
7. Rosenbaum, L. Facing Covid-19 in Italy—Ethics, logistics, and therapeutics on the epidemic's front line. *N. Engl. J. Med.* **2020**, *382*, 1873–1875. [CrossRef]
8. Romeo, N. The Grim Ethical Dilemma of Rationing Medical Care, Explained|How Hospitals Decide Which Covid-19 Patients to Prioritize When Resources Are Scarce. 2020. Available online: https://www.vox.com/coronavirus-covid19/2020/3/31/21199721/coronavirus-covid-19-hospitals-triage-rationing-italy-new-york (accessed on 25 May 2020).

9. Ouyang, H.; Argon, N.T.; Ziya, S. Allocation of intensive care unit beds in periods of high demand. *Oper. Res.* **2020**, *68*, 591–608. [CrossRef]
10. Farrohknia, N.; Castrén, M.; Ehrenberg, A.; Lind, L.; Oredsson, S.; Jonsson, H.; Asplund, K.; Göransson, K.E. Emergency department triage scales and their components: A systematic review of the scientific evidence. *Scand. J. Trauma Resusc. Emerg. Med.* **2011**, *19*, 42. [CrossRef] [PubMed]
11. King, M.A.; Kissoon, N. Triage during pandemics: Difficult choices when business as usual is not an ethically defensible option. *Crit. Care Med.* **2016**, *44*, 1793–1795. [CrossRef] [PubMed]
12. Moore, B.; Bone, E.A. Decision-making in crisis: Applying a healthcare triage methodology to business continuity management. *J. Bus. Contin. Emerg. Plan.* **2017**, *11*, 21–26.
13. Small Business Network (SBN). A Triage Approach to Operational Efficiency. 2017. Available online: https://www.sbnonline.com/article/triage-approach-operational-efficiency/ (accessed on 23 May 2020).
14. Renjen, P. The Heart of Resilient Leadership: Responding to COVID-19. 2020. Available online: https://www2.deloitte.com/us/en/insights/economy/covid-19/heart-of-resilient-leadership-responding-to-covid-19.html (accessed on 28 May 2020).
15. Cerocke, S. How to Conduct a Business Process Triage. 2015. Available online: https://ncet.org/how-to-conduct-a-business-process-triage/ (accessed on 26 May 2020).
16. Fabrizio, A. *Ferrovial 1Q20 Toll Road Revenue Up Despite COVID-19*; Inframation—An Acuris Company: New York, NY, USA, 2020.
17. Shaver, K. Maryland Likely to Be on the Hook for Millions If It Wants to Save the Purple Line Project, Analysts Say. 2020. Available online: https://www-washingtonpost-com.cdn.ampproject.org/c/s/www.washingtonpost.com/local/trafficandcommuting/maryland-likely-to-be-on-the-hook-for-millions-if-it-wants-to-save-the-purple-line-project-analysts-say/2020/06/12/29b40dda-ab39-11ea-a9d9-a81c1a491c52_story.html?outputType=amp (accessed on 14 June 2020).
18. Federal Emergency Management Agency (FEMA). *PDA Pocket Guide*; FEMA: Washington, DC, USA, 2020.
19. Casady, C.B.; Eriksson, K.; Levitt, R.E.; Scott, W.R. (Re) defining public-private partnerships (PPPs) in the new public governance (NPG) paradigm: An institutional maturity perspective. *Public Manag. Rev.* **2020**, *22*, 161–183. [CrossRef]
20. Casady, C.B. Examining the institutional drivers of Public-Private Partnership (PPP) market performance: A fuzzy set Qualitative Comparative Analysis (fsQCA). *Public Manag. Rev.* **2020**, 1–25. [CrossRef]
21. United Nations Economic Commission for Europe (UNECE). *"What are People-First PPPs?"*; UNECE International Center of Excellence: Geneva, Switzerland, 2019.
22. Baxter, D.; Casady, C.B. Proactive and Strategic Healthcare Public-Private Partnerships (PPPs) in the Coronavirus (Covid-19) Epoch. *Sustainability* **2020**, *12*, 5097. [CrossRef]
23. Gulati, R.; Nohria, N.; Wohlgezogen, F. Roaring out of Recession. 2010. Available online: https://hbr.org/2010/03/roaring-out-of-recession (accessed on 28 May 2020).
24. Farquharson, E.; Torres de Mastle, C.; Yescombe, E.R.; Encinas, J. *How to Engage with the Private Sector in Public-Private Partnerships in Emerging Markets*; World Bank: Washington, DC, USA, 2011.
25. Weston, D.C.; Gibson, G.E., Jr. Partnering-project performance in US Army Corps of Engineers. *J. Manag. Eng.* **1993**, *9*, 410–425. [CrossRef]
26. Henisz, W.J.; Levitt, R.E.; Scott, W.R. Toward a unified theory of project governance: Economic, sociological and psychological supports for relational contracting. *Eng. Project Organ. J.* **2012**, *2*, 37–55. [CrossRef]
27. Crowley, L.G.; Karim, M.A. Conceptual model of partnering. *J. Manag. Eng.* **1995**, *11*, 33–39. [CrossRef]
28. Goniewicz, K.; Khorram-Manesh, A.; Hertelendy, A.J.; Goniewicz, M.; Naylor, K.; Burkle, F.M. Current Response and Management Decisions of the European Union to the COVID-19 Outbreak: A Review. *Sustainability* **2020**, *12*, 3838. [CrossRef]
29. Gismondi, A. P3 Projects Moving Ahead Despite Pandemic, Some Accelerated. 2020. Available online: https://canada.constructconnect.com/dcn/news/projects/2020/05/p3-projects-moving-ahead-despite-pandemic-some-accelerated (accessed on 1 June 2020).
30. Sherratt, F.; Sherratt, S.; Ivory, C. Challenging complacency in construction management research: The case of PPPs. *Constr. Manag. Econ.* **2020**, 1–15. [CrossRef]

13

Transmission of Influenza A in a Student Office Based on Realistic Person-to-Person Contact and Surface Touch Behaviour

Nan Zhang and Yuguo Li *

Department of Mechanical Engineering, The University of Hong Kong, Pokfulam Road, Hong Kong, China; zhangnan@hku.hk

* Correspondence: liyg@hku.hk

Abstract: Influenza A viruses result in the deaths of hundreds of thousands of individuals worldwide each year. In this study, influenza A transmission in a graduate student office is simulated via long-range airborne, fomite, and close contact routes based on real data from more than 3500 person-to-person contacts and 127,000 surface touches obtained by video-camera. The long-range airborne, fomite and close contact routes contribute to 54.3%, 4.2% and 44.5% of influenza A infections, respectively. For the fomite route, 59.8%, 38.1% and 2.1% of viruses are transmitted to the hands of students from private surfaces around the infected students, the students themselves and other susceptible students, respectively. The intranasal dose via fomites of the students' bodies, belongings, computers, desks, chairs and public facilities are 8.0%, 6.8%, 13.2%, 57.8%, 9.3% and 4.9%, respectively. The intranasal dose does not monotonously increase or decrease with the virus transfer rate between hands and surfaces. Mask wearing is much more useful than hand washing for control of influenza A in the tested office setting. Regular cleaning of high-touch surfaces, which can reduce the infection risk by 2.14%, is recommended and is much more efficient than hand-washing.

Keywords: influenza A; airborne; fomite; close contact; infection; surface touch; office; mask; hand-washing

---

1. Introduction

Influenza is a highly contagious respiratory illness that causes 1,250,000 deaths annually worldwide [1]. It is estimated that influenza A viruses result in the deaths of approximately half a million individuals worldwide every year [2]. Influenza A viruses exist on many surfaces in our daily lives, such as towels in homes and medical cart items in hospitals [3].

Despite human beings' vast clinical experience, debate about the transmission of influenza continues [4]. The influenza virus is known to be spread from person to person by at least two mechanisms: direct and indirect transfer of respiratory secretions and contact with large droplets that settle onto fomites [5]. Studies have shown that influenza A may be transmitted by inhalation of small airborne particles [6]. Although some evidence was found of animal-to-animal transmission [7], other evidence of person-to-person transmission was based on observational and epidemiological studies [8]. Influenza can also be transmitted by droplet nuclei [9,10]. In addition, other studies have found that the fomite route could be a potential route of influenza transmission [11]. In general, influenza A can be spread via the airborne, droplet and direct and indirect contact routes.

Many simulations of influenza transmission have been conducted in enclosed spaces such as hospitals [12] and air cabins [13], and in large spaces such as cities [14], and even between cities [15]. Large-scale influenza transmission is usually based on macroscopic factors such as human mobility via airplane and other modes of public transport [15]. Microscopic factors such as how people talk or make contact with each other are ignored because of complexity. Most human behaviour, including person-to-person contact and surface touches, are hypothesised even when all transmission routes are considered. However, human behaviour changes with the environment, and large errors may result if all human behaviour is unknown or randomly set. A simulation of influenza A transmission based on realistic data of human behaviour in a confined space is needed to help understand influenza A transmission and to implement effective measures to prevent and control disease.

In this study, we simulated influenza A transmission in a graduate student office by considering three routes: long-range airborne, fomite and close contact (short-range airborne and droplet spray). All student behaviour, including close contact and surface touches in the office, was recorded by video-camera from 9 a.m. to 9 p.m., from 11 to 15 September 2017. The data included more than 3500 close contacts between students and more than 127,000 surface touches. Influenza A transmission was simulated in the office via three routes based on realistic behaviour obtained from these recorded data. We discovered how influenza A virus is transmitted via air, hands, surfaces, mucous membranes and inhalation. We also analysed the efficacy of various strategies for prevention of influenza A via various transmission routes.

2. Materials and Methods

We simulated influenza A transmission via three routes (long-range airborne, fomite and close contact) in a graduate student office in China. The office measured 12 × 8.4 × 2.7 m and included 39 students. All surfaces were grouped into six categories (primary surfaces): private (i.e., the student [*Std*]; body parts), students' belongings (*Bln*), desks (*Dsk*), chairs (*Chr*), computers (*Cpt*) and public facilities (*Pbf*). These primary surfaces were in turn divided into 31 secondary surfaces consisting of 57 types of sub-surfaces with multiple surfaces for each type, giving a total of 1490 basic surfaces (Supplementary Materials: Table S1).

The data for each student's surface touch behaviour were taken from four video-cameras installed on the office ceiling to monitor student behaviour of close contact and surface touch from 9 a.m. to 9 p.m. on five successive weekdays from 11 to 15 September 2017. All students in the office gave informed consent for inclusion before they participated in the study. Five video image analysis assistants were appointed to process the data second by second, recording all visible touch actions made by every student in the office. A surface touch was defined as any contact between a hand or finger and a solid surface or object lasting for 1 s or longer. The information recorded comprised the onset time, duration, and location of each touch, and details of which student had done the touching, which hand had been used, and which surface had been touched. For quality control during the video image analysis, one author (NZ) verified touch actions at two time points, namely the 15th minute and the 45th minute of each of the 60 h. Verification revealed that 67 out of the 1712 touch actions (3.1%) had been incorrectly recorded by the original video analysers.

In the 5-day study period, 127,052 touches by left and right hands on 1490 coded surfaces were recorded. The surfaces had a total exposure to touch of 1,517,958 person·seconds. The students spent 90.74% of their time in the office touching surfaces [16].

In this paper, we used influenza A as an example. Figure 1 illustrates how influenza A is transmitted via the long-range airborne, fomite and close contact routes. When an infected student breathes, talks, coughs or sneezes, the virus is carried in particles and released into the environment. Small droplets disperse in the air. Some floating particles flow outdoors through the ventilation system, some are inhaled by students, some are deposited on surfaces and those still in the air lose viability over time. Large droplets are rapidly deposited on surfaces near the infected student or are directly sprayed onto the hands of the infected person while covering their mouth and nose while coughing or sneezing. The virus will then be transferred to a surface if it is touched by a contaminated hand. A clean hand can also be contaminated if it touches a contaminated surface. Some large droplets with virus on hands can be transferred to the mucous membranes if the student touches his or her own lips, nose or eyes. Some large droplets are resuspended from surfaces to the air because of human activities such as walking. In addition, viruses on hands and surfaces also lose viability over time. Moreover, when an infected student speaks face-to-face with other students, particles are sprayed from the mouth of the infected student. Some small particles will be directly inhaled via the respiratory tract by students who speak with the infected student, and some large particles might be rapidly deposited on their mucous membranes. The inhalation dose and intranasal dose of susceptible students gradually increase, and each student's infection risk can be calculated based on the dose-response parameters of influenza A.

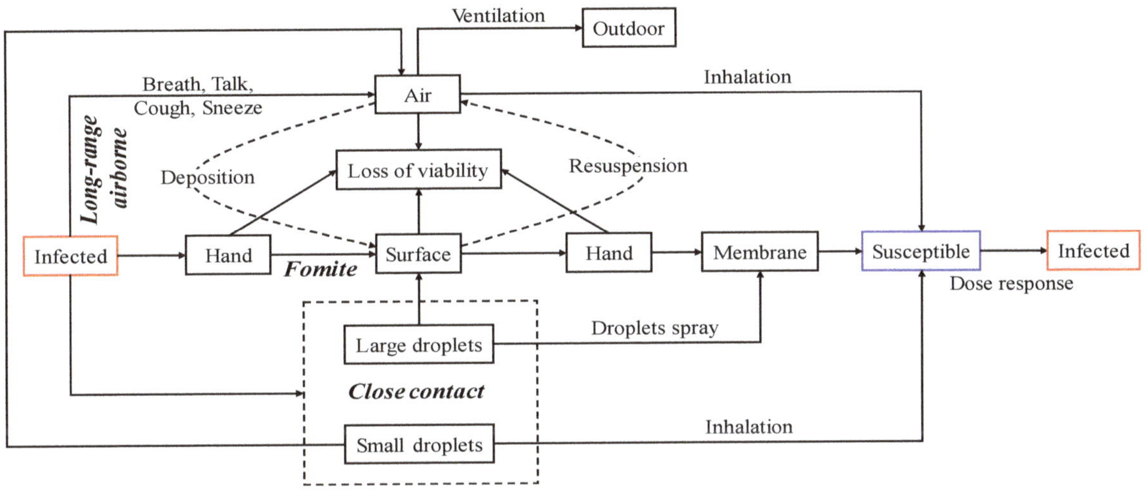

Figure 1. Three routes for influenza A transmission.

All students go to lunch and dinner between 12 a.m. and 1 p.m. and between 5 p.m. and 6 p.m., respectively, every day. In real conditions, all students do not stay in the office all the time. To reduce the randomness caused by their stay duration, all students are assumed to remain in the office from 9 a.m. to 9 p.m. except for lunch and dinner time.

2.1. Parameter Setting

The US Centers for Disease Control and Prevention (CDC) have defined three influenza transmission routes: long-range airborne, fomite (direct and indirect) and close contact (Table 1). Only particles with a diameter of less than 10 μm can penetrate the lungs [17]. Pathogens carried in particles with an aerodynamic diameter (d_a) between 10 and 100 μm are inspired if a person is facing the patient at close range during an expiratory event such as a cough or a talk [18]. More than 99% of the pathogens emitted in a cough are carried by particles with an aerodynamic diameter $d_a > 100$ μm [19], and these particles tend to settle rapidly on surfaces near the point of emission [18].

Table 1. Modes of person-to-person transmission of respiratory viruses [20].

Transmission Route	Definition
Aerosol transmission	Virus is transmitted through the air by aerosols within the inspirable size range or smaller; aerosol particles are small enough to be inhaled into the nasopharynx and distally into the trachea and lung.
Direct transmission	Virus is transferred by contact from an infected person to another person without a contaminated intermediate object (fomite).
Indirect transmission	Virus is transferred by contact with a contaminated intermediate object (fomite).
Droplet spray transmission	Virus is transmitted through the air by droplet sprays (such as those produced by coughing or sneezing); a key feature is deposition of droplets by impaction on exposed mucous membranes.

At the beginning of the simulation, there are 39 students in the office, i.e., one infected student (P_0) and 38 susceptible students (P_1–P_{38}). They touch surfaces and talk with each other based on realistic data on surface touch and interpersonal contacts obtained from the video analysis. In each simulation, all students will select an action, such as with surfaces they touch and with whom they talk, from the database (collected surface touch and close contact data) at each time step (second).

2.2. Long-Range Airborne

Particles of various sizes ae generated by activities such as breathing, talking, coughing and sneezing. We assumed that particles (d_a < 10 μm) uniformly floated in the air of the office. The deposition of these small particles is slight because it requires around an hour in a steady environment [21,22]. In an office setting, the deposition rate will be reduced because of frequent walking by the students. We assumed that the deposition rate was 0.1 min^{-1}, which means that 10% of the particles' volume is deposited uniformly on all surfaces per minute.

Because the difference in the association between the size and number of particles from previous researchers is large, we use the average values from previous studies to assess the total virus quantity in small particles. Summarising the previous studies [23–29], the total volume of small particles (d_a < 10 μm) by breathing (V'_{vb}), talking (V'_{vt}) (counting from 1 to 100, which takes about 100 s), coughing (V'_{vc}) and sneezing (V'_{vs}) are estimated as 1.02 × 10^{-10} mL, 1.47 × 10^{-7} mL, 1.65 × 10^{-7} mL and 1.27 × 10^{-6} mL, respectively. The total volume of large particles (d_a > 10 μm) generated by breathing (V''_{vb}), talking (V''_{vt}), coughing (V''_{vc}) and sneezing (V''_{vs}) are estimated as 0 mL, 5.15 × 10^{-3} mL, 6.15 × 10^{-3} mL and 4.75 × 10^{-2} mL, respectively. Here, we assumed that the size distribution of particles generated by coughing and sneezing was the same. People take an average of 15 breaths per minute, so a breath takes around 4 s [30]. The average frequencies of coughing and sneezing episodes for an influenza A infected person are 22/h [31] and 5/h [32] respectively. A cough takes 1 s, and a sneeze is assumed to take 3 s. Our recorded data show that students in the office spent an average of 10% of their time talking with others. Therefore, the frequency of breathing (f_b), talking (f_t), coughing (f_c) and sneezing (f_s) of an infected person are 21,600 times, 0.8 h (two students on average share the time during talking), 352 times and 80 times per day (talking, coughing and sneezing during 16 h except 8-h sleep). The total volume of droplets generated by an infected person per day (V_V) is calculated by Equation (1).

$$V_v = V\prime_v + V\prime\prime_v = \sum_{i=1}^{4}(V\prime_{vi} + V\prime\prime_{vi})\cdot f_i \approx 6.11\ \text{mL/day} \tag{1}$$

where i = 1 to 4 shows the human activities of breathing, talking, coughing and sneezing, respectively; $V\prime_v$ and $V\prime\prime_v$ are the total volume of small and large droplets generated by an infected person per day, respectively.

We assumed that an infected person's initial viral shedding rate is around 1.5 × 10^7 TCID50/day [19,24,25,31,33], and it changes with time and the severity of infection. Because the amount of virus in a particle is roughly proportional to the particle's volume [34], we considered the virus concentrations in all particles to be the same. The virus concentration (C_v) in all particles is then obtained (C_v = 1 × $10^{6.39}$ TCID50/mL). This value is between the virus concentration in nasopharyngeal fluid (10^2–10^7 TCID50/mL) measured by Douglas [35] and that in saliva (10^4–10^8 TCID50/mL) estimated by Nicas [36].

The ventilation rate (V_{AC}) in offices is usually set to 1 ACH [37]. The respiratory rate (R_R) of a person is around 0.38 m^3/h (0.11 L/s) [38]. The inactivation rate (μ_a) of influenza A in aerosols in the air changes with the relative humidity (RH%) and temperature [39]. We assumed that the relative humidity and temperature in the office were around 50% and 20 °C to 24 °C, respectively; they were not measured. The inactivation rate (μ_a) of influenza A in aerosols in the air is 13.9 day^{-1} [40].

If a susceptible person inhales aerosol that contains influenza A viruses, he or she has a probability of being infected. The infection probability depends on the total inhalation quantity of the virus.

$$IR_I = 1 - \exp(-\alpha_R \times D) \quad (2)$$

where IR_I is the infection risk (probability to be infected), D is the respiratory dose, α_R is the estimated dose-response parameter for exposure to the respiratory tract distal to the head airways from the respirable particle inhalation study, and $\alpha_R = 0.18$ TCID50^{-1} is obtained by influenza A2/Bethesda/10/63 virus aerosol in humans [36].

All values mentioned above are listed in Table 2.

Table 2. Parameters related to long-range airborne.

Parameter	Symbol	Value	Source
Deposition rate	R_D	0.1 min^{-1}	Assumed
Volume of small particles by breathing	V'_{vb}	1.02×10^{-10} mL	[23–29]
Volume of small particles by talking	V'_{vt}	1.47×10^{-7} mL	[23–29]
Volume of small particles by coughing	V'_{vc}	1.65×10^{-7} mL	[23–29]
Volume of small particles by sneezing	V'_{vs}	1.27×10^{-6} mL	[23–29]
Volume of large droplets by breathing	V''_{vb}	0 mL	[23–29]
Volume of large droplets by talking	V''_{vt}	5.15×10^{-3} mL	[23–29]
Volume of large droplets by coughing	V''_{vc}	6.15×10^{-3} mL	[23–29]
Volume of large droplets by sneezing	V''_{vs}	4.75×10^{-2} mL	[23–29]
Frequency of breath	F_b	15 min^{-1}	[30]
Frequency of coughing (infected person)	F_c	22 h^{-1}	[31]
Frequency of sneezing (infected person)	F_s	5 h^{-1}	[32]
Duration per cough	D_c	1 s	Assumed
Duration per sneeze	D_s	3 s	Assumed
Percentage of time on talking with others	P_t	10%	Monitored
Viral shedding rate	R_s	1.5×10^7 TCID50/day	[19,24,25,31,33]
Virus concentration in exhaled particles	C_v	$1 \times 10^{6.39}$ TCID50/mL	Calculated based on [19,23–29,31,33,34]
Ventilation rate in the office	V_{AC}	1 ACH	[37]
Respiratory rate of a person	R_R	0.38 m^3/h	[38]
Inactivation rate of influenza A [1]	μ_a	13.9 day^{-1}	[40]
Dose-response parameter	α_R	0.18 TCID50^{-1}	[36]

[1] The inactivation rate of influenza A in aerosols in the air in the condition of 50% R.H and 20 °C–24 °C.

2.3. Fomite

Large droplets rapidly settle on the ground [41]. In the simulations, we considered that droplets larger than 10 μm ($d_a > 10$ μm) do not remain airborne long enough to become respirable [19]. When an infected student talks, coughs or sneezes, areas 1-m in front of and 0.5-m on both sides of the patient will be contaminated [29]. We assumed that half of the particles are deposited on surfaces that are touched by the infected persons themselves and that the remaining 50% of particles are randomly distributed on the surfaces near the infected persons when they talk, cough and sneeze. If no surface is touched, half of the particles are deposited on the infected student's desktop if he or she sits on his or her own chair; otherwise, half of the particles are deposited on the floor. According to the analysis of human touch behaviour in an office, the touch frequency for each surface is listed in Table 3, and the type and area of each surface are also listed.

Table 3. Detailed information of all sub-surfaces.

Sub-Surf [1]	Surf Type [2]	F [3] (h^{-1})	Area [4] (cm^2)	Hori-Coef [5]	Sub-Surf [1]	Surf Type [2]	F [3] (h^{-1})	Area [4] (cm^2)	Hori-Coef
StdH_1	S	6.32	469	0.5	*Std*H_2	S	19.41	470	0
StdH_3	S	1.01	470	0	*Std*S_1	P	0.28	504	0.5
StdS_2	P	0.34	504	0.5	*Std*A_1	P	1.17	1293	0.5
StdA_2	P	1.35	1293	0.5	*Std*D_1	S	3.76	183	0
StdD_2	S	3.80	183	0	*Std*B_1	P	2.86	2401	0
StdB_2	P	0.99	940	0	*Std*L_1	P	12.64	6592	0
BlnB_1	P	3.05	2600	0.5	*Bln*C_1	N	2.88	500	0
BlnE_1	N	1.94	10	0.5	*Bln*G_1	N	2.71	10	0.5
BlnM_1	N	15.12	200	0.5	*Bln*O_1	P	0.65	7500	0
BlnP_1	P	0.39	2400	0.5	*Cpt*M_1	N	23.61	120	0.5
CptK_1	N	28.98	700	1	*Dsk*T_1	N	20.19	6000	1
DskD_1	St	1.04	90	0.25	*Dsk*F_1	N	0.08	300	1
DskF_2	N	0.14	180	1	*Dsk*F_3	N	0.18	180	1
DskF_4	N	0.06	400	0	*Dsk*F_5	N	0.06	400	0
ChrA_1	N	3.17	200	1	*Chr*A_2	N	3.00	200	1
ChrC_1	P	0.73	1200	1	*Chr*B_1	P	1.56	100	1
ChrB_2	P	0.09	1200	0	*Chr*B_3	P	0.23	1200	0
ChrB_4	P	0.09	80	0	*Chr*B_5	P	0.05	80	0
PbfC_1	N	0.03	5	0	*Pbf*C_2	N	0.01	60	0
PbfP_1	N	<0.01	200	1	*Pbf*P_2	N	0.28	35	0
PbfP_3	N	0.08	100	0	*Pbf*P_4	N	0.51	3200	0
PbfP_5	N	0.09	660	0	*Pbf*D_1	St	0.05	100	0.25
PbfD_2	N	0.04	300	0	*Pbf*D_3	N	0.01	5000	0
PbfO_1	St	<0.01	100	0.25	*Pbf*O_2	St	0.01	1600	0
PbfO_3	N	<0.01	6000	0	*Pbf*W_1	N	0.01	12000	0
PbfW_2	N	0.05	2750	0.2	*Pbf*W_3	N	0.31	12	1
PbfT_1	N	0.18	200	0	*Pbf*R_1	N	0.04	400	0
PbfB_1	N	0.14	10	0.5	*Pbf*K_1	N	0.08	4400	1
PbfH_1	N	0.03	4260	0.4					

[1] Sub-surf: sub-surfaces. The codes of 57 sub-surfaces can be found in Table S1. [2] Surf type: type of surfaces including porous (P), non-porous (N), stainless steel (St) and skin (S). No one wears shorts while in the office, so the hands, head, face and neck are regarded as skin, and other body parts are regarded as porous surfaces. [3] Frequency of each sub-surface to be touched (h^{-1}). [4] Data for the human body's skin area were obtained from [42,43]. The area of the hand does not include the back of the hand. Area for other surfaces was measured or estimated. Therefore, the area considered includes only the parts usually touched by hands; for example, the area of a mouse includes only the top and side surfaces because few people will directly touch its bottom surface. [5] Horizontal coefficient of area. It means that the portion of the area that is horizontal can gather particles caused by deposition. For example, a horizontal coefficient of 1 means that all surface areas are horizontal and are totally exposed to particle deposition (e.g., *Dsk*T1: desktop).

When a hand touches a surface, the total quantity of virus (TCID50) on the hand and on the surface can be calculated based on Equations (3) and (4).

$$\frac{dV_h(t)}{dt} = R_{sh} \cdot A_c \cdot \frac{V_s}{A_S} - R_{hs} \cdot A_c \cdot \frac{V_h}{A_h}, \quad (3)$$

$$\frac{dV_s(t)}{dt} = R_{hs} \cdot A_c \cdot \frac{V_h}{A_h} - R_{sh} \cdot A_c \cdot \frac{V_s}{A_S}, \quad (4)$$

where $V_h(t)$ and $V_s(t)$ are the total quantity of virus ($TCID_{50}$) on a hand and a surface at time t caused by surface touch, respectively; R_{sh} and R_{hs} are the virus transfer rates from surfaces to hands and from hands to surfaces, respectively; A_s, A_h and A_C represent the area of the surface, the hand (palm) and the parts of the hand and the surface that make contact.

The transfer rate between hands and various surfaces directly determines the amount of influenza A that is transmitted via the fomite route. Table 4 lists some values for the transfer rate between hands and surfaces with various materials.

Table 4. [1] Virus transfer rate between hands and surfaces.

Donor	Recipient	Transfer Rate	Donor	Recipient	Transfer Rate
Porous	Hand	3% [44]	Hand	Porous	80% [45]
Non-porous	Hand	7% [46]	Hand	Non-porous	12% [47]
Stainless steel	Hand	7.9% [48]	Hand	Stainless steel	16.1% [49]
Hand	Hand	25.5% [50]			

[1] All surfaces in the office are regarded as composed by materials shown in the Table. In addition, many factors influence the transfer rate, including temperature, humidity, touch duration and dry/wet hand, thus causing some errors here.

Virus can reach the mucous membranes if a student touches his or her mouth, nasopharynx and eyes with a contaminated hand. Studies have shown that the mean rate of all finger contacts with the lips, nostrils and eyes ranges from 0.7 h^{-1} to 15 h^{-1} [36,51]. In this study, we assumed that the frequency of mucous membrane touching is 5 h^{-1}. Therefore, from Table 1, one of four hand-face contacts are hand-mucous membrane contacts. The virus transfer rate from the fingertip to the mucous membranes is set to 35% [52]. The dose-response parameter based on intranasal inoculation of humans $\alpha_I = 5.7 \times 10^{-5}\ TCID_{50}^{-1}$.

Resuspension of microorganisms from the floor, clothing and furniture acts as a secondary source [53]. Resuspended dust comprises up to 60% of the total particulate matter in indoor air [54,55]. The resuspension rate depends on many factors, such as the room height, the relative humidity and the particle size. To simplify the resuspension, we assumed that resuspension rate in the office is $10^{-4}\ h^{-1}$ [56]. Only resuspension between surfaces and the air is considered, while that between skin and the air is ignored because skin is usually moist.

Influenza A virus loses viability on surfaces over time. Porous and non-porous surfaces are both considered because the death rate of the virus differs significantly between the two surfaces [31]. According to a previous study [48], the inactivation rate of influenza A virus on a porous surface such as pyjamas (μ_p) is $1.6 \times 10^{-2}\ min^{-1}$, that on a non-porous surface such as stainless steel (μ_s) is $2.0 \times 10^{-3}\ min^{-1}$ and that on the hand (μ_h) is 1.2 min^{-1}. Inactivation on mucous membranes is not considered here.

Based on the balance between virus generation and disappearance (flew out of the room, lost viability or inhaled by people), the virus quantity in the air and on the surfaces can be calculated (Equations (5) and (6)).

$$\frac{dV_{Air}(t)}{dt} = V_{Ps} + R_{SA} - D_{AS} - \frac{V_{Air}}{V_R} \cdot V_{AC} - \left(1 - e^{-V_{Da}}\right) \cdot V_{Air} - V_I, \quad (5)$$

$$\frac{dV_{Sf}(t)}{dt} = V_{Pl} + D_{AS} - R_{SA} - \left(1 - e^{-V_{Ds}}\right) \cdot V_{sf}(t) + V_{HS} - V_{SH}, \tag{6}$$

where V_{Air} and V_{Sf} are the quantity of virus ($TCID_{50}$) in the air and on surfaces in the office; V_{Ps} and V_{Pl} are the virus generation velocity in small droplets and large droplets, respectively, generated by breathing, talking, coughing and sneezing by the infected student; D_{AS} and R_{SA} are the particle deposition velocity from the air to surfaces and the resuspension velocity from surfaces to the air, respectively; V_R is the room's total volume; V_{AC} is the air change rate; V_{Da} and V_{Ds} are the inactivation rate of virus in the air and on surfaces, respectively; V_{HS} and V_{SH} are the quantity of virus ($TCID_{50}$) transferred from the hands to surfaces and from surfaces to the hands at each step, respectively; and V_I is the inhalation velocity of each student.

2.4. Close Contact

Close contact is usually defined as being within 3 ft (~1 m) of the infector [36]. When two or more students talk, small and large droplets will be sprayed from the infected student's mouth. Large droplets are likely deposited on the mucous membranes of susceptible students, some small droplets are directly inhaled by the students who are talking with the infected student and some of the remaining small droplets are inhaled by others via the long-range airborne route. In this study, a close contact was counted when a face to face contact occurs between any two students who are within 3 ft (~1m). The quantity of virus ($TCID_{50}$) changes via inhalation and deposition on mucous membranes according to factors such as relative height, distance and direction in which the two students were facing and the room's airflow. Here we assumed that 50% of small droplets [18,19] are inhaled by the student who is talking with the infected student and 30% of large droplets are deposited on that student's face (10% of droplets on the face are deposited directly on the mucous membranes). Other small droplets diffuse into the air, and large droplets are deposited on surfaces nearby.

We observed 3526 close contacts between students in an office over the course of 5 days. Figure 2 shows the association between the duration of close contact and percentage of contacts. The frequency of close contact per person is 9.64 h^{-1} per student, including active and passive contacts. Each student spent an average of 9.86% of their time in close contact. The average duration and the mean duration of close contact were 53.8 s and 17 s, respectively.

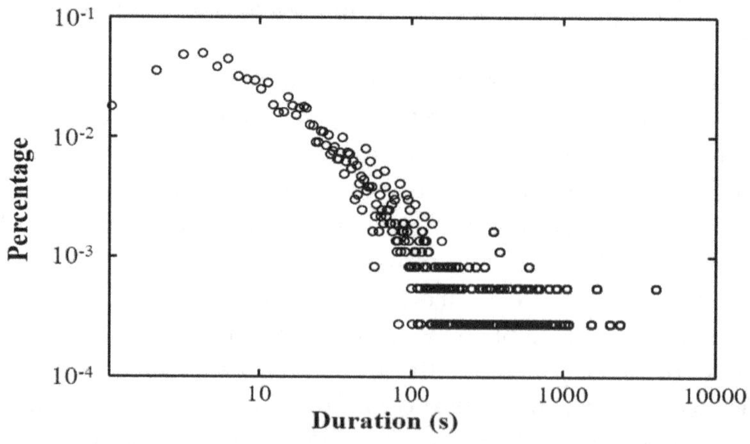

Figure 2. Association between the duration of close contact and the percentage of contacts.

3. Results

3.1. Spatio-Temporal Virus Distribution

Students move, make contact with other students, and touch surfaces in the office. Influenza A virus will be transferred between the hands and surfaces over time. From Figure 3a, the virus on the hands of the infected student increases rapidly and reaches a balance because limited numbers of his or her private surfaces share the virus. The hands of other students (susceptible) will be gradually contaminated, and virus on the hands of susceptible students almost reach a balance after 3 h (12 a.m.). The private surfaces of infected students are highly contaminated, and the quantity of virus ($TCID_{50}$) on the private surfaces of the infected student is almost three orders of magnitude of that on the private surfaces of susceptible students. Public surfaces are dirtier than the private surfaces of susceptible students, and they also play important roles in the spread of infection like hubs in the surface touch network. The cumulative quantity of virus ($TCID_{50}$) on the mucous membranes of susceptible students expresses each student's intranasal dose and gradually increases over time.

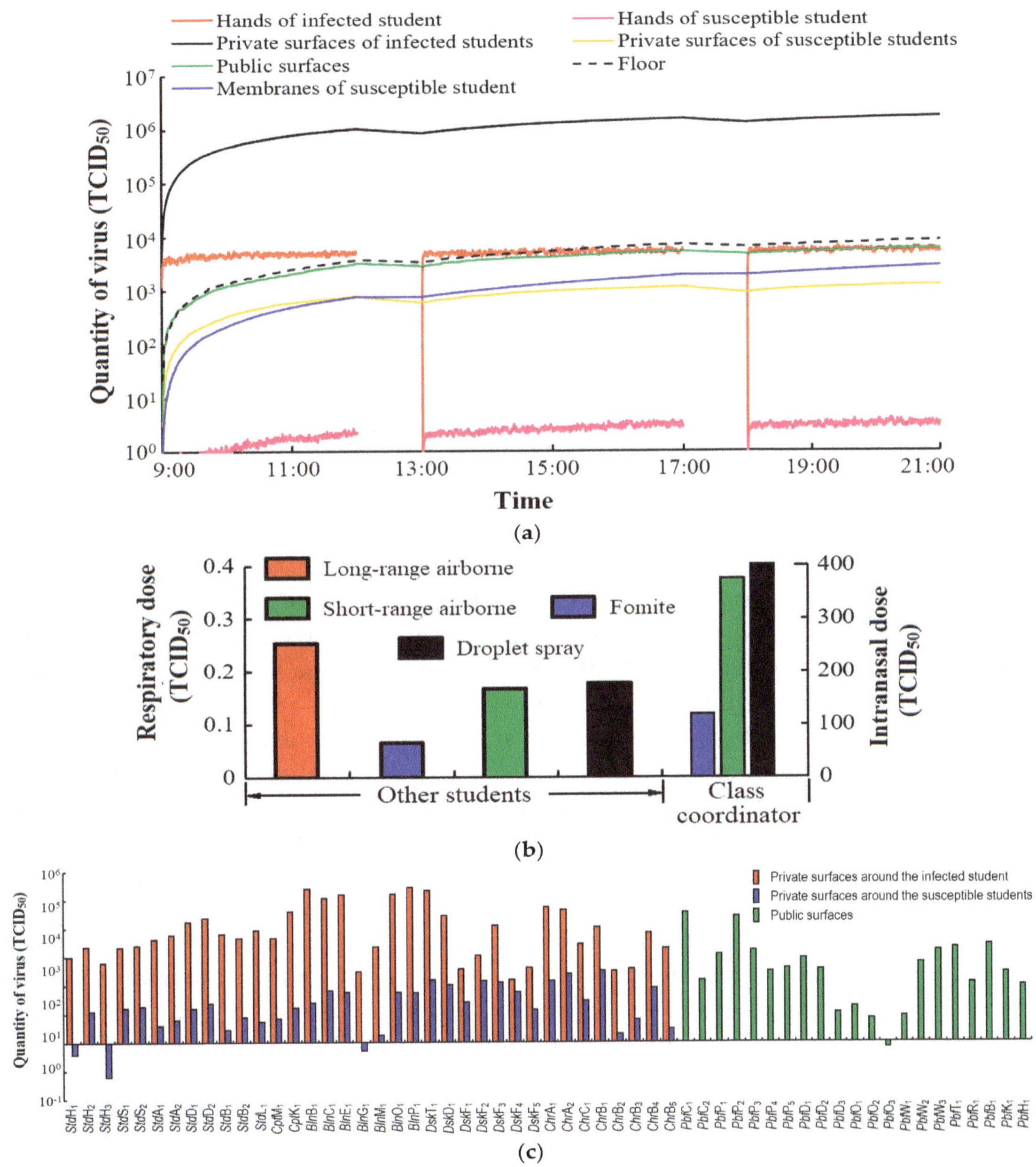

Figure 3. Quantity of virus ($TCID_{50}$) (**a**) on different types of surface [1]; (**b**) absorbed by the class coordinator and other students via various transmission routes (close contact includes both short-range airborne and droplet spray); (**c**) on different types of sub-surfaces after a whole day ($TCID_{50}$ per surface).[1] Quantity of virus ($TCID_{50}$) on private surfaces, hands and mucous membranes of susceptible students are the average value of each student rather than a summation of all susceptible students.

The quantity of virus ($TCID_{50}$) on the floor is relatively low because we assumed that most large droplets generated by talking, coughing and sneezing are deposited on the top surfaces of the desk, if the infected student is sitting in his or her own seat. In a 1-day simulation, we found that the respiratory dose per day of each susceptible student from the long-range and short-range airborne routes are 0.25 and 0.17 $TCID_{50}$, respectively, and the intranasal dose per day from the fomite and droplet spray routes are 63.81 and 185.24 $TCID_{50}$ (Figure 3b). All results are average values from 1000 simulations. Based upon the dose-response parameters from two routes, the total infection risk for each susceptible student during 1 day in the office is 8.75%, of which 54.31%, 4.23% and 44.46% are contributed by the long-range airborne, fomite and close contact routes. The class coordinator usually has more frequent interaction with other students, and we assumed that the probability of the class coordinator touching others' desks and chairs and talking with others is twice that of the other students. The infection risk of the monitor is 13.79% (Figure 3b). The virus distribution on the surfaces of the desks and chairs of the class coordinator and the other students is shown in Figure S1 (Supplementary Materials). The class coordinator has a higher infection risk than the other students. There are 57 types of sub-surfaces, and the final quantity of virus ($TCID_{50}$) on each type of sub-surface ($TCID_{50}$ per surface) is shown in Figure 3c. The quantity of virus ($TCID_{50}$) is much higher on the private surfaces around the infected student (approaching 800 times) than around susceptible students. Keyboards, headphones, desktops, mice and mobile phones are the five most-contaminated private surfaces around the infected student. The top of the seat back, the right chair arm, the desktop, the left chair arm and the top of the left desk's fence are the five most-contaminated private surfaces around the susceptible students. Air conditioning (AC) controllers, printer touch screens, cabinet handles, tissue dispensers and the printer drawer are the dirtiest of all public surfaces. Surfaces with small areas, such as headphones and the buttons on the AC controller usually have a high virus concentration.

3.2. *Infection Spread via the Fomite Route*

The spread of infection can be controlled only after the route of virus transmission is known. Figure 4 shows that 95.1% of virus is transmitted via private surfaces, while only 4.9% is transmitted via public surfaces. In all private surfaces, 59.8% of virus is transmitted via the private surfaces around the infected student, 38.1% of virus is transmitted via the private surfaces around the self and only 2.1% of virus is transmitted via the private surfaces of other susceptible students. The percentage of intranasal doses of susceptible students from the fomites of six primary surfaces—students, their belongings, computers, desks, chairs and public facilities—are 8.0%, 6.8%, 13.2%, 57.8%, 9.3% and 4.9%, respectively. Most virus absorbed by susceptible students comes from desktops, mice, mobile phones, faces, chair arms, keyboards, hands, printer touch screens and the button of the water dispenser. In addition, most virus absorbed by students comes from the private surfaces of infected students and the student himself or herself. The face is dirty, because some large droplets are deposited upon it when two students speak. Few students touch the faces of other students; therefore, the main sources of virus on the face are from the student himself or herself. During disinfection, the red and orange surfaces labelled in Figure 4 should receive more attention because of the high rate of virus transmission through them.

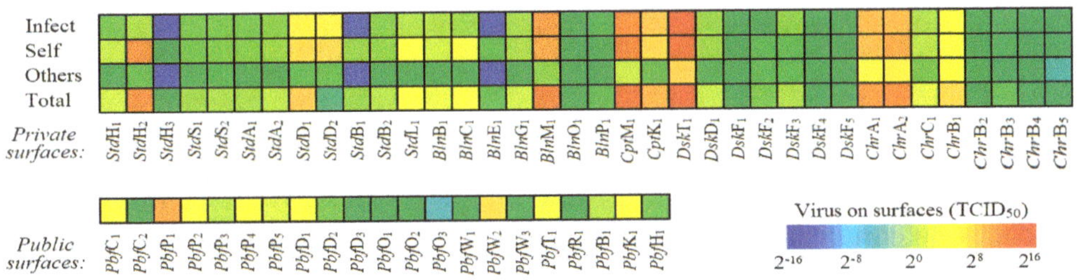

Figure 4. Quantity of virus ($TCID_{50}$) transmitted from various types of sub-surfaces from the private surfaces of the infected student, the student's own private surfaces, the private surfaces of other susceptible students and public surfaces to the hands ($TCID_{50}$).

Many factors influence effectiveness of virus transmission via fomites such as virus inactivation on surfaces and the virus transfer rate between hands and surfaces. With decreasing R_{sh} and increasing R_{hs}, the respiratory dose per student per day gradually increases (Figure 5a). When $R_{sh} > 0.1$, the intranasal dose increases as R_{hs} increases, while when $R_{sh} < 0.1$, the intranasal dose is negative in proportion with R_{hs} (Figure 5b). When R_{sh} is high, the quantity of virus ($TCID_{50}$) on surfaces increases as R_{hs} increases because more viruses are transferred from the hands of the infected student. When susceptible students touch the surfaces, more virus will be transferred from the surfaces to their hands. The intranasal dose of the susceptible students increases. When R_{sh} is very low, it is difficult for the virus to transfer from surfaces to the hands. Although the virus from the hands of the infected student to surfaces increases as R_{hs} increases, the transmission of virus from surfaces to the hands of susceptible students is limited because of small R_{sh}. As R_{hs} increases, more virus is transmitted from the hands of susceptible students to surfaces than from the surfaces to their hands, and the intranasal dose of the susceptible students decreases. In reality, adjustment of R_{sh} and R_{hs} to a specific value can efficiently limit virus transmission via fomites, thus reducing the infection risk, especially in infectious diseases that are transmitted mainly via fomites such as norovirus. From Figure 5c,d, the respiratory dose gradually decreases as R_{sh} increases and as R_{hs} decreases. In contrast, the intranasal dose gradually increases, thus the total quantity of virus ($TCID_{50}$) on surfaces decreases. The amount of virus aerosol in the air as a result of resuspension decreases. Therefore, in most cases, the respiratory dose decreases as intranasal dose increases.

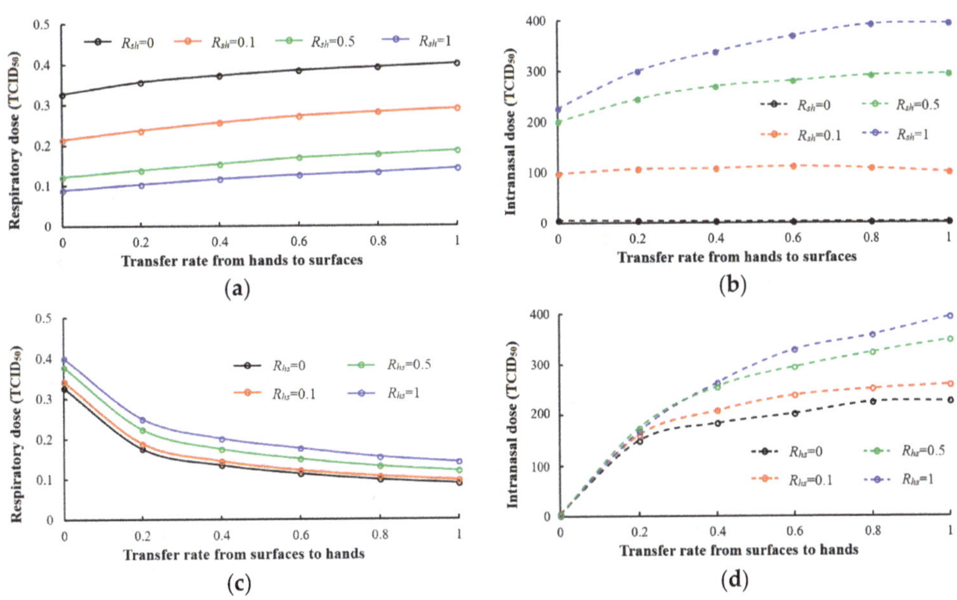

Figure 5. Different transfer rate between surfaces and hands (R_{hs} & R_{sh}). (**a**) Respiratory dose changes with R_{sh}; (**b**) intranasal dose changes with R_{sh}; (**c**) respiratory dose changes with R_{hs}; (**d**) intranasal dose changes with R_{hs}.

3.3. Strategies for Influenza A Prevention

3.3.1. Mask Wearing

Masks have various filtrating resolutions and efficacies. Surgical masks can only prevent large droplets, and N95 masks can prevent both large and small droplets. We hypothesised that 95% of both large and small droplets can be blocked by a tightly worn N95 mask. The particle block efficiency reduces if the mask is not tightly worn. Figure 6a,b show the respiratory and intranasal dose absorbed by susceptible students with different large and small droplets blocking efficiency and mask wearing strategies (the infected or the susceptible students wearing masks). When the blocking efficiency for large droplets (E_{BL}) is reduced from 100% to 30%, the respiratory dose of susceptible students from the long-range airborne route increases from 0.04 to 0.19 $TCID_{50}$. The intranasal dose via fomites and droplet spray increase from 0.01 to 42.53 $TCID_{50}$ and from 0 to 131.79 $TCID_{50}$, respectively (Figure 6b). When $E_{BL} = 100\%$, the intranasal dose comes only from the deposition of small aerosol in the air. Therefore, comparing no mask with wearing mask with 100% E_{BL}, each susceptible student's average infection risk is reduced from 8.75% to 3.82%. When an N95 mask is worn, small droplets can also be filtered. By increasing the mask's blocking efficiency for small droplets (E_{BS}), the respiratory dose via both long-range and short airborne routes decreases (Figure 6a). However, the intranasal dose via the fomite and droplet spray routes remain nearly the same if E_{BS} increases (Figure 6b). When 95% of both small and large droplets are blocked ($E_{BL} = E_{BS} = 95\%$), the infected student's total risk of infection will be reduced from 8.75% to 0.45%.

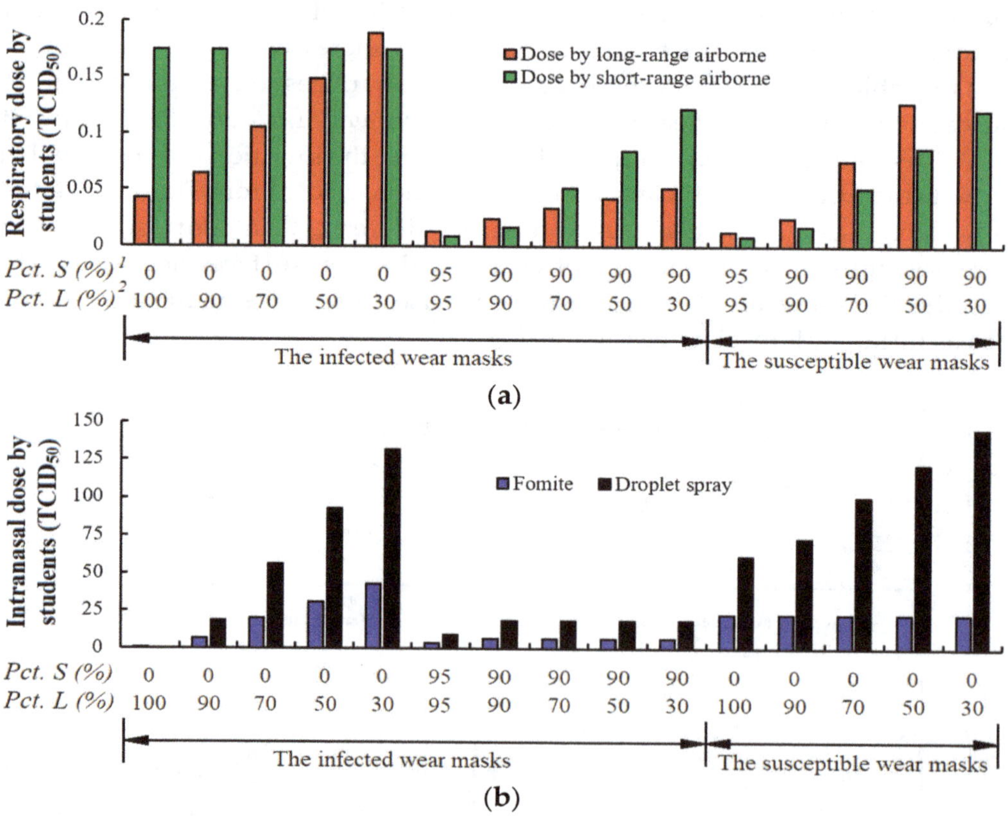

Figure 6. Dose of influenza A virus by susceptible students under different mask wearing strategies and efficiencies. (**a**) Long-range and short-range airborne routes; (**b**) fomite and droplet spray routes.[1] Pct.S (%): Percentage of small particles blocked by masks.[2] Pct.L (%): Percentage of large droplets blocked by masks.

If only susceptible students wear the mask rather than the infected student, the infection risk changes. The respiratory dose via the long-range and short-range airborne routes decreases with increasing E_{BS}. When 95% of both small and large droplets are blocked, the respiratory dose from the airborne route is reduced to 0.02 $TCID_{50}$ (Figure 6a). A mask can block the virus from the hands to the nose and lips because the mask isolates them. When all susceptible students wear masks with high E_{BL}, intranasal dose through fomites can hardly be further reduced. This case differs when only the infected student wears the high-E_{BL} mask. The intranasal dose caused by droplet spray decreases as E_{BL} increases (Figure 6b). The total infection risk will be reduced to 0.87% if all susceptible students tightly wear N95 masks.

3.3.2. Ventilation

It is well known that ventilation can efficiently reduce the risk of infection via the long-range airborne route. It is determined by natural and mechanical ventilation, which are influenced by many factors such as open doors, open windows and AC systems. When the ventilation rate changes from 1 ACH to 4 ACH, the respiratory dose via the long-range airborne route will be reduced from 0.26 to 0.19 $TCID_{50}$, and the general infection risk will be reduced by 1.2% (Figure 7). If the ventilation rate increases to 10 ACH, the infection risk via the long-range airborne route will be less than half under only 1 ACH. With no ventilation, all virus in the air moves out only through inactivation and deposition, and the virus concentration in the air is much higher.

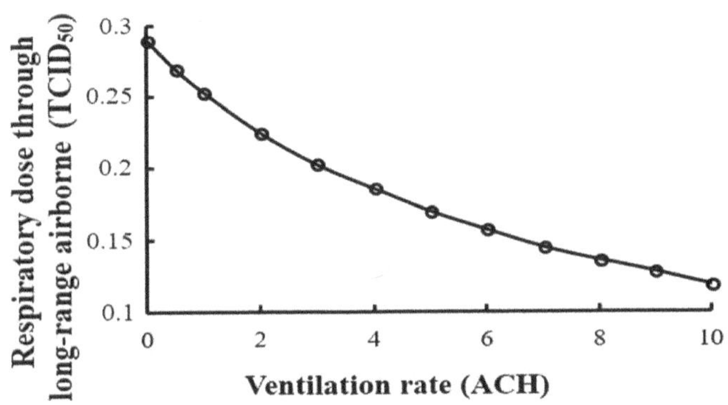

Figure 7. Respiratory dose via the long-range airborne route at various ventilation rates.

3.3.3. Hand Washing

Figure 8 shows how hand washing by the infected student and susceptible students influences the respiratory and intranasal dose. In the simulation, we hypothesised that hands become completely clean (no virus) after hand washing. The infected student's hands usually possess a large quantity of virus ($TCID_{50}$), which will then be transmitted to surfaces and resuspended in the air. As shown in blue and red lines in Figure 8, when the infected student's hand washing frequency is less than 6 times per hour, the decrease in the respiratory and intranasal doses for susceptible students is obvious. If susceptible students wash their hands, rather than the infected student, the infection risk reduction via fomites is slightly higher. If the hand washing frequency is less than 6 times per hour, the intranasal dose reduction via fomites will be obviously limited. Moreover, hand washing by susceptible students hardly reduces the respiratory dose. In general, focusing on the influenza A virus, if the frequency of hand washing is more than twice per hour, very little further improvement can be made in the efficacy for infection risk reduction.

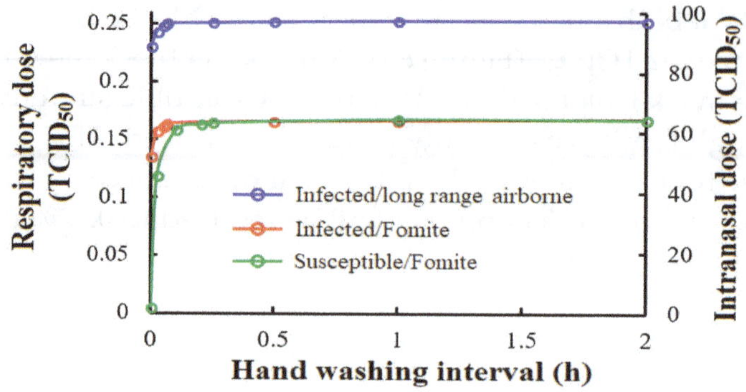

Figure 8. Infection risk reduction by hand washing (Blue and red lines show the respiratory and intranasal doses of the susceptible students when only the infected student washes his or her hands; the green line shows the intranasal dose from susceptible students when only they wash hands).

3.3.4. Surface Cleaning

In the simulation, we hypothesised that surfaces become completely clean (no virus) after surface cleaning. Figure 9a shows how respiratory and intranasal doses change with various strategies of surface cleaning with frequency of 0.5 h^{-1}. No student touches the floor, and a clean floor can only reduce the resuspension of aerosol. Regular desktop cleaning can reduce the respiratory and intranasal dose from 0.26 to 0.14 $TCID_{50}$ and from 65.87 to 35.10 TCID50, respectively (the general infection risk ranges from 8.75% to 6.71%). The cleaning of more surfaces, such as the top five high-touch surfaces and all private surfaces, can slightly reduce the infection risk from 6.71% to 6.61%, and to 6.17%, respectively.

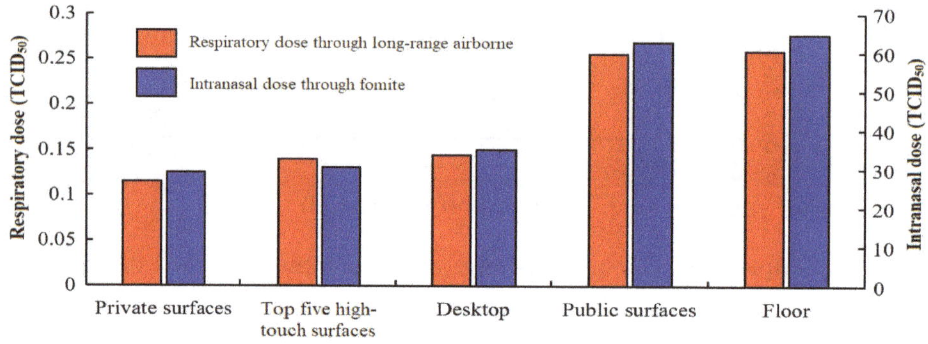

(**a**)

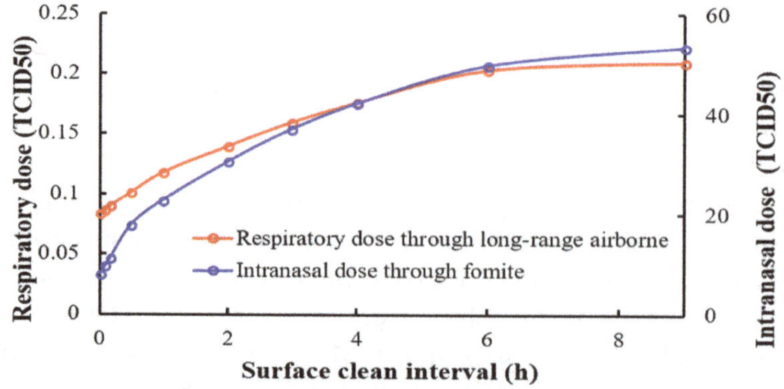

(**b**)

Figure 9. Surface cleaning. (**a**) Various types of surfaces with a cleaning frequency of 0.5 h−1; (**b**) different clean interval for top five high-touch surfaces [1]. [1] Top five high-touch surfaces: desktop, mouse, mobile phone, keyboard and chair arms.

Figure 9b shows that the respiratory and intranasal dose grows logarithmically as the interval at which high-touch surfaces are cleaned increases. If only a regular high-touch surface cleaning is conducted at 3 p.m. each day, the respiratory dose via long-range airborne and the intranasal dose via fomites are 0.16 and 36.97 $TCID_{50}$ (infection risk = 6.97%), respectively. However, if the frequency of surface cleaning is increased to once per hour (surface clean interval = 1 h), the infection risk is reduced to 6.19%. With a continuous decrease in the clean frequency when it is lower than once per hour, the infection risk will be reduced quickly, but the workload is huge.

4. Discussion

In this paper, we studied how influenza A transmits in a graduate student office in one day from 9 a.m. to 9 p.m. through long-range airborne, fomite and close contact (short-range airborne and droplets spray) routes based on real recorded data of contacts between students and surfaces touch. Most parameters set in the simulation are from real recorded data and existing studies.

We found that each susceptible student's average infection risk during a day in the office is 8.75%, of which 54.31%, 4.23%, 33.24% and 11.22% are contributed by the long-range airborne, fomite, short-range airborne and droplet spray routes. However, in an air cabin, focusing on influenza A H1N1, the contributions via the airborne, close contact and fomite routes are 34.30%, 64.98% and 0.72% [13]. In the air cabin, close contact is more frequent because of the high density of passengers. Fomites contribute less due to the low probability of direct touch between the infected and susceptible passengers. The long-range airborne route is less frequent because a high ventilation rate (25 ACH) is set in the air cabin even though the population density is high. Focusing on virus on surfaces, the private surfaces around the infected student had the most virus, because most contaminated droplets are deposited on surfaces around the infected person, and nearby surfaces are also easily touched [18]. The quantity of virus ($TCID_{50}$) on all surfaces stops its rapid increase after 3 h. Virus on the hands of susceptible students always remains at a lower level because the inactivation rate of influenza A on the hands is high. The quantity of virus ($TCID_{50}$) on public surfaces is higher than on private surfaces around the susceptible students. Moreover, some active students such as the class coordinator have more contacts and a higher probability of touching other's private surfaces. We found that the class coordinator's infection risk is almost 1.6 times that of other students.

Approximately 4.2% of the influenza A infection risk comes from fomites. However, for other infectious diseases such as norovirus, which makes more than 85% of the contribution to infection risk [13], and fomite plays an important role. In the office, 95.1% of viruses were transmitted via private surfaces and only 4.9% via public surfaces. The desk is the dirtiest of all private surfaces. In this study, we hypothesised that most contaminated droplets generated by talking, coughing and sneezing are deposited on desks. Desktops, mice, mobile phones and keyboards transmit virus easily. This result accords with previous studies on microbiome [57,58]. Public surfaces are the hubs of the surface touch network [16]. AC controller buttons, printer touch screens and public cabinet handles are highly contaminated. The button of the water dispenser is frequently touched. However, the infected students usually touched the chair arms, cups and seatbacks of other students before getting a cup of water. The virus on hands is diluted, and the total quantity of virus ($TCID_{50}$) on the water dispenser is limited. These high-risk surfaces should be given more attention in infectious disease transmission, especially on some diseases that are highly dependent on fomite, such as norovirus. If we can design an anti-virus material to build all high-touch surfaces, we could efficiently control virus transmission via fomites.

From a virus transfer rate perspective, if we can create a surface that can block virus transmission from surfaces to hands ($R_{sh} = 0$), the virus from fomites could be efficiently controlled. Indeed, the transfer rate between surfaces and hands cannot reach 0 or 1. A material with low R_{sh} can limit virus transmission from surfaces to hands, such as porous materials [44]. Surfaces made with material with a high R_{hs} can absorb more virus from hands of both the infected student and susceptible students. Therefore, the means by which to adjust the virus transfer rate between surfaces and hands by using materials with different R_{sh} and R_{hs} is very helpful to prevent virus transmission via fomites. We found that when $R_{sh} > 0.1$, the intranasal dose increases as R_{hs} increases, while when $R_{sh} < 0.1$, it decreases with R_{hs} in an office setting.

Many strategies, such as mask wearing [59], ventilation [4], hand washing [11] and surface cleaning [60], can limit the spread of influenza A in a confined room. Wearing a mask can control the spread of disease via the long-range airborne, fomite and close contact routes. A high ventilation rate helps to dilute the virus concentration in the air, and the respiratory dose from the long-range airborne route will be obviously reduced. Hand washing can reduce the infection risk directly via fomites and indirectly via the long-range airborne route because of the lower rate of resuspension from surfaces to the air. The same effects are brought by surface cleaning. Mask wearing is much more efficient than hand washing because influenza A is transmitted mainly via the airborne and close contact routes. Mask wearing by the infected student has greater efficiency at reducing the infection risk than simply having the susceptible students wear masks (infection risk of 0.87% vs. 0.45% when an N95 mask is tightly sealed). According to the test in hospitals, tightly sealing a mask to the face can block the entry of 94.5% of total virus and 94.8% of infectious virus [59]. We found that 94.9% of the infection risk can be reduced if an N95 mask is tightly sealed on the infected student, which is very useful in influenza A transmission control. The airborne route is the main route of influenza A virus spread. In a norovirus outbreak, the efficiency of mask-wearing should be reassessed.

Hands play a very important role in the surface touch network, because hands can be contaminated by covering the mouth and nose when coughing and sneezing or by touching contaminated surfaces, and thus can also contaminate surfaces. Some previous studies have shown that hand washing can cut the risk of respiratory infection by 16% [61]. We found that only hand washing is limited to reduce infection risk. When the hand washing frequency is greater than six times per hour, the infection risk can be obviously reduced. However, in the hospital, when all doctors and nurses wear masks, hand washing is more efficient because hands are one of the main ways to spread virus from hospital workers to susceptible people. We also found that if the susceptible students wash their hands (rather than the infected student), the efficiency of infection risk reduction is slightly higher.

Students spent more than 90% of their time in the office touching surfaces. The intranasal dose due to contact between hands and mucous membranes depends on the quantity of viable pathogens on the office's surfaces, the frequency of contact between hands and contaminated surfaces, contact between hands and mucous membranes and the efficiency of pathogen transfer to and from hands-on contact [18]. Regular surface cleaning can reduce the infection risk. Public surfaces are frequently touched, so viruses on public surfaces are diluted by many touches by susceptible students. Public surface cleaning every 2 h is not very efficient because there are few public surfaces in the office. Desktops are among the most contaminated surfaces in the office because the students spent most of their time at their desks. Contaminated droplets are deposited on the desktop when an infected student talks, coughs or sneezes. Students often touch the desktops of other students, because of the high frequency of discussions between students in the office. Cleaning of all private surfaces can reach a better condition (infection risk reduced by 2.56%), but the workload is too large. Therefore, regular cleaning of desktops or high-touch surfaces is suggested if the virus is very severe. In addition, cleaning of high-touch surfaces is much more efficient than hand-washing because high-touch surfaces gathered more virus and because the inactivation rate on surfaces is much lower than on the hands. The results of influenza A simulation based on real data of human behaviour in a confined space is very helpful to help understand the real characteristics of influenza A transmission and to make effective plans to prevent and control diseases.

This work perhaps lacks a direct and strong connection to Health-EDRM (health-related emergency disaster risk management). However, the model that we built and suggestions that we put forward are useful in for controlling infectious diseases transmission, and major outbreaks if infectious diseases can be itself a health-related disaster. Moreover, natural and complex disasters such as floods, tsunamis, and earthquakes can dramatically increase the risk of infectious diseases outbreak including malaria, measles, viral hepatitis, etc. [62,63]. After a serious disaster, many people who have been affected by the disaster will be gathered in an emergency shelter. Risk of infectious disease transmission through different routes can be calculated based on our model, and suggestions we obtained also can guide disaster managers in making efficient emergency plans for infectious disease control and prevention after disasters.

This study has various limitations. All students are assumed to stay in the office at all times except at lunch and dinner time, virus generation is overestimated, and a higher infection risk of susceptible students is calculated. The virus transfer rate between surfaces and hands is influenced by many factors, such as force, area and touch duration. We assumed that each touch between a specific surface and a hand has the same transfer rate. Most particles are deposited on the desktop when the infected student talks, coughs or sneezes, and we did not consider that some private things such as mice, keyboards and cups share the virus on the desk. Therefore, the quantity of virus ($TCID_{50}$) on the desk is overestimated. Moreover, in our simulation, some parameters such as transfer rate between hand and various surfaces are not based on influenza virus due to data unavailability. Heterogeneity exists in the study, and it may result in some errors. The differences in human behaviour by gender are ignored, and relative positions, heights and angles between two students during close contact are not considered. A future study should collect some samples in the office if any students are infected with influenza A. We can then compare the real virus distribution data with our simulation data to verify the accuracy of our model.

5. Conclusions

Influenza A transmission in a graduate student office is simulated via long-range airborne, fomite, and close contact routes based on realistic data of human behaviours. The long-range airborne, fomite and close contact routes contribute to 54.3%, 4.2% and 44.5% of influenza A infections, respectively. For the fomite route, 59.8%, 38.1% and 2.1% of viruses are transmitted to the hands of students from private surfaces around the infected students, the students themselves and other susceptible students, respectively. The private surfaces of infected students are highly contaminated. The quantity of virus ($TCID_{50}$) is much higher on the private surfaces around the infected student (approaching 800 times) than around susceptible students. Keyboards, headphones, desktops, mice and mobile phones are the five most-contaminated private surfaces around the infected student. Public surfaces are dirtier than the private surfaces of susceptible students. The intranasal dose via fomites of the students' bodies, belongings, computers, desks, chairs and public facilities are 8.0%, 6.8%, 13.2%, 57.8%, 9.3% and 4.9%, respectively. The intranasal dose does not monotonously increase or decrease with the virus transfer rate between hands and surfaces, and a specific value setting can optimally limit influenza A virus transmission via fomites Mask wearing is much more useful than hand washing for control of influenza A in the tested office setting, and the total risk can be reduced from 8.75% to 0.45% if an N95 mask is tightly sealed by infected students. Regular cleaning of high-touch surfaces, which can reduce the infection risk by 2.14%, is recommended and is much more efficient than hand-washing.

Author Contributions: Conceptualization, N.Z. and Y.L; Data curation, N.Z.; Formal analysis, N.Z.; Funding acquisition, Y.L.; Investigation, N.Z.; Methodology, N.Z.; Software, N.Z.; Supervision, Y.L.; Writing—original draft, N.Z.; Writing—review & editing, Y.L.

References

1. Monto, A.S.; Whitley, R.J. Seasonal and pandemic influenza: A 2007 update on challenges and solutions. *Clin. Infect. Dis.* **2008**, *46*, 1024–1031. [CrossRef] [PubMed]
2. Englund, J.A. Antiviral therapy of influenza. *Semin. Pediatr. Infect. Dis.* **2002**, *13*, 120–128. [CrossRef] [PubMed]
3. Morens, D.M.; Rash, V.M. Lessons from a nursing home outbreak of influenza A. *Infect. Control Hosp. Epidemiol.* **1995**, *16*, 275–280. [CrossRef] [PubMed]

4. Brankston, G.; Gitterman, L.; Hirji, Z.; Lemieux, C.; Gardam, D.M. Transmission of influenza A in human beings. *Lancet Infect. Dis.* **2007**, *7*, 257–265. [CrossRef]
5. Weinstein, R.A.; Bridges, C.B.; Kuehnert, M.J.; Hall, C.B. Transmission of influenza: Implications for control in health care settings. *Clin. Infect. Dis.* **2003**, *37*, 1094–1101. [CrossRef] [PubMed]
6. Tellier, R. Review of aerosol transmission of influenza A virus. *Emerg. Infect. Dis.* **2006**, *12*, 1657–1662. [CrossRef] [PubMed]
7. Lowen, A.C.; Mubareka, S.; Tumpey, T.M.; García-Sastre, A.; Palese, P. The guinea pig as a transmission model for human influenza viruses. *Proc. Natl. Acad. Sci. USA* **2006**, *103*, 9988–9992. [CrossRef] [PubMed]
8. Moser, M.R.; Bender, T.R.; Margolis, H.S.; Noble, G.R.; Kendal, A.P.; Ritter, D.G. An outbreak of influenza aboard a commercial airliner. *Am. J. Epidemiol.* **1979**, *110*, 1–6. [CrossRef] [PubMed]
9. McLean, R.L. General discussion. *Am. Rev. Respir. Dis.* **1961**, *83*, 36–38.
10. Schulman, J.L.; Kilbourne, E.D. Airborne transmission of influenza virus infection in mice. *Nature* **1962**, *195*, 1129. [CrossRef] [PubMed]
11. Hertzberg, V.S.; Weiss, H.; Elon, L.; Si, W.P.; Norris, S.L. the FlyHealthy Research Team. Behaviors, movement, and transmission of droplet-mediated respiratory diseases during transcontinental airline flights. *Proc. Natl. Acad. Sci. USA* **2018**. [CrossRef] [PubMed]
12. Gilardi, F.; Castelli, G.G.; Vinci, M.R.; Ciofi, D.A.M.; Santilli, V.; Brugaletta, R.; Santoro, A.; Montanaro, R.; Lavorato, L.; Raponi, M.; et al. Seasonal influenza vaccination in health care workers. A pre-post intervention study in an Italian paediatric sospital. *Int. J. Environ. Res. Public Health* **2018**, *15*, 841. [CrossRef] [PubMed]
13. Lei, H.; Li, Y.; Xiao, S.; Lin, C.H.; Norris, S.L.; Wei, D.; Hu, Z.; Ji, S. Routes of transmission of influenza A H1N1, SARS CoV, and norovirus in air cabin: Comparative analyses. *Indoor Air* **2017**, *28*, 394–403. [CrossRef] [PubMed]
14. Chong, K.C.; Goggins, W.; Zee, B.C.Y.; Wang, M.H. Identifying meteorological drivers for the seasonal variations of influenza infections in a subtropical city—Hong Kong. *Int. J. Environ. Res. Public Health* **2015**, *12*, 1560–1576. [CrossRef] [PubMed]
15. Charu, V.; Zeger, S.; Gog, J.; Bjørnstad, O.N.; Kissler, S.; Simonsen, L.; Grenfell, B.T.; Viboud, C. Human mobility and the spatial transmission of influenza in the United States. *PLoS Comput. Biol.* **2017**, *13*, e1005382. [CrossRef] [PubMed]
16. Zhang, N.; Li, Y.G.; Huang, H. Surface touch and its network growth in a graduate student office. *Indoor Air*, under review.
17. Bolashikov, Z.D.; Melikov, A.K. Methods for air cleaning and protection of building occupants from airborne pathogens. *Build. Environ.* **2009**, *44*, 1378–1385. [CrossRef]
18. Nicas, M.; Sun, G. An integrated model of infection risk in a health-care environment. *Risk Anal.* **2006**, *26*, 1085–1096. [CrossRef] [PubMed]
19. Nicas, M.; Nazaroff, W.W.; Hubbard, A. Toward understanding the risk of secondary airborne infection: Emission of respirable pathogens. *J. Occup. Environ. Hyg.* **2005**, *2*, 143–154. [CrossRef] [PubMed]
20. Approaches to Better Understand Human Influenza Transmission (CDC). Available online: https://www.cdc.gov/influenzatransmissionworkshop2010/ (accessed on 1 May 2018).
21. Yang, W.; Elankumaran, S.; Marr, L.C. Concentrations and size distributions of airborne influenza A viruses measured indoors at a health centre, a day-care centre and on aeroplanes. *J. R. Soc. Interface* **2011**, *8*, 1176. [CrossRef] [PubMed]
22. Drossinos, Y.; Housiadas, C. Aerosol flows. In *Multiphase Flow Handbook*; Crowe, C.T., Ed.; CRC Press: Boca Raton, FL, USA, 2006; pp. 6-1–6-58.
23. Duguid, J.P. The size and the duration of air-carriage of respiratory droplets and droplet-nuclei. *Epidemiol. Infect.* **1946**, *44*, 471–479. [CrossRef]
24. Loudon, R.G.; Roberts, R.M. Relation between the airborne diameters of respiratory droplets and the diameter of the stains left after recovery. *Nature* **1967**, *213*, 95–96. [CrossRef]
25. Hayden, F.G.; Fritz, R.; Lobo, M.C.; Alvord, W.; Strober, W.; Straus, S.E. Local and systemic cytokine responses during experimental human influenza A virus infection. Relation to symptom formation and host defense. *J. Clin. Investig.* **1998**, *101*, 643–649. [CrossRef] [PubMed]
26. Zhu, S.; Kato, S.; Yang, J.H. Study on transport characteristics of saliva droplets produced by coughing in a calm indoor environment. *Build. Environ.* **2006** *41*, 1691–1702. [CrossRef]

27. Fabian, P.; McDevitt, J.J.; DeHaan, W.H.; Fung, R.O.P.; Cowling, B.J.; Chan, K.H.; Leung, G.M.; Milton, D.K. Influenza virus in human exhaled breath: An observational study. *PLoS ONE* **2008**, *3*, e2691. [CrossRef] [PubMed]
28. Chao, C.Y.H.; Wan, M.P.; Morawska, L.; Johnson, G.R.; Ristovski, Z.D.; Hargreaves, M.; Mengersen, K.; Corbett, S.; Li, Y.; Xie, X.; et al. Characterization of expiration air jets and droplet size distributions immediately at the mouth opening. *J. Aerosol Sci.* **2009**, *40*, 122–133. [CrossRef]
29. Xie, X.; Li, Y.; Sun, H.; Liu, L. Exhaled droplets due to talking and coughing. *J. R. Soc. Interface* **2009**, *6*, S703. [CrossRef] [PubMed]
30. Sinnreich, R.; Kark, J.D.; Friedlander, Y.; Sapoznikov, D.; Luria, M.H. Five minute recordings of heart rate variability for population studies: Repeatability and age–sex characteristics. *Heart* **1998**, *80*, 156–162. [CrossRef] [PubMed]
31. Atkinson, M.P.; Wein, L.M. Quantifying the routes of transmission for pandemic influenza. *Bull. Math. Biol.* **2008**, *70*, 820–867. [CrossRef] [PubMed]
32. Chen, S.C.; Liao, C.M. Probabilistic indoor transmission modeling for influenza (sub) type viruses. *J. Infect.* **2010**, *60*, 26–35. [CrossRef] [PubMed]
33. Knight, V.; Fedson, D.; Baldini, J.; Douglas, R.G.; Couch, R.B. Amantadine therapy of epidemic influenza A2 (Hong Kong). *Infect. Immun.* **1970**, *1*, 200–204. [PubMed]
34. Couch, R.B.; Gerone, P.J.; Cate, T.R.; Griffith, W.R.; Alling, D.W.; Knight, V. Preparation and properties of a small-particle aerosol of coxsackie A21. *Proc. Soc. Exp. Biol. Med.* **1965**, *118*, 818–822. [CrossRef] [PubMed]
35. Douglas, R. Influenza in man. In *fluenza Virus and Influenza: Kilbourne*; Academic Press, Inc.: New York, NY, USA, 1975; pp. 395–445.
36. Nicas, M.; Jones, R.M. Relative contributions of four exposure pathways to influenza infection risk. *Risk Anal.* **2009**, *29*, 1292–1303. [CrossRef] [PubMed]
37. Zhang, N.; Huang, H.; Su, B.; Ma, X.; Li, Y. A human behavior integrated hierarchical model of airborne disease transmission in a large city. *Build. Environ.* **2018**, *127*, 211–220. [CrossRef]
38. Chen, S.C.; Chang, C.F.; Liao, C.M. Predictive models of control strategies involved in containing indoor airborne infections. *Indoor Air* **2006**, *16*, 469–481. [CrossRef] [PubMed]
39. Weber, T.P.; Stilianakis, N.I. Inactivation of influenza A viruses in the environment and modes of transmission: A critical review. *J. Infect.* **2008**, *57*, 361–373. [CrossRef] [PubMed]
40. Harper, G.J. Airborne micro-organisms: Survival tests with four viruses. *Epidemiol. Infect.* **1961**, *59*, 479–486. [CrossRef]
41. Blachere, F.M.; Lindsley, W.G.; Pearce, T.A.; Anderson, S.E.; Fisher, M.; Khakoo, R.; Meade, B.J.; Lander, O.; Davis, S.; Thewlis, R.E.; et al. Measurement of airborne influenza virus in a hospital emergency department. *Clin. Infect. Dis.* **2009**, *48*, 438. [CrossRef] [PubMed]
42. Yang, J. Numerical and Experimental Study on Physiological Responses in Hot Environments Based on Human-Clothing-Environment System. Ph.D. Thesis, Tsinghua University, Beijing, China, 2015. (in Chinese).
43. Wester, R.C.; Maibach, H.I. Regional variation in percutaneous absorption. *Drugs Pharm. Sci.* **1999**, *97*, 107–116.
44. Sattar, S.A.; Jacobsen, H.; Springthorpe, V.S.; Cusack, T.M.; Rubino, R. Chemical disinfection to interrupt transfer of rhinovirus type 14 from environmental surfaces to hands. *Appl. Environ. Microbiol.* **1993**, *59*, 1579–1585. [PubMed]
45. Mackintosh, C.A.; Hoffman, P.N. An extended model for transfer of micro-organisms via the hands: Differences between organisms and the effect of alcohol disinfection. *Epidemiol. Infect.* **1984**, *92*, 345–355. [CrossRef]
46. Mokhtari, A.; Jaykus, L.A. Quantitative exposure model for the transmission of norovirus in retail food preparation. *Int. J. Food Microbiol.* **2009**, *133*, 38–47. [CrossRef] [PubMed]
47. Lopez, G.U.; Gerba, C.P.; Tamimi, A.H.; Kitajima, M.; Maxwell, S.L.; Rose, J.B. Transfer efficiency of bacteria and viruses from porous and nonporous fomites to fingers under different relative humidity conditions. *Appl. Environ. Microbiol.* **2013**, *79*, 5728–5734. [CrossRef] [PubMed]
48. Bean, B.; Moore, B.M.; Sterner, B.; Peterson, L.R.; Gerding, D.N.; Balfour, H.H. Survival of influenza viruses on environmental surfaces. *J. Infect. Dis.* **1982**, *146*, 47–51. [CrossRef] [PubMed]

49. Ansari, S.A.; Sattar, S.A.; Springthorpe, V.S.; Wells, G.A.; Tostowaryk, W. Rotavirus survival on human hands and transfer of infectious virus to animate and nonporous inanimate surfaces. *J. Clin. Microbiol.* **1988**, *26*, 1513–1518. [PubMed]
50. Pancic, F.; Carpentier, D.C.; Came, P.E. Role of infectious secretions in the transmission of rhinovirus. *J. Clin. Microbiol.* **1980**, *12*, 567–571. [PubMed]
51. Hendley, J.O.; Wenzel, R.P.; Gwaltney, J.M., Jr. Transmission of rhinovirus colds by self-inoculation. *N. Eng. J. Med.* **1973**, *288*, 1361–1364. [CrossRef] [PubMed]
52. Rusin, P.; Maxwell, S.; Gerba, C. Comparative surface-to-hand and fingertip-to-mouth transfer efficiency of gram-positive bacteria, gram-negative bacteria, and phage. *J. Appl. Microbiol.* **2002**, *93*, 585–592. [CrossRef] [PubMed]
53. Prussin, A.J.; Marr, L.C. Sources of airborne microorganisms in the built environment. *Microbiome* **2015**, *3*, 78. [CrossRef] [PubMed]
54. Alshitawi, M.S.; Awbi, H.B. Measurement and prediction of the effect of students' activities on airborne particulate concentration in a classroom. *HVAC&R Res.* **2011**, *17*, 446–464.
55. Ocak, Y.; Kılıçvuran, A.; Eren, A.B.; Sofuoglu, A.; Sofuoglu, S.C. Exposure to particulate matter in a mosque. *Atmos. Environ.* **2012**, *56*, 169–176. [CrossRef]
56. Qian, J.; Ferro, A.R. Resuspension of dust particles in a chamber and associated environmental factors. *Aerosol Sci. Technol.* **2008**, *42*, 566–578. [CrossRef]
57. Fierer, N.; Lauber, C.L.; Zhou, N.; McDonald, D.; Costello, E.K.; Knight, R. Forensic identification using skin bacterial communities. *Proc. Natl. Acad. Sci. USA* **2010**, *107*, 6477–6481. [CrossRef] [PubMed]
58. Meadow, J.F.; Altrichter, A.E.; Green, J.L. Mobile phones carry the personal microbiome of their owners. *PeerJ* **2014**, *2*, e447. [CrossRef] [PubMed]
59. Noti, J.D.; Lindsley, W.G.; Blachere, F.M.; Cao, G.; Kashon, M.L.; Thewlis, R.E.; McMillen, C.M.; King, W.P.; Szalajda, J.V.; Beezhold, D.H. Detection of infectious influenza virus in cough aerosols generated in a simulated patient examination room. *Clin. Infect. Dis.* **2012**, *54*, 1569. [CrossRef] [PubMed]
60. Kramer, A.; Schwebke, I.; Kampf, G. How long do nosocomial pathogens persist on inanimate surfaces? A systematic review. *BMC Infect. Dis.* **2006**, *6*, 130. [CrossRef] [PubMed]
61. Rabie, T.; Curtis, V. Handwashing and risk of respiratory infections: A quantitative systematic review. *Trop. Med. Int. Health* **2006**, *11*, 258–267. [CrossRef] [PubMed]
62. Jafari, N.; Shahsanai, A.; Memarzadeh, M.; Loghmani, A. Prevention of communicable diseases after disaster: A review. *J. Res. Med. Sci.* **2011**, *16*, 956–962. [PubMed]
63. Kouadio, I.K.; Aljunid, S.; Kamigaki, T.; Hammad, K.; Oshitani, H. Infectious diseases following natural disasters: Prevention and control measures. *Expert Rev. Anti-Infect. Ther.* **2012**, *10*, 95–104. [CrossRef] [PubMed]

14

Research Methods and Ethics in Health Emergency and Disaster Risk Management: The Result of the Kobe Expert Meeting

Myo Nyein Aung [1], Virginia Murray [2,*] and Ryoma Kayano [3]

1 Advanced Health Science Institute and Faculty of International Liberal Arts, Juntendo University, Hongo 2-1-1, Bunkyo-ku, Tokyo 113-8421, Japan; myo@juntendo.ac.jp
2 Head of Global Disaster Risk Reduction, Public Health England, Wellington House, 133-155, Waterloo Road, London SE1 8UG, UK
3 World Health Organization Centre for Health Development, 1-5-1 Wakinohama-kaigandori, Chuo-ku, Kobe 651-0073, Japan; kayanor@who.int
* Correspondence: Virginia.Murray@phe.gov.uk

Abstract: In October 2018, at Asia Pacific Conference for Disaster Medicine (APCDM), an expert meeting to identify key research needs was organized by the World Health Organization (WHO) Centre for Health Development (WHO Kobe Centre (WKC)), convening the leading experts from Asia Pacific region, WHO, WHO Thematic Platform for Health Emergency and Disaster Risk Management (Health-EDRM) Research Network (TPRN), World Association for Disaster and Emergency Medicine (WADEM), in collaboration with Asia Pacific Conference for Disaster Medicine (APCDM) and Japan International Cooperation Agency (JICA). International experts, who were pre-informed about the meeting, contributed experience-based priority issues in Health-EDRM research, ethics, and scientific publication. Two moderators, experienced in multi-disciplinary research interacted with discussants to transcribe practical issues into related methodological and ethical issues. Each issue was addressed in order to progress research and scientific evidence in Health-EDRM. Further analysis of interactive dialogues revealed priorities for action, proposed mechanism to address these and identified recommendations. Thematic discussion uncovered five priority areas: (1) the need to harmonize Health-EDRM research with universal terms and, definitions via a glossary; (2) mechanisms to facilitate and speed up ethical review process; (3) increased community participation and stakeholder involvement in generating research ideas and in assessing impact evaluation; (4) development of reference materials such as possible consensus statements; and (5) the urgent need for a research methods resource textbook for Health-EDRM addressing these issues.

Keywords: health emergency and disaster risk management (Health-EDRM); Sendai Framework for Disaster Risk Reduction; WHO Thematic Platform for Health-EDRM; research methods; ethics; glossary

---

1. Introduction

At the Asia Pacific Conference for Disaster Medicine (APCDM) [1], October 2018, an expert meeting to identify key research needs in major research areas was organized by the World Health Organization (WHO) Centre for Health Development (WHO Kobe Centre (WKC), convening the leading experts from Asia Pacific region, WHO, WHO Thematic Platform for Health Emergency and Disaster Risk Management (Health-EDRM) Research Network (TPRN), World Association for Disaster and Emergency Medicine (WADEM). An expert meeting was conducted along with aseries of progresses in scientific aspects of the implementation of the 2015 Sendai Framework on Disaster

Risk Reduction (SFDRR) [2], the resulting document of the Third UN World Conference on Disaster Risk Reduction (WCDRR), included the establishment of TPRN [3,4] and following journal papers on recommended Health-EDRM research activities [5,6]. Through the expert meeting and related review of literature and existing projects and activities, key research needs in five major Health-EDRM research areas were identified.

The Health-EDRM Network identified one major area of work that is important to address was clarity in relevant 'Research Methods and Ethics'. The broad intersection of health and disaster risk reduction has resulted in an area of work now known as Health-EDRM which encompasses emergency and disaster medicine, disaster risk reduction, community health resilience, health system resilience, and impact of changing climate on health. Public health response during and after disasters has traditionally been focused on protecting populations from immediate threats [7]. Health-EDRM research involves the systematic analysis and management of health risks in emergencies and disasters by reducing the health risks and vulnerability. The complexity of undertaking research in disasters, and complying with ethical standards for these research, is critical but often much more difficult to ensure. This paper summarizes the outcome of the discussions and the proposed actions needed to support the delivery of Health-EDRM research.

2. Material and Methods

Prior to the meeting a range of international experts contributed experience-based priority issues in Health-EDRM research, ethics and scientific publication. It is of note that even in 1997, Stallings was able to state that " ... *it is the context of research not the methods that makes disaster research unique*" [8]. The lead discussant, the rapporteur, and the other experts who participated to the discussion primarily aimed to identify priorities in scientific evidence on Research Methods and Ethics in Health Emergency and Disaster Risk Management Research focused on questions and issues to fill these gaps. In addition to identifying knowledge gaps, experts also aimed to assess knowledge-to-practice gaps in order to better integrate current expertise and research in this area into each phase of disaster risk management. Following a preliminary literature review and expert consultations, a series of questions that were thought to be very important to address for building better understanding of research methods and ethics in Health-EDRM included

(a) What are the definitions of research methods and technical terms for Health-EDRM?
(b) How can impact evaluation methods for intervention and qualitative—quantitative mixed methods be standardized?
(c) How can the publication process for Health-EDRM research become more systematic and effective?

Those participated in discussion were leading experts in Health-EDRM as well as country experts in disaster and emergency, and came from multiple disciplines such as public health, emergency medicine, nursing, and health care management. They discussed major issues in Health-EDRM research from practitioner viewpoints and different regional perspectives. Each issue was addressed by active discussion of participants with the aim of addressing priorities and actions on how to progress research and scientific evidence in Health DRM. Interactive dialogues noted simultaneously into minutes of discussion were further analyzed by the moderators into the gaps, proposed mechanism to overcome the gaps and to provide a summary of recommendations.

3. Results and Discussion

Experts from different parts of the globe participated in this thematic group discussion. The findings from this discussion were wide ranging. It was noted that research findings from disaster research is not easily translated into different contexts of the many countries around the world, and there were challenges and difficulties in implementing practices in addressing national health system, cultural and religious issues before, during, and after interventions. These issues were difficult to address without more complete and systematic evidence to inform Health-EDRM policy and practice. Although translating research findings into policy is the ambition of many researchers and practitioners in order to develop evidence-based policies, there are issues of how much researchers can communicate with policy makers in comparison to the opportunities to facilitate policy makers' uptake of research findings. A key strategy to overcome this barrier is stakeholders' involvement and community participation since the development of research ideas in designing phase of the research project. For example, research in disaster affected area might recruit participants who were disasters casualties and there should be rules and regulation especially listing ethical 'don't's such as providing food as an incentive for participation in the research. For instance, food is sometimes used as incentive for the participation in the research, in some context. However, in the disaster and emergency situation, food is the basic need provided as the humanitarian aid regardless of participation in the research. Thus, if food is used as incentives for research recruiting such persons, it might be forcing someone to participate in the research, in the fear that they cannot receive food supply. Therefore, it is not appropriate to use food as incentives in Health-EDRM research.

Thematic discussion in the meeting uncovered five priority areas: (1) the need to harmonize Health-EDRM research with universal terms and definitions via a glossary; (2) mechanisms to facilitate and speed up ethical review process; (3) development of reference materials such as possible consensus statements; (4) increased community participation and stakeholder involvement in generating research ideas and in assessing impact evaluation; and (5) and the urgent need for a textbook for Health-EDRM research addressing these and other issues. Discussions also agreed that there was a need to harmonize definitions in Health-EDRM research with universal terms, and the development of a glossary of definitions. Such a glossary could promote common understanding and common usage of concepts, terms, and aims for Health-EDRM. If undertaken by WHO, the glossary might have the additional advantage of being translated into the WHO official languages. Even though the United Nations Office for Disaster Risk Reduction (UNISDR) convened an Open-ended Intergovernmental Expert Working Group (OIEWG) to report on indicators with recommended terminology relating to disaster risk reduction, which was delivered in 2016 [9], and adopted by the UN General Assembly on 2 February 2017 and updated the 2009 UNISDR Terminology on Disaster Risk Reduction [10]; however, not all the necessary Health-EDRM terms were included in these or other terminologies.

The need to find mechanisms to facilitate and speed up ethical review process was addressed and the need to quicken the review process for disaster research ethics was noted as being complex and very dynamic. A basic requirement was to agree on methodological terms and should reflect research undertaken in the spectrum of disaster chronology such from preparedness and risk reduction, to emergency management, and to post disaster rehabilitation. One key suggestion was the requirement to reduce the review time for ethical approval with, wherever possible, with pre-agreed ethical approval. As Chan et al. (2019) pointed out their recent Lancet editorial that "research stakeholders have a responsibility to protect the interests of communities involved in research, achieving this is rarely straightforward in emergencies" [11]. From the discussion that it would require international consensus among the professionals and researchers, possibly using as good practice models the CONSORT (Consolidated Standards of Reporting Trials) statement for randomized controlled trials [12,13] and STROBE (STrengthening the Reporting of OBservational studies in Epidemiology) statement for cohort studies [14,15]. Additional models of good practice such as the Guidance for Managing Ethical Issues in Infectious Disease Outbreaks [16] and the Health Emergency and Disaster Risk Management fact sheet on ETHICS [17] were thought to be practical and helpful examples. More data on these topics to address Health-EDRM were considered to be of importance. Once a research proposal can fit in a standardized check list, the ethical committee should be able to agree the research proposed via an expedited channel.

Such activities could be part of the development of reference materials such as possible consensus statements. Such consensus statement provide a checklist of methodology details which allows researcher to check the proposal themselves. Ethical committee can quickly assessthe quality assurance and safety through the list, speeding up the approval. Therefore, it is very essential step to develop a consensus for disaster research.

The call for increased community participation and stakeholder involvement in generating research ideas and in assessing impact evaluation was considered and the need to listen to the voice of the affected and their community leaders and local representatives is increasingly critical. However, relatively few Health-EDRM reports on community participation and stakeholder involvement in generating research ideas were shared in the discussion. There are examples of where research to address stakeholder involvement in health research, such as the recent report from Kapiriri (2018) [18], but it is not from emergency or disaster research. Very little has been published definitively on this area.

Much more is described in the quest of methodological rigour for impact evaluation. The experts brain-stormed how can impact evaluation apply quantitative methods in additional to commonly applied case-studies in disaster research.

Impact evaluation is usually applied to see how a research programme works well in a particular setting. It is a term understood readily by multiple stakeholders whereas it dictates how to measure the outcome an intervention in basic research methodology. There are many methodological tools to measure how an intervention brought about changes in comparison to pre-existing situation or in comparison to naïve control group. A proposed intervention should be tested by efficacy and effectiveness trials before it comes into the guidelines and practice. It was considered that the synthesis of evidence would be primarily through the process of systematic reviewing and, if appropriate, modelling and cost effectiveness decision analysis [19]. The efficacy depends on how the intervention is planned to measure (design), how accurate are the measurement tools (validity and reliability) whereas the effectiveness will inform how robust is the intervention in the real world setting. Furthermore, the scalability of intervention will be challenged by the economic, social, and political context and the resource need. It would be important to follow process recommended where possible by organisations and their reports of activities that are already engaged in working in this area such as WHO [20,21], UK Medical Research Council [22], Organisation for Economic Co-operation and Development [23], and the Humanitarian Policy Group at the Overseas Development Institute and its Good Practice Review [24] with its chapter on Monitoring and Evaluation [25,26].

Diverse research methods from case studies, natural experiment designs and randomized controlled trials can be applied in impact monitoring and evaluation. For example, clinical epidemiology is a discipline to determine clinical outcomes applying tools of epidemiology. Likewise, epidemiological tools can be selected to match where and how they would be applied in Health-EDRM research but are often less easy to monitor and evaluate as they are used in more difficult environments. Through the synergy of Health-EDRM experts and the discussion on research methods, designs, and tools, it might be possible to encourage selection and use of more appropriate mechanisms. Events to gather such multidisciplinary professionals such as international workshops are important opportunity to generate the list of strategic research methodology tools. Relatively few resources for disaster risk reduction and management research methods have been identified and some excellent examples are cited below [27–32]. However most of these do not specifically address the full range of Health-EDRM research domains. Therefore, it is considered that there is relatively little currently that reflects the wide needs of Health-EDRM researchers, practitioners, and policy makers. Therefore, a text book linked to a website for easy updating is needed and such a resource could be tentatively entitled "research methods for health emergency and disaster risk management". This would be a rewarding endeavor and would be beneficial to the establishment of the WHO Thematic Platform for Health Emergency and Disaster Risk Management Research Network.

4. Conclusions

It is hoped this paper on key issues in research methods and ethics in health emergency and disaster risk management will contribute to the identification and implementation of concrete solutions that foster the creation and the use of knowledge for research and ethics building resilience before, during, and after disasters. In the discussion, issues were raised on potential gap areas in the disaster research methodology: impact evaluations; Consensus on the definitions; development of common research statements like the CONSORT or STROBE for disaster research; how research findings in disaster research can be translated into different contexts of the many countries around the world; and the need to develop the textbook in disaster research methodology to help guide international researchers.

As for other major Health-EDRM research areas, research and ethics requires collaboration between experts, decision-makers, practitioners, and communities in order to facilitate coordinated response when and where it is most needed. It is critical a text book is created to provide a reference which would be fundamental and global contribution to the establishment of the WHO Thematic Platform for Health Emergency and Disaster Risk Management Research Network.

Author Contributions: Conceptualization, R.K. and V.M.; Methodology, M.N.A. and V.M.; Writing—Original Draft Preparation, M.N.A. and V.M.; Writing—Review & Editing, V.M., M.N.A. and R.K.; Project Administration, R.K.

Acknowledgments: The authors thank all the meeting participants who contributed to achieving the results (alphabetical order of their last name): Jonathan Abrahams (WHO), Francis Archer (Monash University, Australia), Sarah Louise Barber (WHO), Emily YY Chan (The Chinese University of Hong Kong, China), Shinichi Egawa (Tohoku University, Japan), Paul Farrell (WADEM), Teodoro Herbosa (University of the Philippines, Philippines), Sonoe Mashino (University of Hyogo, Japan), Toshiyuki Ojima (Hamamatsu University School of Medicine, Japan), Philip Schluter (University of Canterbury, New Zealand), Shiori Usami (Kumamoto University, Japan).

References

1. Asian Pacific Conference for Disaster Medicine. 2018. Available online: http://www.apcdm2018.org/index.html (accessed on 28 January 2019).
2. Sendai Framework for Disaster Risk Reduction 2015–2030. Available online: https://www.unisdr.org/we/inform/publications/43291 (accessed on 28 January 2019).
3. World Health Organization. WHO Thematic Platform for Health Emergency and Disaster Risk Management. Available online: http://www.who.int/hac/techguidance/preparedness/WHO-Thematic-Platform-Health-EDRM-Terms-Reference-2018.pdf?ua=1 (accessed on 28 January 2019).
4. World Health Organization. WHO Thematic Platform for Health Emergency and Disaster Risk Management Research Network. Available online: http://www.who.int/hac/techguidance/preparedness/WHO-Thematic-Platform-Health-EDRM-Research-Network-2018.pdf?ua=1 (accessed on 3 March 2019).
5. Chan, E.Y.Y.; Murray, V. What are the health research needs for the Sendai Framework. *Lancet* **2017**, *390*, e35–e36. Available online: https://www.thelancet.com/journals/lancet/article/PIIS0140-6736(17)31670-7/fulltext (accessed on 28 January 2019). [CrossRef]
6. Lo, S.T.T.; Chan, E.Y.Y.; Chan, G.K.W.; Murray, V.; Abrahams, J.; Ardalan, A.; Kayano, R.; Yau, J.C.W. Health Emergency and Disaster Risk Management (Health-EDRM): Developing the Research Field within the Sendai Framework Paradigm. *Int. J. Disaster Risk Sci.* **2017**, *8*, 145–149. [CrossRef]
7. Aitsi-Selmi, A.; Murray, V. The Sendai framework: Disaster risk reduction through a health lens. *Bull. World Health Organ.* **2015**, *93*, 362. Available online: https://www.who.int/bulletin/volumes/93/6/15-157362.pdf (accessed on 1 January 2019). [CrossRef] [PubMed]
8. Stallings, R.A. Methods of Disaster Research: Unique or Not? *Int. J. Mass Emerg. Disasters March* **1997**, *15*, 7–19. Available online: http://ijmed.org/articles/408/download/ (accessed on 1 January 2019).
9. United Nations General Assembly. Report of the Open-Ended Intergovernmental Expert Working Group on Indicators and Terminology Relating to Disaster Risk Reduction A/71/644. 2016. Available online: https://www.preventionweb.net/files/50683_oiewgreportenglish.pdf (accessed on 3 March 2019).
10. United Nations International Strategy for Disaster Reduction (UNISDR). UNISDR Terminology on Disaster Risk Reduction. 2009. Available online: https://www.unisdr.org/files/7817_UNISDRTerminologyEnglish.pdf (accessed on 1 January 2019).

11. Chan, E.Y.; Wright, K.; Parker, M. Health-emergency disaster risk management and research ethics. *Lancet* **2019**, *393*, 112–113. [CrossRef]
12. Schulz, K.F.; Altman, D.G.; Moher, D. CONSORT 2010 statement: Updated guidelines for reporting parallel group randomised trials. *BMJ* **2010**, *340*, c332. [CrossRef] [PubMed]
13. CONSORT Website: Consolidated Standards of Reporting Trials and Encompasses Various Initiatives Developed by the CONSORT Group to Alleviate the Problems Arising from Inadequate Reporting of Randomized Controlled Trials. Available online: http://www.consort-statement.org/ (accessed on 29 January 2019).
14. Vandenbroucke, J.P.; von Elm, E.; Altman, D.G.; Gotzsche, P.C.; Mulrow, C.D.; Pocock, S.J.; Poole, C.; Schlesselman, J.J.; Egger, M. Strengthening the Reporting of Observational Studies in Epidemiology (STROBE): Explanation and elaboration. *Int. J. Surg.* **2014**, *12*, 1500–1524. [CrossRef] [PubMed]
15. STROBE Website: Strengthening the Reporting of Observational Studies in Epidemiology (STROBE) Statement: Guidelines for Reporting Observational Studies. 2014. Available online: https://www.strobe-statement.org/index.php?id=strobe-home (accessed on 29 January 2019).
16. World Health Organization. WHO Guidelines on Ethical Issues in Public Health Surveillance. 2017. Available online: http://apps.who.int/iris/bitstream/10665/255721/1/9789241512657-eng.pdf (accessed on 20 January 2019).
17. World Health Organization; Public Health England. Health Emergency and Disaster Risk Management ETHICS. 2017. Available online: https://www.who.int/hac/techguidance/preparedness/risk-management-ethics-december2017.pdf?ua=1 (accessed on 20 January 2019).
18. Kapiriri, L. Stakeholder involvement in health research priority setting in low income countries: The case of Zambia. *Res. Involv. Engagem.* **2018**, *4*, 41. [CrossRef] [PubMed]
19. National Institute for Health and Care Excellence (NICE). Research Recommendations Interim Process and Methods Guide. 2015. Available online: https://www.nice.org.uk/Media/Default/About/what-we-do/Research-and-development/Research-Recommendation-Process-and-Methods-Guide-2015.pdf (accessed on 29 January 2019).
20. World Health Organization. The WHO Strategy on Research for Health. 2012. Available online: https://www.who.int/phi/WHO_Strategy_on_research_for_health.pdf (accessed on 3 March 2019).
21. World Health Organization. *Monitoring and Evaluating Digital Health Interventions: A Practical Guide to Conducting Research and Assessment*; World Health Organization: Geneva, Switzerland, 2016; Available online: https://apps.who.int/iris/bitstream/handle/10665/252183/?sequence=1 (accessed on 1 January 2019).
22. Medical Research Council. Developing and Evaluating Complex Interventions. 2019. Available online: https://mrc.ukri.org/documents/pdf/complex-interventions-guidance/ (accessed on 20 January 2019).
23. Organisation for Economic Co-operation and Development (OECD). Outline of Principles of Impact Evaluation. 2006. Available online: http://www.oecd.org/dac/evaluation/dcdndep/37671602.pdf (accessed on 20 January 2019).
24. Twigg, J. Disaster Risk Reduction Good Practice Review. Humanitarian Policy Group, Overseas Development Institute, 2015. Available online: https://goodpracticereview.org/wp-content/uploads/2015/10/GPR-9-web-string-1.pdf (accessed on 20 January 2019).
25. Twigg, J. Disaster Risk Reduction Good Practice Review. Chapter 18 Monitoring and Evaluation, Humanitarian Policy Group, Overseas Development Institute, 2015. Available online: https://goodpracticereview.org/wp-content/uploads/2015/10/GPR_9_Chapter_18.pdf (accessed on 20 January 2019).
26. World Health Organization. *WHO Evaluation Practice Handbook*; World Health Organization: Geneva, Switzerland, 2013; ISBN 978-92-4-154868-7. Available online: https://apps.who.int/iris/bitstream/handle/10665/96311/9789241548687_eng.pdf?sequence= (accessed on 20 January 2019).
27. Rodríguez, H.; Donner, W.; Trainor, J.E. (Eds.) *Handbook of Disaster Research*, 2nd ed.; Springer: New York, NY, USA, 2018; Available online: https://www.springer.com/gb/book/9783319632537 (accessed on 1 January 2019).
28. Oliver-Smith, A.; Alcántara-Ayala, I.; Burton, I.; Lavell, A. *Forensic Investigations of Disasters (FORIN): A Conceptual Framework and Guide to Research*; IRDR FORIN Publication: Beijing, China, 2016.
29. Stallings, R.A. Methods of Disaster Research. Xlibris, 2003. Available online: https://www.xlibris.com/bookstore/bookdetail.aspx?bookid=SKU-0016862003 (accessed on 1 January 2019).

30. Phillips, B.D. *Qualitative Disaster Research*; Oxford University Press: Oxford, UK, 2014; Available online: https://global.oup.com/academic/product/qualitative-disaster-research-9780199796175?cc=gb&lang=en& (accessed on 29 January 2019).
31. Norris, F.; Galea, S.; Friedman, M.; Watson, P. *Methods for Disaster Mental Health Research*; Guildford Press: New, York, NY, USA, 2006; Available online: https://zodml.org/sites/default/files/Methods_for_Disaster_Mental_Health_Research.pdf (accessed on 29 January 2019).
32. Oakes, J.M.; Kaufman, J.S. (Eds.) *Methods in Social Epidemiology*; John Wiley & Sons: Hoboken, NJ, USA, 2017; Volume 16.

Health Vulnerability Index for Disaster Risk Reduction: Application in Belt and Road Initiative (BRI) Region

Emily Yang Ying Chan [1,2,3,*], Zhe Huang [1], Holly Ching Yu Lam [1], Carol Ka Po Wong [1] and Qiang Zou [4]

1 Collaborating Centre for Oxford University and CUHK for Disaster and Medical Humanitarian Response (CCOUC), JC (Jockey Club) school of Public Health and Primary Care, Faculty of Medicine, Chinese University of Hong Kong, Hong Kong, China; huangzhe@cuhk.edu.hk (Z.H.); hollylam@cuhk.edu.hk (H.C.Y.L.); wongcarol@cuhk.edu.hk (C.K.P.W.)

2 Nuffield Department of Medicine, University of Oxford, Oxford OX3 7BN, UK

3 François-Xavier Bagnoud Center for Health & Human Rights, Harvard University, Boston, MA 02138, USA

4 Institute of Mountain Hazards and Environment, Chinese Academy of Science, Chengdu 610041, China; zouqiang@imde.ac.cn

* Correspondence: emily.chan@cuhk.edu.hk

Abstract: Despite the importance of health vulnerability in disaster risk assessment, most of the existing disaster vulnerability indicators only emphasize economic and social vulnerability. Important underlying health risks such as non-communicable disease are not included in vulnerability measures. A three-phase methodology approach was used to construct a disaster risk model that includes a number of key health indicators which might be missing in global disaster risk analysis. This study describes the development of an integrated health vulnerability index and explains how the proposed vulnerability index may be incorporated into an all-hazard based disaster risk index in the Belt and Road Initiative (BRI), also known as the "Silk Road Economic Belt", region. Relevant indicators were identified and reviewed in the published literature in PubMed/Medline. A two-stage dimension reduction statistical method was used to determine the weightings of relevant dimensions to the construction of the overall vulnerability index. The proposed final health vulnerability index included nine indicators, including the proportion of the population below 15 and above 65 years, under-five mortality ratio, maternal mortality ratio, tuberculosis prevalence, age-standardized raised blood pressure, physician ratio, hospital bed ratio, and coverage of the measles-containing-vaccine first-dose (MCV1) and diphtheria tetanus toxoid and pertussis (DTP3) vaccines. This proposed index, which has a better reflection of the health vulnerability in communities, may serve as a policy and implementation tool to facilitate the capacity-building of Health-Emergency Disaster Risk management (Health-EDRM).

Keywords: Health vulnerability; Health-EDRM; disaster risk; Silk Road Economic Belt; map; Belt and Road Initiative

---

1. Introduction

Disasters have brought huge losses in human health and the economy globally. According to Economic Losses, Poverty & Disasters, 1998–2017 issued by the Centre for Research on the Epidemiology of Disasters and United Nations Office for Disaster Risk Reduction in 2018, climate-related and geophysical disasters alone have taken lives from 1.3 million people, and have affected 4.4 billion people in the world between 1998–2017. The report also highlighted a global direct economic loss of USD 2908 billion due to disasters within the same period [1]. Asia, similar to previous years, suffered from the highest disaster occurrence (more than 40% of the total) [2], while China, India, Indonesia, and the Philippines were four of the top five countries that were most frequently hit by natural disasters over the last decade [3]. Due to climate change, both the frequency and intensity of disasters have been predicated to increase in the 21st century [4]. Relevant risk assessment tools and disaster risk reduction plans are important for saving lives and reducing losses in the future.

Understanding disaster risk in all its dimensions is the first priority for Disaster Risk Reduction action in the Sendai Framework, which was the first major agreement endorsed by the United Nations (UN) General Assembly on Disaster Risk Reduction for policies and practices for disaster risk management [5]. Disaster risk can be conceptualized as a function of hazard, exposure, and vulnerability [6]. According to UNISDR [7], risk is defined as the harmful consequences resulting from interactions between hazards, exposure, and vulnerable conditions. Hazard refers to dangerous phenomena that may cause negative health impacts; exposure refers to the people who are present in hazard zones and subject to potential health losses; vulnerability refers to the characteristics and circumstances of a community that make it susceptible to the damaging effects of a hazard. Disaster risk assessment can be understood as quantifying these three components among the population.

There are major technical gaps in how to describe vulnerability, particularly to health risks, when constructing disaster risk indexes [8]. Existing vulnerability indicators/indexes mostly focus on economic and social vulnerability [9–11]. Most health vulnerability indexes were developed after 2010, and were related to human health vulnerability toward climate-related disasters such as heat wave [12–14], flooding [15], dengue fever [16], and climate change [17]. In addition, as the data used for index construction were largely based on the country's own capacity in data collection, multi-country comparisons are often difficult, as countries may have different data collection methods and capacities. The Index For Risk Management (INFORM), a collaborative work with the United Nations, and the World Risk Index, a joint work with the Integrated Research on Disaster Risk (IRDR), are sophisticated global disaster risk indexes that have accounted for health vulnerability [18,19]. However, the current indexes do not include important health-affecting factors such as chronic diseases. Chronic disease is an important aspect to be considered in disaster risk management, as discontinuous treatment and medicine, which is possible during a disaster event, can lead to adverse health consequences among chronic disease patients. For instance, the provision of insulin may sustain the well-being and survival of diabetes patients [20].

Under the influence of globalization, the spread of health risks is borderless, and the prevention and control of health emergencies (e.g., disasters) need to be managed collaboratively. China's Belt and Road Initiative (BRI), also known as the "Silk Road Economic Belt", was initiated in 2013 and aimed to connect the Asian, European, and African continents and their adjacent seas, and establish and strengthen partnerships among the countries along the Belt and Road [21]. Among these BRI countries, various types of disasters occur frequently, and the widespread damage and destruction caused by disasters seriously disrupts the functioning of a society, and poses a major socio-economic development challenge for the Belt and Road Initiative region. The BRI also provides a health cooperation platform to handle regional health emergencies, offers medical assistance, and disseminates experience in the field of health care [22]. Understanding disaster risk and vulnerability for the countries along the Belt and Road is crucial for resource allocation. Yet, current available health vulnerability indexes may not apply to the countries within Belt and Road Initiative.

Health-Emergency Disaster Risk Management (Health-EDRM) is an academic paradigm representing the intersection of health and disaster risk reduction that covers the systematic analysis and management of health risks surrounding emergencies and disasters [23]. This study falls into the primary Health-EDRM intervention category (prevention/preparedness) in the system (country) level.

The objective of this paper is to describe the development of a health vulnerability index that aims to be incorporated into the vulnerability index, and might be applied to the use of the all-hazard based disaster risk index in the BRI region. The developed index described in this study used open access data and proposed indicators that are available in most countries and make disaster risk comparison between countries possible. The proposed method can also be adopted by regions or populations that were not included in this study. The findings from this study provide evidence to support disaster risk reduction in the BRI regions, and serve as a basis for the development of a population-based disaster risk assessment tool.

2. Materials and Methods

A three-phase methodology approach was used to develop the final disaster risk model. Phase 1 of the approach focuses on the development of the health vulnerability index, which includes an extensive literature review to identify the relevant published indicators to construct health vulnerability. Phase 2 involves a two-stage dimension reduction statistical method to identify the weighting for the indicators that were included for the health vulnerability index development. Phase 3 aims to create the final disaster risk index by combining the three main component indexes (health vulnerability index, exposure, and hazard index), which can be described in the following equation: Risk = Exposure × Hazard × Vulnerability [6]. The health vulnerability index is combined with existing exposure and hazard indexes to form a disaster risk index at the national level. The exposure and hazard indexes were based and accessed through the Institute of Mountain Hazards and Environment at the Chinese Academy of Science (http://english.imde.cas.cn). As the mechanisms and the development of the two indexes were out of the scope of this study, they were not included in this paper's discussion.

2.1. *Phase I*

Data Scoping and Variable Selection

Variable selection criteria include: (1) any indicator that is conceptually relevant to health vulnerability or may capture the Health-EDRM risks of the community; (2) indicators that have been identified/suggested in relevant literatures or organizations (e.g., the World Health Organization (WHO), UN, INFORM model [18] and World Risk Index [19]), and (3) indicators that are available for open access from reliable sources (e.g., WHO and the World Bank) for all of the study regions. Since subsequent factor analysis cannot be performed with missing values, countries with missing values were excluded in the subsequent analysis. The countries/areas along the BRI region and countries/areas included in the analysis were listed in the supplementary material A1.

2.2. *Phase II*

Statistical Model for the Health Vulnerability Index

As this study made no assumption on the weighting for indicators, in order to determine the weightings and explore the importance of the underlying dimensions to the overall vulnerability, a two-stage dimension reduction statistical method was used. This method also increases robustness [10] and allows monitoring changes in the weighting of indicators over time. In stage one, factor analysis (FA) was used as the primary statistical procedure for dimension reduction. The observed and correlated indicators were assumed to be adequately explained by a lower number of unobserved and uncorrelated factors. Stage two modeling was based on the result of FA; the selected health indicators were used to produce a more compact representation of the indicators (factors).

Stage 1: Selected indicators are normalized and included in the FA analysis. The matrix of factor loadings was estimated via the maximum likelihood method, and the number of factors that is extracted should contribute cumulatively to the explanation of the overall variance by more than 60% [24]. The Chi-square test was used to examine whether the number of factors, k, are sufficient to account for the observed covariance [25]. A non-significant Chi-square test result ($p \geq 0.05$) indicates that k is sufficient to explain the observed covariance. The explanation power increases when k increases. To obtain the most efficient model, the smallest k that yielded a non-significant Chi-square test was chosen. The initial k tried was one, and then, k was increased by one at a time. Then, the process is repeated until the p-value of the Chi-square test ≥ 0.05 [25]. Factors identified from FA are sometimes expressed as a compound with a relative large number of non-zero weighting indicators, which may make factor interpretation hard. To make interpretations of factors easier, Varimax rotation [26] was conducted to obtain as few large loadings and as many near-zero loadings as possible.

Stage 2: The development of the Health Vulnerability Index (HVI) is based on the latent factors derived from the FA. Each latent factor has factor loading on every health indicator, measuring the correlation between the health factor and the health indicator. The construction of the weights of the selected health indicators is from the rotated matrix of factor loadings [24,27]: (1) the proportion on each latent factor of the total unit variance was extracted; (2) the intermediate weights of all of the health indicators were calculated from the factor loadings corresponding to the latent factor; (3) the proportion on each latent factor is multiplied by the intermediate weights of all the health indicators on each latent factor to generate the weights for all the selected health indicators. Finally, the weights were multiplied by the corresponding standardized health indicator, and were added together for every country's HVI. A higher value indicates a more vulnerable country. The HVI value of each country involved was categorized into five HVI clusters using the equal interval method for data presentation in the form of a vulnerability map. A five-level scale was selected, as it provides a good balance between risk-level differentiation and clarity, and has been widely adopted in risk-level presentations [28,29]. R version 3.4.1 and ArcMap version 10.4.1 were used.

2.3. *Phase III*

Disaster Risk Index Model

Exposure and Hazard

The exposure and hazard index were provided by the working dataset of The Institute of Mountain Hazards and Environment at The Chinese Academy of Science. The exposure index was estimated by using the population density data from the Socioeconomic Data and Applications Center [30] as a proxy. For hazard, the frequency of natural disaster was applied. Both indexes were in a pixel-based format, and can be illustrated using a map.

Disaster Risk Index

Raster values from the Exposure index, the Hazard index, and the Vulnerability index were multiplied to generate the final Risk index. Since both the exposure and the hazard indexes are pixel-based data, the vulnerability index was transformed from the country-based format to the pixel-based using ArcMap before combining with the other two indexes to form the final risk index.

$$\text{Calculation of Risk (Risk} = \text{Exposure} \times \text{Hazard} \times \text{Vulnerability)} \quad (1)$$

Logarithm transformations were applied for skewed data, including the exposure index and the hazard index. The log-transformed indexes and the vulnerability index were then transformed to a 0–1 scale using min–max normalization. The final disaster risk index was calculated by multiplying the three transformed components with equal weight (Formula (1)) [18,19]. The results were presented in the form of map in a scale with five risk levels.

3. Results

3.1. *Key Indicators of Vulnerability*

Based on the three evaluation criteria, nine health indicators were identified and included in the final index development. Table 1 describes the key health indicators included.

Table 1. Key indicators of health vulnerability and their relevance.

Dimension of Health Vulnerability	Indicator	Conceptual Relevance to Health Vulnerability
Vulnerable age [a]	1. Population ages 0–14 and population ages 65 and above (% of total)	Extreme age groups (children and elderly) are known to be more vulnerable to health risks and less likely to be resilient when a disaster strikes. This is an important component in the "dependency ratio". They are more likely to accumulate post-disaster health and service needs.
Premature mortality [b]	2. Under-five mortality rate (probability of dying by age five per 1000 live births)	Leading indicator of health in the United Nation (UN)'s Sustainable Development Goals (SDGs). It is closely linked to maternal health.
Preventable mortality [b]	3. Maternal mortality ratio (per 100,000 live births)	Leading indicator of health in the UN's Sustainable Development Goals (SDGs). In addition to preventable deaths, this indicator reflects the capacity of health systems to effectively prevent and address the complications occurring during pregnancy and childbirth.
Vaccination gap for measles [b]	4. Measles-containing-vaccine first-dose (MCV1) immunization coverage gap among one-year-olds (%)	Standard Expanded Program on Immunization (EPI) for common preventable Childhood Communicable Diseases for children <one year old. Coverage may be used to monitor immunization services as well as guide disease eradication and elimination efforts, and are a good indicator of health system performance. MCV1: Measles is one of the most contagious and mortality-causing diseases in displaced camps. DTP3: Tetanus is common preventable infection associated with injury/wound.
Vaccination gap for diphtheria, tetanus, and pertussis [b]	5. Diphtheria tetanus toxoid and pertussis (DTP3) immunization coverage gap among 1-year-olds (%)	
Chronic diseases status [b]	6. Raised blood pressure (SBP $\geq$140 OR DBP $\geq$90), age-standardized (%)	A proxy indicator for chronic non-communicable disease. Hypertension and heart disease are some of the leading causes of mortality and morbidity globally. Disease status and potential activity limitations among adults can impair one's ability to prepare, respond, or recover from a disaster.
Infectious disease [b]	7. Incidence of tuberculosis (per 100,000 population per year)	Tuberculosis (TB) is the second leading infectious cause of death, and one of the most burden-inflicting diseases in the world. SDGs include ending the TB epidemic by 2030. The incidence of tuberculosis gives an indication of the burden of TB in a population.
Coping capacity [b]	8. Hospital beds (per 10,000 population)	Health systems resources indicate the level of access to care and the provision of quality medical care, which are highly correlated with live-saving and health status.
	9. Physicians' density (per 1000 population)	

Source: [a] Data collected from the World Bank; [b] Data collected from the World Health Organization. DBP: diastolic blood pressure; SBP: systolic blood pressure.

The Health Vulnerability Index was constructed for the 147 countries along the Belt and Road region. Indicators one, six, and seven are related to population structure and health status; indicators four and five are used to monitor immunization services, which are good indictors of health system performance; indicators two and three are leading indicators of the level of child and maternal health, as well as the overall development in countries; and indictors eight and nine measure the availability of healthcare, and are important indicators of disaster coping capacity. The correlations between the nine health indicators were shown in Figure 1. All of the correlations presented are statistically significant (all p-values < 0.01).

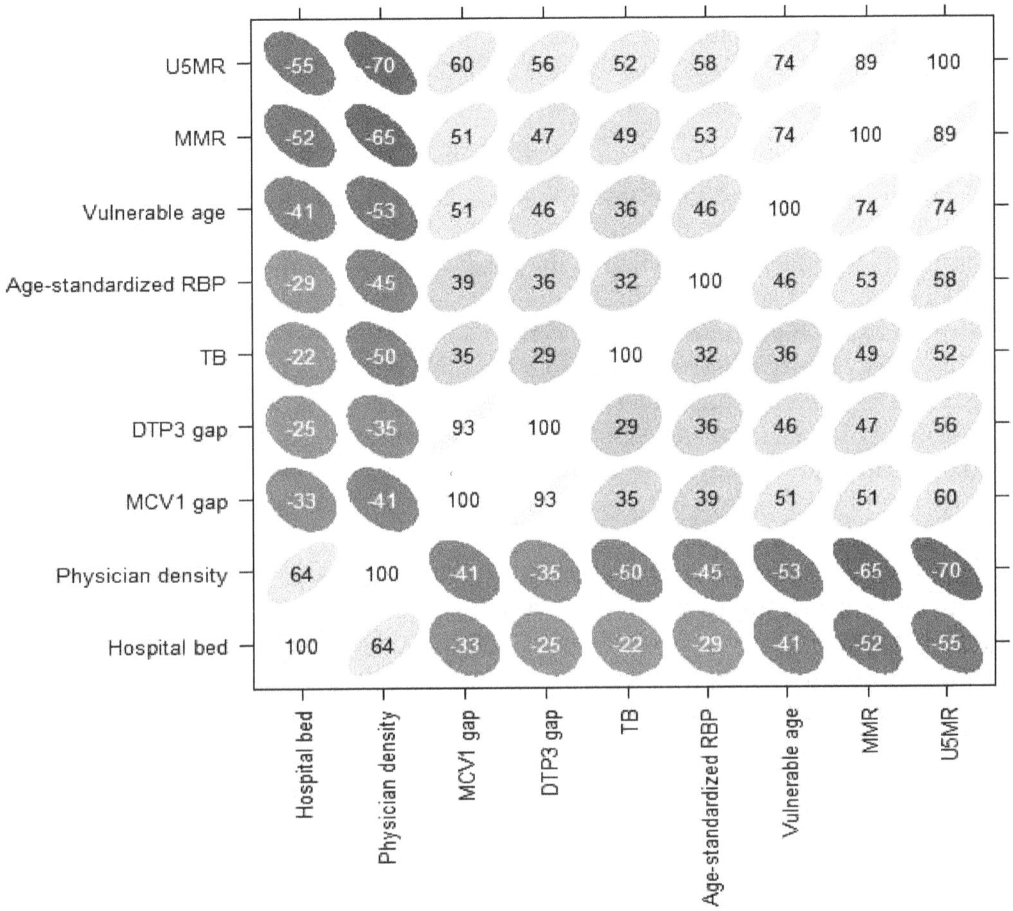

Figure 1. Correlation matrix of the proposed nine health indicators. Note: The figure depicts each correlation by an ellipse whose shape tends toward a line with a slope of one (or −1) for correlation coefficients near one (or −1), and toward a circle for a correlation coefficient near zero. In addition, 100 times the correlation coefficient is printed inside the ellipse (significance level at $\alpha = 0.05$).

3.2. *Underlying Dimensions of Health Vulnerability*

The results of the Chi-square test for the sufficiency of the number of factors suggested that a three-factor solution was adequate to account for the observed covariances in the data among the 147 countries. Both of the eigenvalues of the three-factor solution were larger than one, and the three factors counted for about 71% of the total variance. Factor loadings after rotation are shown in Figure 2.

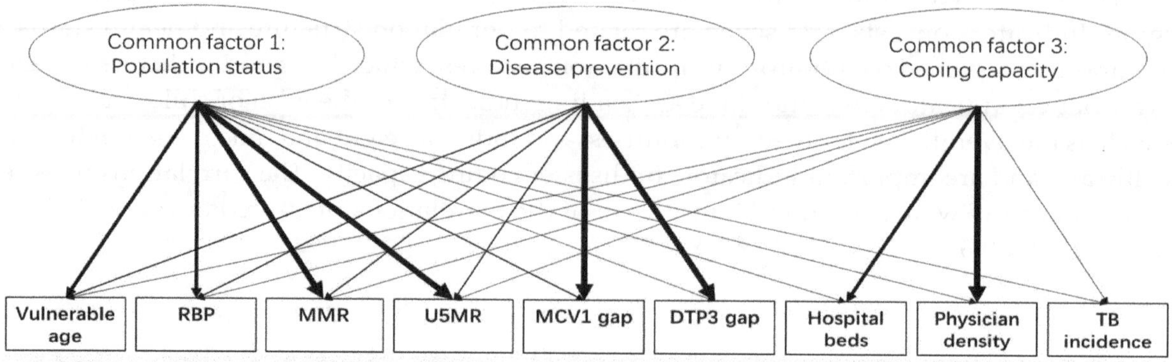

	Vulnerable age	RBP	MMR	U5MR	MCV1 gap	DTP3 gap	Hospital beds	Physician density	TB incidence
Factor 1	0.67	0.47	0.84	0.80	0.29	0.26	-0.34	-0.34	0.37
Factor 2	0.28	0.22	0.22	0.32	0.92	0.90	-0.13	-0.15	0.18
Factor 3	0.28	0.28	0.35	0.41	0.19	0.14	-0.55	-0.93	0.38

Figure 2. Factor loadings of the three latent factors. Note: Factor loadings are printed under the corresponding indicator. They are also indicated by the thickness of the arrow linking the factor and the indicator: the thicker the arrow, the higher the factor loading. Arrows are not shown if the absolute value of the factor loading is less than 0.2. Vulnerable age: people aged 0–14 or/and 65+ (%); RBP: Age-standardized raised blood pressure prevalence (%); MMR: Maternal mortality ratio (per 100,000 live births); U5MR: Under-five mortality rate (per 1000 live births); MCV1 gap: MCV1 Coverage Gap (%); DTP3 gap: DTP3 Coverage Gap (%); Hospital beds: Hospital beds density (per 10,000 population); Physician density: Physicians density (per 1000 population); TB incidence: Incidence of tuberculosis (per 100,000 population).

Since factor one is dominated by the maternal mortality ratio (per 100,000 live births) (MMR, 0.84) and the under-five mortality rate (per 1000 live births) (U5MR, 0.80), and moderately affected by vulnerable age (0.67) and age-standardized raised blood pressure prevalence (RBP) (0.47), this factor was labeled the "population status" factor. The second factor has its highest loadings on the measles-containing-vaccine first-dose (MCV1) gap (0.92) and diphtheria tetanus toxoid and pertussis (DTP3) gap (0.90), which was labeled the "disease prevention" factor. The third factor was highly correlated with physician density (0.92) and moderately with hospital beds (0.90), so it was labeled the "coping capacity" factor.

3.3. *Factor Scores of Countries*

The estimated scores of factors one to three for each country were calculated and categorized into five levels, as shown in Figure 3. Considering factor one, which reflects population status, Sierra Leone, Chad, and the Central African Republic are the most vulnerable countries, whilst Ukraine was shown to be the least vulnerable among all of the studied countries. For the second factor, Equatorial Guinea and Ukraine are prominent, because they had low MCV1 and DTP3 immunization coverage. For factor three, Thailand, the Solomon Islands, and Indonesia were at the highest end of the scale.

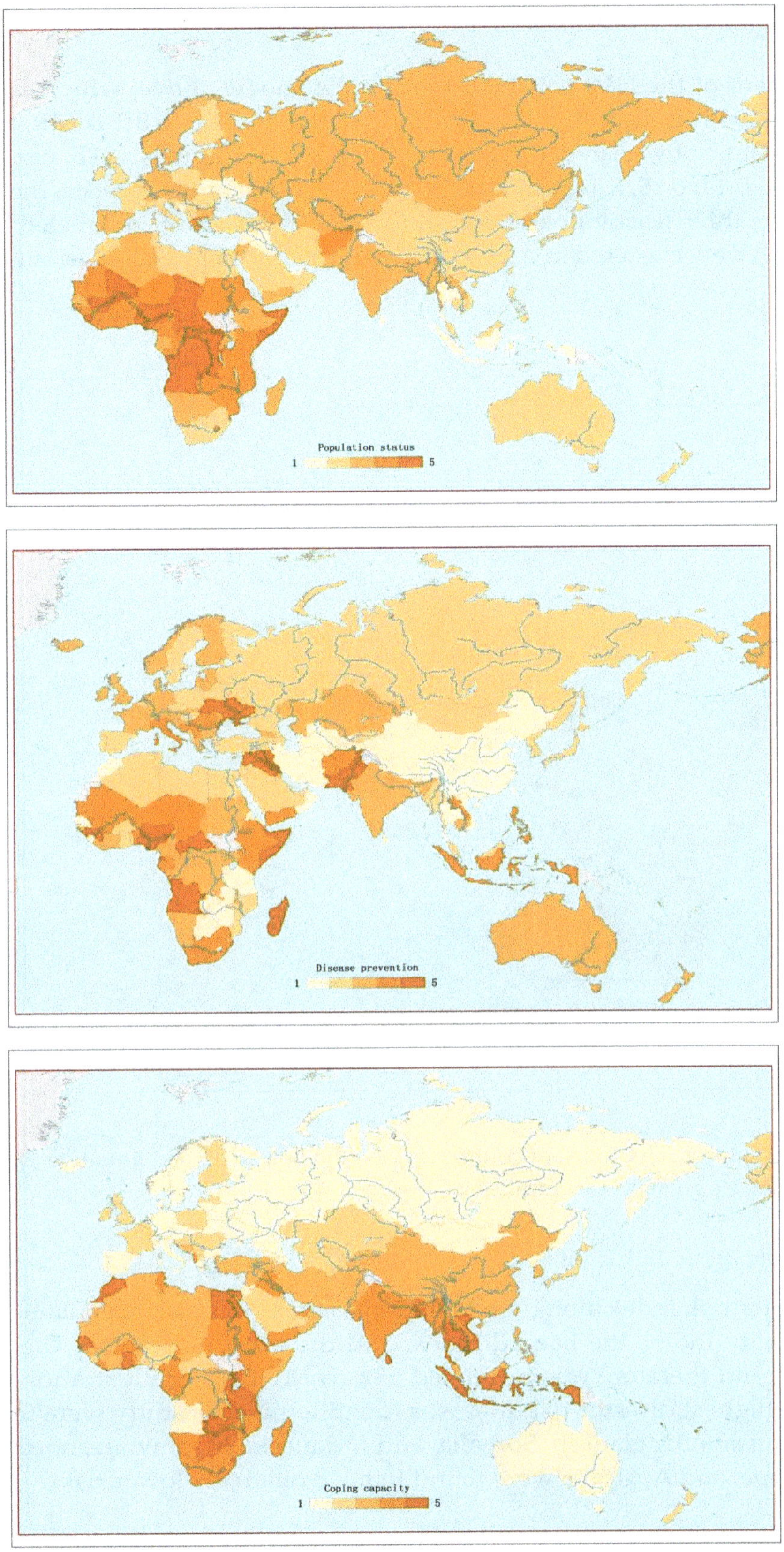

Figure 3. Factor scores of countries along the Belt and Road Initiative (BRI) region. Note: deeper color indicates a higher factor score and greater vulnerability.

3.4. *Health Vulnerability Index of Countries*

The development of the HVI was based on the FA model above, which captured the relative weights of the six health indicators. Weights for vulnerable age, RBP, MMR, U5MR, MCV1 gap, DTP3 gap, hospital beds, physician density, and incidence of tuberculosis (TB, per 100,000 population) were 0.10, 0.05, 0.14, 0.14, 0.15, 0.14, 0.07, 0.16, and 0.05, respectively. Greece, the Republic of Korea, and Belarus were the three least vulnerable countries, whereas countries labeled in the darkest color (the most vulnerable) were clustered in Africa, such as Somalia, the Central African Republic, and Chad (Figure 4).

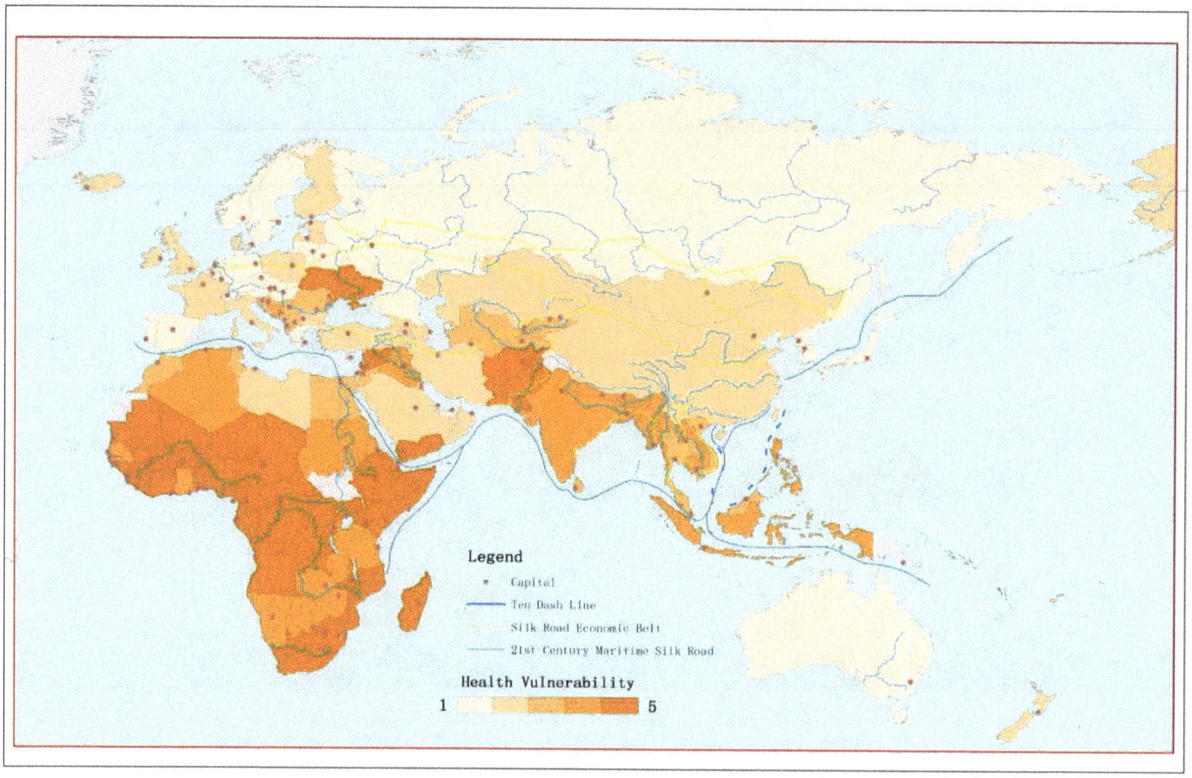

Figure 4. Health Vulnerability Index of countries along the Belt and Road Initiative (BRI) region. Note: deeper color indicates greater vulnerability.

3.5. *Disaster Risk Mapping in Silk Road*

The final disaster risk index along the Belt and Road region were calculated by combining the proposed vulnerability index, the hazard index, and the exposure index. The final index was in pixel-based format, and therefore was presented in a world map for illustration (Figure 5). The top five areas with the highest disaster risk that was identified in this study were in locations near the Philippines, Afghanistan, Bangladesh, Somalia, and Indonesia. Meanwhile, northwest China, North Africa, eastern Europe, and Australia were found to have relatively lower risks.

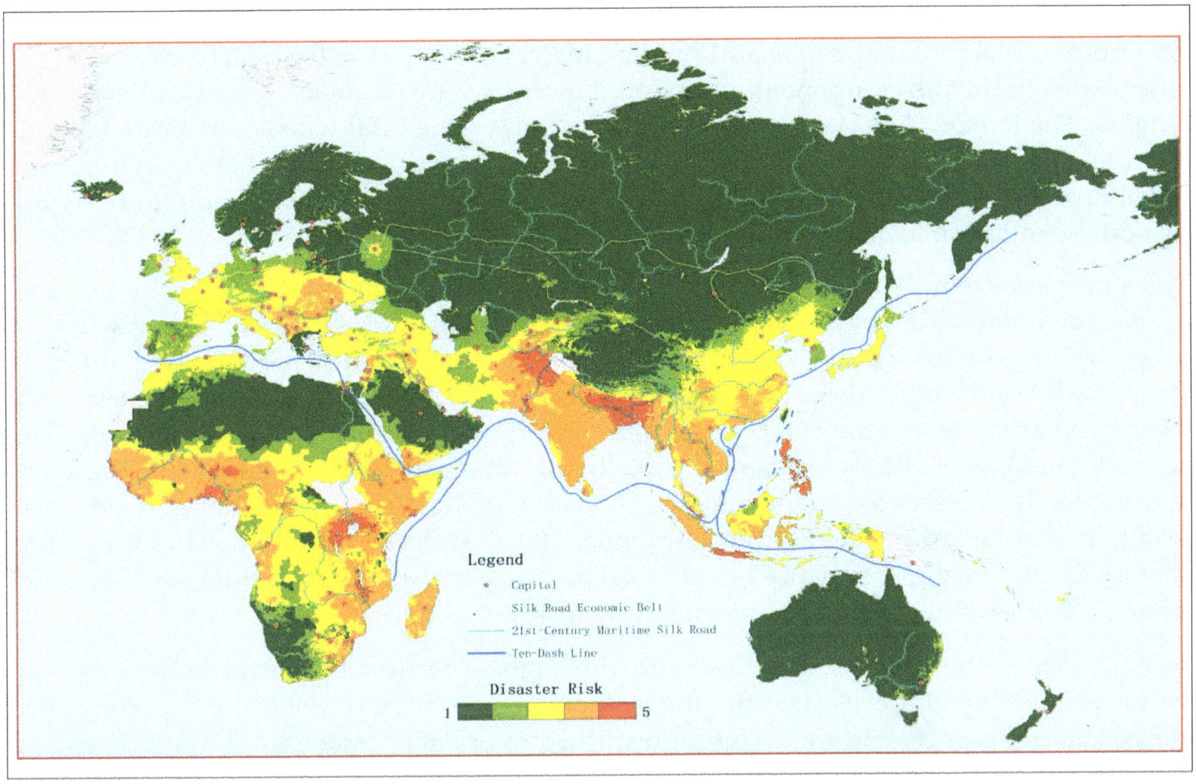

Figure 5. Health disaster risk of countries along the Belt and Road Initiative (BRI) region.

4. Discussion

This paper presents a three-phase methodology approach for disaster risk assessment that incorporated health vulnerability dimensions into an existing hazard-based disaster risk map development. The proposed health vulnerability assessment index covers seven health dimensions, including infectious disease, chronic disease, maternity, under five years old, healthcare services, immunization, and the dependency ratio. Under these seven dimensions, nine indicators were used for formulating the vulnerability index, namely: (1) proportion of population below 15 years and above 65 years, (2) under-five mortality ratio, (3) maternal mortality ratio, (4) prevalence of tuberculosis, (5) the age-standardized raised blood pressure, (6) physician ratio, (7) hospital bed ratio, and (8) coverage of the MCV1 and (9) DTP3 vaccines. Then, the vulnerability index that was formed was combined with an existing disaster risks index from the Institute of Mountain Hazards and Environment at The Chinese Academy of Science.

Based on the formula established in this study and the public data mentioned in the Methods session, Greece, the Republic of Korea, and Belarus were found to be the three least vulnerable countries, while Somalia, the Central African Republic, and Chad were the three most vulnerable countries. After combining the vulnerability index with the exposure and hazard indexes, areas close to the Philippines, Afghanistan, Bangladesh, Somalia, and Indonesia were shown to have the highest disaster risk among the 147 study countries along the BRI region.

The Index For Risk Management (INFORM) and the World Risk Index are global disaster risk indexes that have incorporated health related components for vulnerability. INFORM is a global risk assessment index that is a collaboration of the Inter-Agency Standing Committee Task Team for Preparedness and Resilience and the European Commission and is adopted in the Global Risk Map (https://globalriskmap.terria.io/About.html) (including 190 countries). These included tuberculosis prevalence, HIV prevalence, malaria death rate, and under-five mortality as vulnerability indicators, and have included physician density as a capacity-coping indicator. The World Risk Index (171 countries considered) presented by Birkmann and Welle, and the Integrated Research on Disaster Risk (IRDR) team [19], have combined susceptibility, lack of coping, and adaptive capacity within vulnerability. They considered a dependency ratio for susceptibility, physicians, and hospital beds ratio for coping capacity, and private and public medical expenditure for adaptive capacity. Table 2 below compares the health components considered in the two mentioned indexes and those included in this index. The INFORM model and the Word Risk Index were built with sophisticated calculations and variables from different aspects in risk assessments such as health-related components, economic status, political environment, and infrastructure. Yet, many important health vulnerability burdens such as non-communicable diseases were not included.

The study aims to advance the current disaster risk assessment to include health vulnerability, which will inevitably affect population vulnerability in times of crisis. Thus, the discussion here focused on health-related components. The index proposed in this study has included indicator(s) of seven important health components in disaster risk assessment. Specifically, although chronic diseases have been cited as the most important causes of mortality and morbidity [31], attention has yet to be placed on global disaster risk assessment. People living with chronic diseases usually highly rely on long-term medicine for disease management. Unstable medicine access during and after disasters may lead to preventable adverse health consequences for the affected individual and the community. Considering the increasing prevalence of chronic diseases globally, related factors are suggested to be included as a vulnerability indicators in estimating disaster risks.

Table 3 shows the top 10 countries with the highest vulnerability/lowest coping capacity obtained from the three indexes. Despite the lack of consideration of the socio-economic, political, and infrastructural aspects and the different health components considered in the proposed index, five out of the 10 countries also appeared in top 10 from the other two indexes. This suggested that the health dimension is a strong determinant for disaster risk vulnerability. It is of note that although South Sudan was shown to be the most vulnerable with least coping capacity in the INFORM model, due to the missing data for South Sudan in the dataset that was used in this study (WHO and the World Bank), South Sudan was not included in this analysis. Ukraine was the most vulnerable country in Europe according to this study. Its vulnerability was mainly due to the country's low vaccination rate, which was almost the lowest among all of the studied countries in the dataset. Since this study only accounted for health-related aspects calculating vulnerabilities, rather than other factors such as economic and political factors, Ukraine was found to be more vulnerable for disaster risk compared to the INFORM and the World Risk Indexes. The relatively higher coping capacity for European countries might reflect the better socio-economic status in these countries.

Vulnerability made substantial contributions to understandings and conceptualizations of disaster risk. When populations are exposed to natural disasters, vulnerable groups such as young children, older people, and people with mobility problems have more difficulties in evacuations, and might have a higher immediate risk of injuries. After extreme natural events, people might lose their homes and have to stay closely together in temporary shelters where hygiene and living conditions are usually compromised. In communities with low vaccination rates, outbreaks of infectious diseases might happen. Chronic diseases, as well as mental and psychological problems, also create health concerns and add extra stress to the healthcare system. Efficient medical services are important for handling immediate and indirect health needs in affected areas. Delayed or insufficient medical support to the affected people would increase fatality and morbidity. This could be due to the non-perfect healthcare system in local areas with poor coping capacity. Thus, this study proposed to include health vulnerability in estimating disaster risks. The results of this study have shown that populations with higher vulnerability were under higher overall risks than populations with lower vulnerability, given that they have comparable hazards and exposures. For example, both Japan and Bangladesh were prone to earthquakes (hazard), and were densely populated (exposure). However, after considering the vulnerability index proposed in this study, area near Bangladesh has a higher overall disaster risk than Japan.

Table 2. Health-related components considered in the Index For Risk Management (INFORM) model, the World Risk Index, and the index developed in this study.

Components	INFORM	World Risk Index	The Proposed Index
Infectious diseases	Tuberculosis prevalence		Tuberculosis prevalence
	Estimate % of adults (>15) living with HIV		
	Malaria death rate		
Chronic diseases			Age-standardized raised blood pressure
Maternal outcome	Maternal mortality		Maternal mortality
Children under five	Under-five mortality		Under five mortality
	Malnutrition in children under five		
Medical services and access	Physician ratio	Physicians ratio	Physicians ratio
		Hospital beds ratio	Hospital beds ratio
	Per capita expenditure on private and public health care	Public medical expenditure; private medical expenditure	
Immunization	Measles immunization coverage		Coverage of two the MCV1 and DTP3 vaccine
Dependency ratio		Proportion of population <15 years old and >65 years old	Proportion of population <15 years old and >65 years old

Table 3. The top 10 countries with the highest vulnerability/lowest coping capacity from the INFORM model, the World Risk Index, and the proposed index developed in this study.

Top 10 Countries/Regions with Highest Vulnerability/Capacity	INFORM		World Risk Index	The Proposed Index
	Coping Capacity	Vulnerability	Vulnerability Including Susceptibility, Coping Capacities, and Adaptive Capacities	Vulnerability
1	**South Sudan**	**South Sudan**	**Chad**	**Somalia**
2	**Somalia**	**Somalia**	Eritrea	**Central African Republic**
3	**Chad**	**Central African Republic**	Afghanistan	**Chad**
4	**Central African Republic**	**Democratic Republic of the Congo**	Haiti	Equatorial Guinea
5	**Democratic Republic of the Congo**	**Chad**	**Niger**	Nigeria
6	Yemen	Yemen	**Central African Republic**	**Guinea**
7	Guinea-Bissau	Syria	Liberia	**Sierra Leone**
8	Eritrea	Afghanistan	**Sierra Leone**	Mali
9	Liberia	Haiti	Mozambique	**Niger**
10	Togo	Sudan	**Guinea**	**Democratic Republic of the Congo**

The study has several limitations. Firstly, due to the study focus, vulnerability (including adaptive and coping capacity) related to other aspects such as sociodemographic and political aspects were not included for this specific model. Secondly, this study applied factor analysis in determining the underlying constructs of the selected predictors. It is important to highlight that factor analysis does not explain the cause of the convertibility [32]; the factors presented in this study were based on the understandings and experience in the field and the references considered. Despite the sample size that was used for this factor analysis being less than the common agreed size of 200 [32] due to the limited number of countries, it was larger than the suggested minimum size of 100 [32], which should provide considerable power for the analysis. Finally, the results presented were based on the 147 countries along the Belt and Road region; the reported vulnerability ranking is subject to change when different countries are considered.

Thirdly, this proposed index is highly driven by data availability and accuracy. Although the disability rate is another important health determinant in disasters that is advocated by WHO, due to the lack of data, disability was not included in this analysis. Similarly, this study can only include a few indicators as proxies for each health dimension due to the limitation of data. This study did not impute missing data due to simplicity and accuracy. Therefore, the number of missing data would be more than those used in the compared indexes. The accuracy of the results of this analysis was highly dependent on the accuracy of the open access data. Data from different organizations may not be consistent due to inconsistency in collection methods, study periods, calculations, imputation methods, or even data sources. Results should be read with caution.

In addition, although the use of all-hazard approach intended to include all disaster types for the hazard index, the health vulnerability index may face constrains in covering the whole disaster spectrum. For instance, physician density may be an important health indicator for coping capacity during disease outbreaks; however, it may be less relevant to injury risk and health vulnerability during and after tsunamis.

According to the WHO, disaster risk management involving health components can avoid or reduce relevant health impacts [33]. While disaster risk assessment is one of the important components of risk management, hazard, vulnerability and capacity are the three elements that were most commonly considered in disaster risk assessment [33]. Among various dimensions of human vulnerability, low sociodemographic status, female gender, large dependency ratio, chronic diseases and disability are risk factors for disaster-associated mortality and morbidity [33]. Some current risk assessment indexes indicated vulnerability or coping capacity by using sociodemographic factors such as age, poverty, ethnic minority and education level [34,35] while some of them also included health-related variables [18,19].

However, not many existing global based disaster risk assessment model considered underlying non-communicable diseases patterns. A country specific vulnerability index for wildfire from the Environmental Protection Agency, the United State, considered chronic diseases such as asthma, diabetes, hypertension and obesity [36]. This study suggests the inclusion of chronic disease in addition to the health-variables considered in current disaster risk assessment tools (World Risk Index, INFORM) and demonstrated how health-related vulnerability could be added into existing risk assessment tools using a relative simple statistical method and open access data. The results of this study could be served as a basis for future development of disaster risk assessment model or adding a health related component to the existing one.

Specifically, the BRI counties are undergoing rapid socio-economic development. Lifestyle changes and westernized diets may increase the prevalence of chronic diseases such as diabetes and cardiovascular diseases [22]. The index presented in this paper may provide a more comprehensive health-related disaster risk assessment tool which may of the Belt and Road Imitative countries. This would help in improving Health-EDRM capacity planning, resources distribution and arrangement for the regions.

5. Conclusions

This paper presents a health vulnerability index that aims to enhance disaster risk assessment for disaster risk reduction. The suggested health vulnerability index covers seven health vulnerability dimensions, including infectious disease, maternal mortality, under-five mortality, healthcare services, immunization, the dependency ratio, and chronic disease. This new index incorporated important health dimensions such as chronic diseases into the existing hazard-based disaster risk mapping approach.

Attention has to be paid specifically to the health vulnerability, which is associated with population living with chronic diseases. As more comprehensive health-related disaster risk assessments emerge, policy makers and program planners may engage in better resources and capacity planning, distribution, and arrangement to address the needs of Health-EDRM in the disaster-affected regions along the Belt and Road Initiative countries.

Author Contributions: Conceptualization, E.Y.Y.C.; Methodology, Z.H. and Q.Z.; Software, Q.Z.; Validation, Z.H. and H.C.Y.L.; Formal Analysis, Z.H.; Data Curation, Z.H., C.K.P.W.; Writing—Original Draft Preparation, E.Y.Y.C., Z.H. and H.C.Y.L.; Writing—Review & Editing, E.Y.Y.C., Z.H., H.C.Y.L., C.K.P.W. and Q.Z.; Project Administration,

Acknowledgments: The authors thank Prof. Peng Cui for his support and advice in this collaborating project and study outcome discussions.

References

1. CRED & UNISDR. Economic Losses, Poverty & Disasters, 1998–2017. 2018. Available online: https://www.unisdr.org/files/61119_credeconomiclosses.pdf (accessed on 10 December 2018).
2. CRED. Natural disasters in 2017: Lower mortality, Higher Cost. 2018. Available online: https://cred.be/sites/default/files/CredCrunch50.pdf (accessed on 17 December 2018).
3. Guha-Sapir, D.; Hoyois, P.H.; Wallemacq, P.; Below, R. *Annual Disaster Statistical Review 2016: The Numbers and Trends*; Centre for Research on the Epidemiology of Disasters (CRED): Brussels, Belgium, 2017.
4. IPCC (Intergovernmental Panel on Climate Change). Climate Change 2014: Impacts, Adaptation, and Vulnerability. 2014. Available online: http://www.ipcc.ch/report/ar5/wg2/ (accessed on 11 December 2018).
5. UN (United Nations). Sendai Framework for Disaster Risk Reduction 2015–2030. 2015. Available online: https://www.unisdr.org/files/43291_sendaiframeworkfordrren.pdf (accessed on 14 December 2018).
6. Kron, W. Flood Risk = hazard• values• vulnerability. *Water Int.* **2005**, *30*, 58–68. [CrossRef]
7. UNISDR. *Terminology on Disaster Risk Reduction*; UNISDR: Geneva, Switzerland, 2009.
8. Chan, E.Y.Y.; Murray, V. What are the health research needs for the Sendai Framework? *Lancet.* **2017**, *390*, e35–e36. [CrossRef]
9. Brooks, N.; Adger, W.N.; Kelly, P.M. The determinants of vulnerability and adaptive capacity at the national level and the implications for adaptation. *Glob. Environ. Chang.* **2005**, *15*, 151–163. [CrossRef]
10. Cutter, S.L.; Carolina, S.; Boruff, B.J.; Carolina, S.; Shirley, W.L.; Carolina, S. Social Vulnerability to Environmental Hazards n. *Soc. Sci. Q.* **2003**, *84*, 242–261. [CrossRef]
11. UNDP (United Nations Development Programme). *Reducing Disaster Risk: A Challenge for Development*; United Nations Development Programme: New York, NY, USA, 2004.
12. Reid, C.E.; O'neill, M.S.; Gronlund, C.J.; Brines, S.J.; Brown, D.G.; Diez-Roux, A.V.; Schwartz, J. Mapping community determinants of heat vulnerability. *Environ. Health Perspect.* **2009**, *117*, 1730. [CrossRef] [PubMed]
13. Wolf, T.; McGregor, G. The development of a heat wave vulnerability index for London, United Kingdom. *Weather Clim. Extrem.* **2013**, *1*, 59–68. [CrossRef]
14. Zhu, Q.; Liu, T.; Lin, H.; Xiao, J.; Luo, Y.; Zeng, W.; Zeng, S.; Wei, Y.; Chu, C.; Baum, S.; et al. The spatial distribution of health vulnerability to heat waves in Guangdong Province, China. *Glob. Health Action* **2014**, *7*, 25051. [CrossRef] [PubMed]
15. Phung, D.; Rutherford, S.; Dwirahmadi, F.; Chu, C.; Do, C.M.; Nguyen, T.; Duong, N.C. The spatial distribution of vulnerability to the health impacts of flooding in the Mekong Delta, Vietnam. *Int. J. Biometeorol.* **2016**, *60*, 857–865. [CrossRef] [PubMed]

16. Pastrana, M.E.; Brito, R.L.; Nicolino, R.R.; de Oliveira, C.S.; Haddad, J.P. Spatial and statistical methodologies to determine the distribution of dengue in Brazilian municipalities and relate incidence with the health vulnerability index. *Spat. Spatio-Temporal Epidemiol.* **2014**, *11*, 143–151. [CrossRef] [PubMed]
17. Malik, S.M.; Awan, H.; Khan, N. Mapping vulnerability to climate change and its repercussions on human health in Pakistan. *Glob. Health* **2012**, *8*, 31. [CrossRef] [PubMed]
18. Inter-Agency Standing Committee (IASC) and the European Commission. Interpreting and Applying the INFORM Global Model. 2015. Available online: http://www.inform-index.org/LinkClick.aspx?fileticket=M-RXb0tKsjs%3d&tabid=101&portalid=0&mid=447 (accessed on 17 December 2018).
19. Welle, T.; Birkmann, J. The world risk index–an approach to assess risk and vulnerability on a global scale. *J. Extrem. Events* **2015**, *2*, 1550003. [CrossRef]
20. Chan, E.Y.Y. *Public Health Humanitarian Responses to Natural Disasters*; Routledge: London, UK, 2017.
21. NDRC (National Development and Reform Commission). Vision and Actions on Jointly Building Silk Road Economic Belt and 21st-Century Maritime Silk Road. 2015. Available online: http://http://en.ndrc.gov.cn/newsrelease/201503/t20150330_669367.html (accessed on 16 December 2018).
22. Hu, R.; Liu, R.; Hu, N. China's Belt and Road Initiative from a global health perspective. *Lancet Glob. Health.* **2017**, *5*, e752–e753. [CrossRef]
23. Lo, S.T.T.; Chan, E.Y.Y.; Chan, G.K.W.; Murray, V.; Ardalan, A.; Abrahams, J. Health Emergency and Disaster Management (H-EDRM): Developing the research field within the Sendai Framework paradigm. *Int. J. Disaster Risk Sci.* **2017**. [CrossRef]
24. Nardo, M.; Saisana, M.; Saltelli, A.; Tarantola, S.; Hoffman, A.; Giovannini, E. *Handbook on Constructing Composite Indicators*; OECD: Paris, France, 2008.
25. Everitt, B.; Hothorn, T. *An Introduction to Applied Multivariate Analysis with R*; Springer Science & Business Media: New York, NY, USA, 2011.
26. Kaiser, H.F. The varimax criterion for analytic rotation in factor analysis. *Psychometrika* **1958**, *23*, 187–200. [CrossRef]
27. Li, V.O.; Han, Y.; Lam, J.C.; Zhu, Y.; Bacon-Shone, J. Air pollution and environmental injustice: Are the socially deprived exposed to more PM 2.5 pollution in Hong Kong? *Environ. Sci. Policy.* **2018**, *80*, 53–61. [CrossRef]
28. UNEP/UNISDR. Global Risk Data Platform. 2013. Available online: https://preview.grid.unep.ch (accessed on 1 November 2018).
29. Shi, P.; Kasperson, R. *World Atlas of Natural Disaster Risk*; Springer: Heidelberg, Germany, 2015.
30. SEDAC (Socioeconomic Data and Applications Center). UN-Adjusted Population Density, v4. Available online: http://beta.sedac.ciesin.columbia.edu/data/set/gpw-v4-population-density-adjusted-to-2015-unwpp-country-totals/maps (accessed on 15 December 2018).
31. WHO (World Health Organization). Global Health Risks: Mortality and Burden of Disease Attributable to Selected Major Risks. 2009. Available online: https://www.who.int/healthinfo/global_burden_disease/GlobalHealthRisks_report_full.pdf (accessed on 17 December 2018).
32. Trninić, V.; Jelaska, I.; Štalec, J. Appropriateness and limitations of factor analysis methods utilized in psychology and kinesiology: Part, I.I. *Fizička Kultura*, 2013; 67, 1–7.
33. WHO (World Health Organization). Emergency Risk Management for Health—Overview. 2011. Available online: http://www.who.int/hac/techguidance/preparedness/risk_management_overview_17may2013.pdf?ua=1 (accessed on 10 December 2018).
34. Ciurean, R.L.; Schröter, D.; Glade, T. Conceptual frameworks of vulnerability assessments for natural disasters reduction. In *Approaches to Disaster Management*; IntechOpen: London, UK, 2013.
35. Matyas, D.; Pelling, M. *Disaster Vulnerability and Resilience: Theory, Modelling and Prospective*; Foresight: London, UK, 2012.
36. Rappold, A.G.; Reyes, J.; Pouliot, G.; Cascio, W.E.; Diaz-Sanchez, D. Community vulnerability to health impacts of wildland fire smoke exposure. *Environ. Sci. Technol.* **2017**, *51*, 6674–6682. [CrossRef] [PubMed]

16

Differences in Sense of Belonging, Pride and Mental Health in the Daegu Metropolitan Region due to COVID-19: Comparison between the Presence and Absence of National Disaster Relief Fund

Young-Jae Kim, Jeong-Hyung Cho and E-Sack Kim *

Department of Physical Education, Chung-Ang University, Seoul 06974, Korea; yjkim@cau.ac.kr (Y.-J.K.); cheer1007@naver.com (J.-H.C.)
* Correspondence: dlaehkgg@naver.com

Abstract: Korea's Daegu Metropolitan City once had the second highest rate of COVID-19 infection after Wuhan in China. Following the outbreak, the government provided the first national disaster relief fund to citizens as financial aid. This study investigated whether the sense of regional belonging, pride, and mental health among 550 citizens of Daegu differed between the times before and after COVID-19, based on the presence or absence of the disaster relief fund. Frequency analysis, descriptive statistical analysis, and *t*-tests were conducted using the SPSS 25.0 program. Results showed that the sense of belonging was higher after COVID-19 than before, while pride was lower. Individuals who received the disaster relief fund showed higher levels of regional belonging and pride with statistical significance. The prevalence of melancholy and depression increased after COVID-19, but the presence or absence of the fund did not lead to a significant difference. Thus, in case of a future national disaster level, provision of the disaster relief fund can raise the sense of regional belonging and pride, in order to elicit communication among local residents toward overcoming difficulties. Furthermore, during challenging disaster situations, central and local governments should provide diverse programs for the citizens' mental health care.

Keywords: COVID-19; Daegu; sense of belonging; pride; mental health; disaster relief fund

---

1. Introduction

The high infectivity of COVID-19, first confirmed in China at the end of 2019, led to an exponential increase in the rates of incidence and infection [1]. COVID-19 has now spread across the world, adversely affecting the political, economic, psychological, and social states in each country [2].

The government of the Republic of Korea recently raised the COVID-19 national crisis level to "serious" [3], and the World Health Organization (WHO) has declared COVID-19 a global pandemic [4].

For a certain period in Korea, the COVID-19 incidence rapidly fell in comparison to other countries, and the daily lives of people seemed to return to normal [5]. However, the 31st patient confirmed to have COVID-19 on 18 February 2020, in Daegu Metropolitan City (Daegu) in Korea led to approximately 5300 additional confirmed patients within 15 days [6]. This spread of infection resulted in the United States raising the travel alert level to the highest phase, at 4, to prohibit trips to Daegu [7]. The rapid spread of COVID-19, however, turned out not just to be a situation in Daegu, Korea; the large number of confirmed cases in New York in the United States and the sudden rise in mortality paralyzed the city [8], and led to shortage of mortuaries in the city's hospitals [9].

Daegu in Korea was designated as a disaster area, due to the large-scale spread of COVID-19. For the first time, the city provided "disaster relief funds" to citizens after the outbreak of COVID-19 [10].

The funds were determined to prioritize the class that had difficulty receiving national welfare for COVID-19 [11].

However, the households that exceed the standard of the national health insurance premium by 100%, teaching staff and employees of public institutions are not eligible for disaster relief funds [12]. Daegu has offered prepaid cards, local currency, and gift cards that could only be used to help the financially distressed citizens and the local economy during the COVID-19 pandemic. This has been contributing to the revitalization of the local economy [13].

According to Park [14], overcoming regional economic difficulties is one of the ways of making citizens feel a sense of stability and a sense of belonging. Park [15] also stated that feeling proud of contributing to the restoration of a local market by using local currency leads to a sense of belonging to and affection for the community, and provides a chance to change the social atmosphere depressed by COVID-19 in a positive way.

The local residents of a city with a high number of confirmed COVID-19 cases may suffer from subsequent psychological trauma [16]. Such emotional damage could reduce residents' sense of regional belonging, as well as solidarity [17]. Thus, the basic data of the residents' sense of belonging and pride are necessary for those in regions, including Daegu, where COVID-19 incidence is high.

A terrifying aspect of COVID-19 is the ambiguity of the information regarding the factors related to the propagation, latency, geographical range, infection frequency, and actual mortality. In fact, an incorrect piece of information could induce anxiety and fear in people, which has a direct negative influence on mental health [18,19]. To understand the psychological and emotional impact of a pandemic, feelings like fear and rage have to be considered. The feeling of fear is a basic human psychological response to a potentially threatening incidence [20]. Nonetheless, continuing fear could exert harmful influence on mental health [21]. National disasters, such as the Ebola virus, severe acute respiratory syndrome outbreaks, and earthquakes, have been shown to have a negative influence on mental health [22–24]. When combating infectious diseases, fear increases the levels of anxiety and stress in healthy individuals, while aggravating the symptoms in those already suffering from a mental disorder, thus deteriorating their health further [25].

Quality of life and health are influenced by the balance between work and life, suggesting that quality of life could be enhanced when a healthy mind and lifestyle achieve harmony [26]. Hence, maintaining the quality of life at an adequate level is likely to improve the defense mechanism against stress and produce emotional stability [27].

A study on mental health among citizens of Hong Kong after the COVID-19 outbreak reported that mental health was influenced by COVID-19 [28]. The continuous spread of COVID-19 has resulted in a deterioration of the quality of life of Daegu citizens, and several people are experiencing reduced mental health [29]. Therefore, this study aimed to determine the necessary factors to aid people when a national disaster occurs, such as in the case of Daegu, while examining the needs of people during the spread of COVID-19. Furthermore, the sense of belonging, pride, and mental health as experienced by the citizens of Daegu was investigated, as Daegu is the city with the largest number of COVID-19 cases in Korea, and the differences based on the presence or absence of the national disaster relief fund was examined.

2. Materials and Methods

2.1. Study Design

This study analyzes the difference between the present and the past with group infection, based on the data of "Social Indices of Daegu in 2018" [30] and "Regional Health Statistics at a glance, 2008–2018" [31], published in the Daegu area before the COVID-19. A comparison between the presence and absence of national disaster relief fund. The data collection period was from 8 May to 13 May 2020.

2.2. Participants

A survey was conducted among Daegu residents aged 19–65 years, excluding adolescents and older adults. Convenience sampling was used, and a self-reported questionnaire was administered. The survey (550 sheets) was conducted online through EMBRAIN, the top survey company in Korea. Consent for participation was obtained from each participant using a preliminary question set, before conducting the survey. The study design was reviewed and approved by the Institutional Review Board at Chung-Ang University (1041078-202005-HRSB-119-01).

2.3. Measurement

To investigate the differences in pride, sense of belonging, and mental health among Daegu citizens with respect to COVID-19, the following measurement tools were used. The questionnaire required 10 min on average for completion.

2.3.1. Indicators of Sense of Belonging and Pride

To measure regional pride of Daegu citizens and its levels, a scale was developed, based on "Social Indices of Daegu in 2018" [30]. The sub-categories of a sense of belonging and pride were comprised of a total of two questions: one question about a sense of belonging as a Daegu citizen and one question about satisfaction. Based on the four-point Likert scale, the scale of a sense of belonging and pride contains four sentences regarding a sense of belonging: "Very strong sense of belonging", "A little sense of belonging", "Little no sense of belonging", and "No sense of belonging at all". There were also four sentences regarding pride: "Very strong sense of pride", "A little sense of pride", "Little no sense of pride", and "No sense of pride at all".

2.3.2. Indicators of Mental Health

Indicators of the mental health status of the citizens were based on the "Regional Health Statistics at a glance, 2008–2018" [31] survey conducted by the Ministry of Health and Welfare and the Korea Centers for Disease Control. The sub-category of mental health was comprised of one question on average daily sleep time and stress awareness, one question on the experience of the feeling of melancholy, and nine questions on the prevalence of depression. The sleep time diagnosis consisted of average daily sleep time was measured. The stress was composed of a four-point scale, and the degree of stress perceived by individuals was indicated. The melancholy experience was usually composed of yes or no, as a question about melancholy. Among the questions, the one regarding depression prevalence used the standardized Korean version of the nine-item Patient Health Questionnaire (PHQ-9), which is a screening tool for depression comprised of nine questions, based on the Diagnostic and Statistical Manual of Mental Disorders, 4th edition [32]. Based on the diagnosis of the prevalence of depression, 0 = "not at all", 1 = "several days", 2 = "more than half the days", and 3 = "nearly every day" were the criteria used to diagnose the prevalence of depression. The total score ranged 0 from 27, and a higher score means a higher incidence of depression [32]. The tool has been reported to have better sensitivity (88%) and specificity (88%) than the Self-Rating Depression Scale and Beck Depression Inventory, which are the most commonly used depression indicators. PHQ-9 has also been found to be valid, with a high level of reliability in the measurement of the severity of depression [33]. Despite the small number of questions that require less time for completion, the PHQ-9 has been reported as a more accurate diagnostic tool for depression in numerous recent studies [34]. This assumes significance in the present time, when almost half of the patients with depression remain undiagnosed, owing to insufficient consultation time in overcrowded outpatient clinics, or wherein most depression patients are examined primarily for physical symptoms like pain or reduced physical functions, rather than psychological ones [35]. In the present study, the Cronbach's alpha coefficient of the PHQ-9 was 0.88.

2.4. Data Analysis

All data in this study were analyzed using SPSS version 25.0 (IBM, Armonk, NY, USA), after a process of coding and data cleaning. For demographic factors, cross-analysis and descriptive statistical analysis were performed, and the results compared in order to analyze the mean and standard deviation from the "Social Indices of Daegu in 2018" and the "Regional Health Statistics at a Glance, 2008–2018". to ensure the required level of confidence in each tool, Cronbach's α values were computed. Lastly, in order to identify the differences according to provision of the national disaster relief fund, an independent t-test was carried out.

3. Results

Table 1 displays the characteristics of the participants. This study targeted 285 females (51.8%) and 265 males (48.2%), which means more females participated in the study. Also, 138 people in their 20s (25.1%) occupied the highest proportion of the subjects, and it was followed by 137 in their 40s (24.9%). There were statistically significant differences in age, monthly household income, and sense of pride depending on national disaster relief funds. Also, there were significant differences in national disaster relief funds depending on the PHQ-9 scores of the subjects.

Table 1. Demographic characteristics (n = 550).

Variable	Total	WDRF [1]	WODRF [2]	p-Value
n	550	264	286	
Gender				
Male, n (%)	265 (48.2)	128 (48.3)	137 (51.7)	0.891
Female, n (%)	285 (51.8)	136 (47.7)	149 (52.3)	
Age, mean (SD)	38.33 (10.64)	38.09 (10.66)	38.54 (10.64)	
20s, n (%)	138 (25.1)	69 (50.0)	69 (50.0)	
30s, n (%)	190 (34.5)	88 (46.3)	102 (53.7)	
40s, n (%)	137 (24.9)	73 (53.3)	64 (46.7)	0.017
50s, n (%)	66 (12.0)	21 (31.8)	45 (68.2)	
60–65 years n (%)	19 (3.5)	13 (68.4)	6 (31.6)	
Marital Status				
Single, n (%)	285 (51.8)	131 (46.0)	154 (54.0)	
Married, n (%)	249 (45.3)	123 (49.4)	126 (50.6)	0.365
Widowed or divorced, n (%)	16 (2.9)	10 (62.5)	6 (37.5)	
Education				
Under high school, n (%)	52 (9.5)	29 (55.8)	23 (44.2)	
College (2-year), n (%)	124 (22.5)	62 (50.0)	62 (50.0)	
University (4-year), n (%)	307 (55.8)	149 (48.5)	158 (51.5)	0.228
Master's degree, n (%)	54 (9.8)	20 (37.0)	34 (63.0)	
PhD degree, n (%)	13 (2.4)	4 (30.8)	9 (69.2)	
Monthly household income [a]				
Under ₩ 1,000,000, n (%)	22 (4.0)	17 (77.3)	5 (22.7)	
₩ 1,000,000–1,990,000, n (%)	32 (5.8)	23 (71.9)	9 (28.1)	
₩ 2,000,000–2,990,000, n (%)	118 (21.5)	68 (57.6)	50 (42.4)	
₩ 3,000,000–3,990,000, n (%)	90 (16.4)	47 (52.2)	43 (47.8)	0.000 *
₩ 4,000,000–4,990,000, n (%)	84 (15.3)	35 (41.7)	49 (58.3)	
₩ 5,000,000–5,990,000, n (%)	86 (15.6)	39 (45.3)	47 (54.7)	
₩ 6,000,000–6,990,000, n (%)	50 (9.1)	17 (34.0)	33 (66.0)	
₩ $\geq$ 7,000,000, n (%)	68 (12.4)	18 (16.5)	50 (73.5)	

Table 1. *Cont.*

Variable	Total	WDRF [1]	WODRF [2]	*p*-Value
Sleep time, mean (SD)	6.77(1.16)	6.77 (1.20)	6.76 (1.13)	0.946
Stress levels				
I feel a lot of stress frequently	57 (10.4	28 (49.1)	29 (50.9)	
I feel stress a lot	176 (32.0)	84 (47.7)	92 (52.3)	0.713
I feel stress a little	281 (51.1)	138 (49.1)	143 (50.9)	
I do not feel stress	36 (6.5)	14 (38.9)	22 (61.1)	
Melancholy				
Yes	104 (18.9)	55 (52.9)	49 (47.1)	0.268
No	446 (81.1)	209 (46.9)	237 (53.1)	
PHQ-9				
PHQ-9 score 0-4 (minimal)	266 (48.4)	117 (44.0)	149 (56.0)	
PHQ-9 score 5–9 (mild)	173 (31.5)	88 (50.9)	85 (49.1)	
PHQ-9 score 10–14 (moderate)	77 (14.0)	46 (59.7)	31 (40.3)	0.004
PHQ-9 score 15–19 (moderately severe)	23 (4.2)	5 (21.7)	18 (78.3)	
PHQ-9 score 20–27 (severe)	11 (2.0)	8 (72.7)	3 (27.3)	
Sense of belonging				
Very strong sense of belonging	68 (12.4)	36 (52.9)	32 (47.1)	
A little sense of belonging	282 (51.3)	141 (50.0)	141 (50.0)	0.174
Little no sense of belonging	163 (29.6)	75 (46.0)	88 (54.0)	
No sense of belonging at all	37 (6.7)	12 (32.4)	25 (67.6)	
Sense of pride				
Very strong sense of pride	41 (7.5)	27 (65.9)	14 (34.1)	
A little sense of pride	163 (29.6)	82 (50.3)	81 (49.7)	0.012
Little no sense of pride	259 (47.1)	124 (47.9)	135 (52.1)	
No sense of pride at all	87 (15.8)	31 (35.6)	56 (64.4)	

Notes: [1] WDRF: with disaster relief fund; [2] WODRF: without disaster relief fund; [a] South Korean 10.000 won (USD 1 = KRW 1203.00). The *p*-values were calculated from chi-square tests and *t*-tests, as appropriate. * Significant difference noted in the comparison between four groups ($p < 0.05$).

Table 2 includes a descriptive statistics analysis to determine the sleep time, stress level, melancholy and depression prevalence, sense of belonging, and sense of pride among Daegu citizens before and during COVID-19. Looking at the results, it was found that in 2016, the sleep time was at 6.6 h in 2016 and 6.8 h in the case of COVID-19. The stress level was 23.3% in 2018 and 42.4% with the current COVID-19. The depression was at 3.4% in 2018 and at 18.9% during COVID-19. The prevalence of depression was 1.9% in 2018 and 5.8% as of the emergence of COVID-19.

For the sense of belonging as a citizen of Daegu, "Very strong sense of belonging" was the lowest, at 5.9% in 2018—as of COVID-19, it was 12.4%. "A little sense of belonging" was at 47.2% in 2018, and 51.3% as of COVID-19. "Little no sense of belonging" was at 36.9% in 2012 and 2016, and 29.6% during COVID-19. "No sense of belonging at all" was at 2.0% in 2012, and 6.7% with COVID-19. Regarding pride, the "Very strong sense of pride" response was the lowest, at 5.6% in 2016 and currently at 7.5% during COVID-19. "A little sense of pride" was at 39.8% in 2018, and 29.6% during COVID-19. "Little no sense of pride" was at 43.0% in 2016, and COVID-19 responses were at 47.1%. Lastly, "No sense of pride at all" had 3.2% in 2012 and 15.8% with COVID-19.

Table 2. The mean and standard deviation (SD) of the mental health indicators, sense of belonging, and pride among Daegu citizens before and during COVID-19 (n = 550).

Items	2012	2014	2016	2018	COVID-19
Sleep time (hours), mean (SD)	6.7	6.7	6.6	6.7	6.8 (1.16)
Stress levels, % (n)	27.2	26.0	26.6	23.3	42.4 (233)
Melancholy, mean (SD)	5.6	5.4	4.9	3.4	18.9 (0.39)
Depression prevalence, mean (SD)				1.9	5.8 (5.05)
Sense of belonging					
Very strong sense of belonging, % (n)	9.9	8.3	7.1	5.9	12.4 (68)
A little sense of belonging, % (n)	51.2	49.2	50.8	47.2	51.3 (282)
Little no sense of belonging, % (n)	36.9	38.7	36.9	41.2	29.6 (163)
No sense of belonging at all, % (n)	2.0	3.8	5.2	5.8	6.7 (37)
Sense of pride					
Very strong sense of pride, % (n)	7.7	7.5	5.6	5.9	7.5 (41)
A little sense of pride, % (n)	47.2	43.0	45.8	39.8	29.6 (163)
Little no sense of pride, % (n)	42.0	45.5	43.0	48.0	47.1 (259)
No sense of pride at all, % (n)	3.2	4.1	5.6	6.3	15.8 (87)

Table 3 shows the independent t-test to determine whether each parameter showed differences according to provision of the disaster relief fund. It shows that all parameters exhibited differences between the presence and absence of the fund (sense of pride: $t = 3.06$, $p = 0.002$; sense of belonging: $t = 2.01$, $p = 0.045$).

Table 3. The differences between presence and absence of the national disaster relief fund (n = 550).

Items	Mean (SD) WDRF [1] (n = 264)	Mean (SD) WODRF [2] (n = 286)	Effect Size	t-Value	p-Value
PHQ-9, mean (SD)	1.85 (0.97)	1.74 (0.95)	0.12	1.40	0.163
Depression prevalence *	1.67 (0.57)	1.62 (0.55)	−0.09	1.01	0.312
Stress levels *	2.52 (0.76)	2.55 (0.78)	−0.04	−0.45	0.650
Melancholy *	1.79 (0.41)	1.83 (0.38)	−0.10	−0.10	0.269
Sense of belonging	2.76 (0.74)	2.62 (0.80)	0.17	2.01	0.045
Sense of pride	2.39 (0.83)	2.18 (0.80)	0.26	3.06	0.002

Notes: p-values were analyzed using the independent t-test. [1] WDRF: with disaster relief fund; [2] WODRF: without disaster relief fund. * Depression prevalence, stress levels, and melancholy each showed no significant difference.

The independent t-test to determine whether each parameter showed differences, according to provision of the disaster relief fund, showed that none of the parameters showed a difference between presence and absence of the fund, with the following results: depression prevalence, $t = 1.01$, $p = 0.312$; stress levels, $t = -0.454$, $p = 0.650$; and melancholy, $t = -0.106$, $p = 0.269$.

4. Discussion

This study aimed to investigate whether COVID-19 had led to differences in the sense of regional belonging, pride, and mental health among the citizens of Daegu, and to analyze the differences based on the presence or absence of the national disaster relief fund. The findings are discussed as follows.

First, the sense of regional belonging was found to have increased after COVID-19 when compared to the time before. Daegu was pointed out as the source of the explosive spread of COVID-19 by the general public, who criticized the citizens of Daegu and posted various expressions of hate on online portal sites and communities, holding them responsible for the COVID-19 outbreak incessantly [36]. Such accusations and discriminating behaviors from people in other regions are thought to have led to the increased sense of belonging among the people of Daegu. In the same context, as the people in other regions blamed the citizens of Daegu, the increased social sharing among the local residents enhanced the regional identity, and subsequently, the regional belonging. Daegu has endured a number of disasters in the past, such as a gas explosion and metro fire, and in each case, the disaster was overcome by the united efforts of the citizens [37]. This is presumed to be the reason behind the increased sense of regional belonging among the citizens of Daegu after COVID-19.

Individuals who received the national disaster relief fund were found to have higher awareness of regional belonging. Financial difficulties in households are being relieved by the disaster relief fund provided by the government [38]. It is thus presumed that the fund is financially aiding small business owners and socially disadvantaged groups to help them overcome the difficult time [39], and individuals who received the fund are consequently showing higher awareness of regional belonging [40]. The disaster relief fund was reported to have a positive influence on the quality of life of the working poor and people with disabilities, who are able to make less than half their original profits owing to the COVID-19 outbreak [41]. Thus, in a prolonged national disaster situation, as is the case of COVID-19, with consequently reduced social and economic activities, providing the national disaster relief fund to citizens, starting with small business owners and the socially disadvantaged, was found to have led to higher awareness of regional belonging among the citizens. Such an increase in regional belonging is likely to strengthen the solidarity among local residents, and the resulting social unity would help the citizens overcome the difficult situation, based on the strong confidence regarding the region, in case of a national disaster in the future.

The regional pride among the citizens of Daegu was shown to have decreased from 2018 after the arrival of COVID-19. This finding contradicts a previous study [42]. It has been reported that the number of additional confirmed patients have substantially decreased in Daegu, Korea—a city that had faced the first phases of COVID-19 outbreak outside China. In reality, however, Daegu is viewed by its citizens as a city where such a social difficulty or disaster may occur again at any time, even though might have overcome the COVID-19 situation, which consequently led to the fall in their regional pride.

This study shows that individuals who received national disaster relief funds had a higher level of pride. According to a previous study, the people of Daegu show high levels of unity, justice, and resourcefulness [43]. This is thought to have increased an already high level of regional pride among the citizens when the national disaster relief fund was provided. Thus, based on an already high level of regional pride, the sense of community among the citizens of Daegu is likely to have increased, and the fund is thought to have further increased their regional pride. Thus, the national disaster relief fund provided to the citizens of Daegu has led to trust towards the region, owing to regional characteristics like conservative ideas, loyalty, and exclusivity; such trust may serve as the basis for communication among local residents, which would help characterize Daegu as a city that can overcome any disaster in the future.

The rate of experiencing melancholy and depression among the citizens of Daegu after COVID-19 was shown to have increased. In addition, no significant difference was found for these parameters with respect to provisions of the disaster relief fund, based on the results of the *t*-test. This indicates that the presence or absence of the fund did not have a significant impact on people's mental health, and that COVID-19 itself is presumed to have had a negative influence on the mental health of the citizens. Hence, the reduced mental health compared to the past is thought to have resulted from the social isolation, staying indoors, and altered daily activities caused by COVID-19. Indicators such as melancholy, depression, and anxiety among the citizens of Hong Kong after COVID-19 showed far higher values than the time before, which is consistent with the results in this study [28]. The continuous increase in the level of melancholy due to COVID-19 among Daegu citizens has even led to coining of the term "Corona Blues", combining the coronavirus and melancholy (blues) [44]. The level of melancholy is thought to have increased in line with the increased anxiety among Daegu citizens, due to the rapid spread of COVID-19, which once led to as high as 741 confirmed patients a day. The social distancing from friends and family due to COVID-19 has led many people to suffer from melancholy [45]. In addition, the changed economic and social values and relationships after COVID-19 are exerting an influence on the psychological stress in people [46]. The findings of these previous studies were partially in agreement with those of the present study. Uncertain situations about COVID-19 have resulted in increased stress and anxiety about not maintaining daily life [47]. In the future, therefore, when a focused disaster situation occurs in a single city as in the case of Daegu, various methods should be sought to reduce the levels of melancholy and stress among the citizens for their mental health care through the use of different media, including phone and the internet, or through a national program developed for the emotional stability of the citizens.

This study has several limitations, as follows. First, the data of the study were gathered online with the use of a professional survey company. For this reason, the way of responding might be influenced by using a computer and computer skills. Second, this is a cross-sectional study, which means it is impossible to observe temporary changes in respondents' sense of belonging, pride, and mental health. Third, the study results cannot apply to other regions and groups in Korea for generalization. Fourth, although giving national disaster relief funds may influence a sense of belonging and pride, these can be boosted by more diverse psychological and social factors. That is why it is impossible to generalize the levels of a sense of belonging and pride revealed in this study.

5. Conclusions

This study examined the differences in the sense of regional belonging, pride, and mental health among the citizens of Daegu, due to COVID-19, between the times before and after COVID-19, and based on the presence or absence of the national disaster relief fund.

The level of regional belonging among the citizens increased after COVID-19, but the level of pride decreased. Regarding differences according to provision of the national disaster relief fund, all parameters of belonging and pride significantly increased among individuals who received the fund. This was thought to be due to the enhanced regional identity, based on the characteristics of Daegu citizens, which involve conservative ideas, local patriotism, loyalty, exclusivity, and faithfulness, combined with the social convention to overcome a difficult situation together. Therefore, in a challenging national situation, providing the disaster relief fund to the citizens is anticipated to raise the sense of regional belonging and pride to enhance regional identity and elicit communication among local residents, whereby the challenge can be overcome.

Furthermore, the citizens of Daegu were found to have experienced melancholy more frequently after COVID-19, and the depression prevalence was also higher compared to the time before COVID-19. In line with this, to protect the mental health of individuals in a national disaster, such as COVID-19, every local government should take initiatives to enhance the mental health of the citizens, and in a narrower sense, a way to enhance the mental health should be sought through the provision of aids to each household, so that the family members can acquire emotional stability.

Author Contributions: Conceptualization, Y.-J.K. and E.-S.K.; methodology, Y.-J.K., J.-H.C. and E.-S.K.; validation, Y.-J.K. and E.-S.K.; formal analysis, Y.-J.K., J.-H.C. and E.-S.K.; investigation, Y.-J.K. and E.-S.K.; data curation, Y.-J.K. and E.-S.K.; writing—original draft preparation, Y.-J.K.; writing—proofreading and editing, Y.-J.K., J.-H.C. and E.-S.K. Both authors have read and agreed to the published version of the manuscript. All authors have read and agreed to the published version of the manuscript.

References

1. Ornell, F.; Schuch, J.B.; Sordi, A.O.; Kessler, F.H.P. "Pandemic fear" AND COVID-19: Mental health burden and strategies. *Braz. J. Psychiatry* **2020**, *42*, 232–235. [CrossRef]
2. Van Bavel, J.J.; Baicker, K.; Boggio, P.S.; Capraro, V.; Cichocka, A.; Cikara, M.; Drury, J. Using social and behavioural science to support COVID-19 pandemic response. *Nat. Hum. Behaviour.* **2020**, *4*, 460–471. [CrossRef] [PubMed]

3. Phase VI Pandemic, the Highest Alert Level, and the Second Declaration after the Swine Flu in 2009. Available online: http://www.donga.com/news/article/all/20200223/99833909/1 (accessed on 27 May 2020).
4. Grasselli, G.; Pesenti, A.; Cecconi, M. Critical care utilization for the COVID-19 outbreak in Lombardy, Italy: Early experience and forecast during an emergency response. *JAMA* **2020**, *323*, 1545–1546. [CrossRef] [PubMed]
5. "COVID-19 Will End Soon," says President Moon. Available online: https://news.joins.com/article/23705968 (accessed on 27 May 2020).
6. Choi, S.; Ki, M. Estimating the reproductive number and the outbreak size of COVID-19 in Korea. *Epidemiology and Health* **2020**, *42*, E2020011. [CrossRef]
7. Lee, H.S. "Travel Regulations May be Reinforced on 'Certain Countries' of High COVID-19 Incidence," said President Trump. Available online: http://news.chosun.com/site/data/html_dir/2020/03/03/2020030301684.html (accessed on 27 May 2020).
8. Yin, H.; Liu, Z.; Kammen, D.M. Impacts of Early Interventions on the Age-Specific Incidence of COVID-19 in New York, Los Angeles, Daegu and Nairobi. *medRxiv* **2020**. [CrossRef]
9. How South Korea Successfully Battled COVID-19 While the U.S. Didn't. Available online: https://www.healthline.com/health-news/what-south-korea-has-done-correctly-in-battling-covid-19 (accessed on 28 May 2020).
10. Daegu to Offer Emergency Aid to Virus-Battered Households, Businesses. The Korea Herald. Available online: http://www.koreaherald.com/view.php?ud=20200323000744 (accessed on 28 May 2020).
11. Businebusiney-in-Battling-Covid-19s Angeles, Daeg Ohmynews. Available online: http://www.ohmynews.com/NWS_Web/View/at_pg.aspx?CNTN_CD=A0002621873 (accessed on 25 June 2020).
12. Daegu City Deciding to Give 500,000 to 900,000 Won to Recipients, Who Belong to Median-Income Households or Below. Available online: http://www.ohmynews.com/NWS_Web/View/at_pg.aspx?CNTN_CD=A0002625088 (accessed on 25 June 2020).
13. "The Emergency Relief Fund will be Provided in a Pre-Paid Card for Reviving the Local Economy" says the Mayor of Daegu. Available online: https://www.yna.co.kr/view/AKR20200326101400053 (accessed on 28 May 2020).
14. [Park Myeong Ho's Financial News Column] To Get Over the Corona Pandemic. Available online: https://www.idaegu.co.kr/news/articleView.html?idxno=309440 (accessed on 29 May 2020).
15. To Make a Meaningful Use of Chid Care Points and Disaster Relief Funds. Available online: http://www.ohmynews.com/NWS_Web/View/at_pg.aspx?CNTN_CD=A0002642483. (accessed on 25 June 2020).
16. Jung, S.J.; Jun, J.Y. Mental Health and Psychological Intervention Amid COVID-19 Outbreak: Perspectives from South Korea. *Yonsei Med. J.* **2020**, *61*, 271–272. [CrossRef] [PubMed]
17. Two Months with COVID-19 Shed Your Anxiety as Deep Sleep, Singing, Sun-Bathing are the Health Boosters. Available online: https://www.seoul.co.kr/news/newsView.php?id=20200318018003&wlog_tag3=naver. (accessed on 27 May 2020).
18. Malta, M.; Rimoin, A.W.; Strathdee, S.A. The coronavirus 2019-nCoV epidemic: Is hindsight 20/20? *EClinicalMedicine* **2020**, *20*, 100289. [CrossRef] [PubMed]
19. Cascella, M.; Rajnik, M.; Cuomo, A.; Dulebohn, S.C.; Di Napoli, R. Features, evaluation and treatment coronavirus (COVID-19). In *Statpearls*; StatPearls Publishing: Treasure Island, Finland, 2020.
20. Garcia, R. Neurobiology of fear and specific phobias. *Learn. Mem.* **2017**, *24*, 462–471. [CrossRef]
21. Shin, L.M.; Liberzon, I. The neurocircuitry of fear, stress, and anxiety disorders. *Neuropsychopharmacology* **2010**, *35*, 169–191. [CrossRef]
22. Shultz, J.M.; Baingana, F.; Neria, Y. The 2014 Ebola outbreak and mental health: Current status and recommended response. *JAMA* **2015**, *313*, 567–568. [CrossRef]
23. Zhang, Z.; Shi, Z.; Wang, L.; Liu, M. One year later: Mental health problems among survivors in hard-hit areas of the Wenchuan earthquake. *Public Health* **2011**, *125*, 293–300. [CrossRef]
24. Mak, I.W.C.; Chu, C.M.; Pan, P.C.; Yiu, M.G.C.; Chan, V.L. Long-term psychiatric morbidities among SARS survivors. *Gen. Hosp. Psychiatry* **2009**, *31*, 318–326. [CrossRef] [PubMed]
25. Shigemura, J.; Ursano, R.J.; Morganstein, J.C.; Kurosawa, M.; Benedek, D.M. Public responses to the novel 2019 coronavirus (2019-nCoV) in Japan: Mental health consequences and target populations. *Psychiatry Clin. Neurosci.* **2020** *74*, 281. [CrossRef]

26. Sánchez-Hernández, M.I.; González-López, Ó.R.; Buenadicha-Mateos, M.; Tato-Jiménez, J.L. Work-Life Balance in Great Companies and Pending Issues for Engaging New Generations at Work. *Int. J. Environ. Res. Public Health* **2019**, *16*, 5122. [CrossRef]
27. Cook, L.H.; Shinew, K.J. Leisure, work, and disability coping: "I mean, you always need that 'in'group". *Leis. Sci.* **2014**, *36*, 420–438. [CrossRef]
28. Choi, E.P.H.; Hui, B.P.H.; Wan, E.Y.F. Depression and Anxiety in Hong Kong during COVID-19. *Int. J. Environ. Res. Public Health* **2020**, *17*, 3740. [CrossRef]
29. Panic Disorder, Claustrophobia ... Citizens of Daegu Suffering from Concerns of Anxiety. Available online: https://www.hankookilbo.com/News/Read/202003011523782150 (accessed on 26 May 2020).
30. 2018 Daegu Community Survey Report. Available online: http://stat.daegu.go.kr/statsPublication/dgSocialSurvey.do (accessed on 10 May 2020).
31. 2008–2018 Regional Health Statistics at a Glance. Available online: https://chs.cdc.go.kr/chs/stats/statsMain.do (accessed on 10 May 2020).
32. Kroenke, K.; Spitzer, R.L.; Williams, J.B. The PHQ-9: Validity of a brief depression severity measure. *J. Gen. Intern. Med.* **2001**, *16*, 606–6132. [CrossRef]
33. Kim, S.R.; Shin, H.C.; Lee, D.C.; Kim, C.H.; Seong, E.J.; Lee, G.H.; Kim, J.Y. The Utility of PHQ-2/PHQ-9 Serial Test for the Screening of Major Depressive Disorder in Primary Health Care. *Korean Soc. Stress Med.* **2011**, *19*, 405–410.
34. Thibault, J.M.; Steiner, R.W. Psychiatric Briefs. *Prim. Care Companion J. Clin. Psychiatry* **2004**, *6*, 270.
35. Beck, A.T.; Ward, C.H.; Mendelson, M.; Mock, J.; Erbaugh, J. An inventory for measuring depression. *Arch. Gen. Psychiatry* **1961**, *4*, 561–571. [CrossRef] [PubMed]
36. Kim, J.S. "I am Disgusted at Anyone from Daegu" Hatred for the Region Brings More Horrors than Corona Virus. Available online: https://news.joins.com/article/23767330 (accessed on 28 May 2020).
37. [A Diary of a Corona Warrior] My 60-Year-Old Mum, Right Before retirement, Took Off Her Nurse Uniform to Put on the Armor. Available online: https://news.joins.com/article/23719357 (accessed on 29 May 2020).
38. 7 out of 10 Citizens Said, "Emergency Disaster relief Fund is Helpful.". Available online: http://www.ohmynews.com/NWS_Web/Event/Special/opinion_poll_2019/at_pg.aspx?CNTN_CD=A0002642570&CMPT_CD=P0010&utm_source=naver&utm_medium=newsearch&utm_campaign=naver_news (accessed on 26 May 2020).
39. Raschky, P.A.; Schwindt, M. On the Channel and Type of Aid: The Case of International Disaster Assistance. *Eur. J. Political Econ.* **2012**, *28*, 119–131. [CrossRef]
40. [LG Hello Vision] The Disaster Relief Fund has Revitalized the Markets. Available online: http://news.lghellovision.net/news/newsView.do?soCode=SC50000000&idx=276836 (accessed on 27 May 2020).
41. "We can Finally Breathe" A Month after Disaster Relief Fund. Available online: http://www.hani.co.kr/arti/politics/politics_general/944246.html#csidx200cbb47c3727c7b89d877092c9beb0 (accessed on 26 May 2020).
42. This South Korean City Once had the Biggest Coronavirus Outbreak Outside of China. Available online: https://www.weforum.org/agenda/2020/04/south-korean-daegu-china-coronavirus-covid19-cases-virus/ (accessed on 28 May 2020).
43. Yoon, S.G.; Kim, M.H. A Study on the Identity of the Citizens of Daegu Metropolitan and North Gyeongsang Regions. *Inst. East-West Thought* **2007**, *3*, 33–64.
44. Regular Briefing on the COVID-19 Response (10 April 2020). Available online: https://www.idaegu.co.kr/news/articleView.html?idxno=307979 (accessed on 27 May 2020).
45. Jiloha, R.C. COVID-19 and Mental Health. *Epidemiol. Int.* **2020**, *5*, 7–9. [CrossRef]
46. An Analysis on the Panic of Filipinos During COVID-19 Pandemic in the Philippines. Available online: https://www.researchgate.net/profile/Christian_Jasper_Nicomedes/publication/340081049_An_Analysis_on_the_Panic_of_Filipinos_During_COVID-19_Pandemic_in_the_Philippines/links/5e7606aa299bf1892cfc4dd3/An-Analysis-on-the-Panic-of-Filipinos-During-COVID-19-Pandemic-in-the-Philippines.pdf (accessed on 27 May 2020).
47. Li, S.; Wang, Y.; Xue, J.; Zhao, N.; Zhu, T. The Impact of COVID-19 Epidemic Declaration on Psychological Consequences: A Study on Active Weibo Users. *Int. J. Environ. Res. Public Health* **2020**, *17*, 2032. [CrossRef] [PubMed]

17

Factors Associated with Urban Risk-Taking Behaviour during 2018 Typhoon Mangkhut

Evan Su Wei Shang [1,2], Eugene Siu Kai Lo [1], Zhe Huang [1,2], Kevin Kei Ching Hung [1,3] and Emily Ying Yang Chan [1,2,3,4,*]

1 Collaborating Centre for Oxford University and CUHK for Disaster and Medical Humanitarian Response (CCOUC), The Chinese University of Hong Kong, Hong Kong, China; evanshang98@link.cuhk.edu.hk (E.S.W.S.); euglsk@cuhk.edu.hk (E.S.K.L.); huangzhe@cuhk.edu.hk (Z.H.); kevin.hung@cuhk.edu.hk (K.K.C.H.)

2 JC School of Public Health and Primary Care, The Chinese University of Hong Kong, Hong Kong, China

3 Accident & Emergency Medicine Academic Unit, The Chinese University of Hong Kong, Prince of Wales Hospital, Hong Kong, China

4 Nuffield Department of Medicine, University of Oxford, Oxford OX37BN, UK

* Correspondence: emily.chan@cuhk.edu.hk

Abstract: Although much of the health emergency and disaster risk management (Health-EDRM) literature evaluates methods to protect health assets and mitigate health risks from disasters, there is a lack of research into those who have taken high-risk behaviour during extreme events. The study's main objective is to examine the association between engaging in high-risk behaviour and factors including sociodemographic characteristics, disaster risk perception and household preparedness during a super typhoon. A computerized randomized digit dialling cross-sectional household survey was conducted in Hong Kong, an urban metropolis, two weeks after the landing of Typhoon Mangkhut. Telephone interviews were conducted in Cantonese with adult residents. The response rate was 23.8% and the sample was representative of the Hong Kong population. Multivariable logistic regressions of 521 respondents adjusted with age and gender found education, income, risk perception and disaster preparedness were insignificantly associated with risk-taking behaviour during typhoons. This suggests that other factors may be involved in driving this behaviour, such as a general tendency to underestimate risk or sensation seeking. Further Health-EDRM research into risk-taking and sensation seeking behaviour during extreme events is needed to identify policy measures.

Keywords: typhoon; hurricane; cyclone; strong wind levels; natural disaster; Health-EDRM; urban; risk-taking behaviour; sensation seeking

---

1. Introduction

Asia is particularly at risk of tropical cyclones, also known as typhoons in the western Pacific, with around half of worldwide tropical cyclones recorded and more than 90% of cyclone-related deaths being from this region [1]. Typhoon Mangkhut, the fourth supertyphoon in the 2018 Pacific typhoon season, started east of Guam in September 2018 and caused devastating damage to the Philippines [2] and South China [3]. In Hong Kong, tropical cyclone warning signal No. 10 (the highest signal for Hong Kong) was hoisted for 10 h, with the highest wind speed exceeding 150 km/h, just lower than the respective records held by Typhoon York in 1999 and Typhoon Ellen in 1983 [4]. Although there were no deaths reported directly due to the typhoon, more than 60,000 trees had reportedly fallen and around 13,500 households experienced a power outage for more than 24 h in Hong Kong [5]. Record breaking storm surges coupled with high waves caused flooding in various coastal areas, despite not being at high tide, with hundreds of stranded or damaged vessels. These occurrences highlighted the increasing environmental hazards and potential health risks faced by coastal communities around the world as typhoons become more frequent and severe through climate change [6].

Health emergency and disaster risk management (Health-EDRM) is a field which involves the systematic analysis and management of health risks surrounding emergencies and disasters. By reducing risk and vulnerabilities and improving preparedness, response and recovery measures, the impact of disasters can be minimised [7]. Health-EDRM focuses on increasing the resilience of individuals, households and communities through education interventions, promotion of disaster risk reduction and supporting mechanisms in place to mitigate impacts of disasters [8]. These can include accessible disaster warning and information, protection of key health services and securing the basic needs of the population. By understanding the causes and factors in play regarding disaster risk, Health-EDRM provides evidence to drive future interventions and policy decisions.

A previous study on urban disaster preparedness in Hong Kong discovered that only 20.6% of respondents chose the correct action to take while major disaster warnings were in force (such as staying in a safe place until heavy rain has passed) [9]. However, few studies investigate individuals intentionally performing risk-taking behaviour during natural disasters. Research on 'storm chasers' (those who intercept severe convective storms for sport or for scientific research) [10] in the United States has examined individual perception of recreational storm chasing to dispel its myths [11], operational methods of storm chasing tour groups [12] and sensation seeking traits associated with tour participants [13]. There is a lack of research into such behaviour outside of the United States, especially in urban areas directly impacted by meteorological disasters. Various studies by Zuckerman on sensation seeking have identified its dimensions [14] and relationships to different aspects through the sensation seeking scale (SSS) [15]. A meta-analysis into sex differences in sensation seeking showed that men scored higher than women using Zuckerman's SSS-V and could be explained by evolutionary psychology and through a cultural socialisation perspective [16]. Furthermore, a review of behavioural and biological correlates of sensation seeking also found males significantly outscored females on total sensation seeking in different western countries and sensation seeking typically decreases with increasing age after adolescence [17]. Education and occupation were less associated with sensation seeking, particularly for females. The review also highlighted high sensation seekers perceived risks in the environment as less threatening compared to low sensation seekers and did not perceive engaging in high-risk behaviours would lead to negative consequences.

This article is an extension of the cross-sectional study investigating risk perception, household preparedness, and self-reported short-term impacts of typhoons after Typhoon Mangkhut [18]. Our previous published paper highlighted 16.0% of respondents reportedly left their homes when the warning signal was T8 or above, when the typhoon was at the height of strength. This behaviour will henceforth be referred to as risk-taking behaviour during typhoons (RBDT). Out of those respondents, a majority (74.7%) performed RBDT for non-essential reasons. The previous article also found that men and younger respondents were more likely to execute non-essential RBDT. Using the same dataset, the objectives of the current study are to expand on these findings and investigate other factors that may be related to RBDT, namely (1) to identify the sociodemographic characteristics of those who left their homes when the storm was at its height of strength (i.e., the warning signal was T8 or above); and (2) to explore the associations between sociodemographic factors other than age and gender, risk perception, household preparedness, and RBDT for non-essential purposes. The study findings will offer further insight into risk-taking behaviour during natural disasters to guide future interventions and policy on preventing such unnecessary high-risk behaviour.

2. Materials and Methods

A computerized digit dialling population-based household telephone survey was conducted from 17 September 2018 to 2 October 2018, right after the date of Typhoon Mangkhut landing in Hong Kong.

Random digit dialling and the last birthday method [19] (interviewer would seek the household member whose birthday was the closest to the interview date) were used to ensure randomization in the study. Hong Kong residents who understood Cantonese and were 18 years old or older were interviewed. In total, 2500 landline numbers were called, and 521 respondents were successfully recruited (Figure 1). The response rate was 23.8% (response rate: 521 (final sample size) /2188 (eligible persons)). Please refer to the previous published study for study design [18].

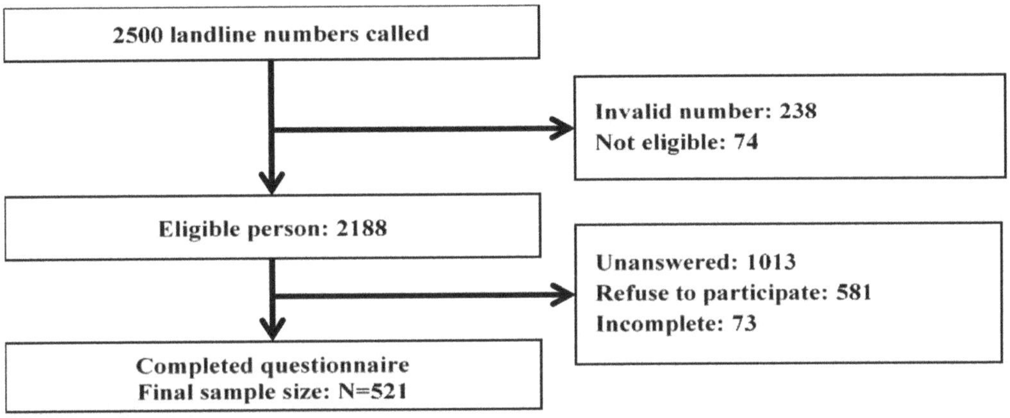

Figure 1. The recruitment details in the telephone survey.

This study investigates the associations between non-essential RBDT and the sociodemographic factors of education and income; indicators of risk perception including perception of Hong Kong being susceptible to disasters, perception of the impact of Typhoon Mangkhut compared to expectations and concern for the safety of oneself and family members; indicators of household preparedness including food and water reserves prepared routinely or specifically for Typhoon Mangkhut.

This paper considers the act of going outside during the strongest typhoon winds as risk-taking (RBDT) or high-risk behaviour, regardless of the reasoning. Those who go outside for work or emergency related purposes would be considered as engaging in socially acceptable or understandable risk-taking behaviour. This article focuses on active risk-taking behaviour, where individuals remove themselves from areas of safety to head into areas posing health risks, and does not investigate passive risk-taking behaviour, such as failure to act, evacuate or engage in other safety-seeking behaviour. This is because there are potentially different motivating factors, rationale and mechanisms involved in these two types of behaviour and research has found that passive risks are associated with a lower risk perception than equivalent active risks [20]. Previous literature has investigated passive risks associated with disasters and relevant methods to protect passive risk, but there is a lack of research into active risk-taking behaviour.

To clarify, the respondents were asked whether they left their homes to go outside during Typhoon Mangkhut while the typhoon warning signal T8 or above was in force. Those who left their home to address any perceived urgent and unexpected situations that required immediate action to prevent further deterioration, such as "due to injury or disease", were classified as having 'emergency' reasons. Those who did not have to manage such pressing issues or work-related duties but left their home for other reasons, such as "eating a meal or watching a movie", were categorized as having 'non-emergency' reasons. This paper will hence refer to RBDT due to 'non-emergency', also referred to as non-emergency and non-occupational reasons in our previous published paper, as non-essential reasons. Verbal informed consent was obtained at the beginning of the interview. The ethical approval of this study was obtained from the Survey Behavioural Research Committee at the Chinese University of Hong Kong (SBRE-18-075).

Descriptive chi-square (or X^2) tests were used to compare the study population and the respondents who reported going outdoors during Typhoon Mangkhut. We conducted univariate analyses to identify associations between sociodemographic characteristics, risk perception, disaster preparedness factors and the risk-taking behaviour. Multivariable logistic regression was performed to identify factors related to going outdoors during strong typhoon winds for 'non-emergency' reasons, using variables with at least marginal statistical association in the univariate analysis ($p < 0.10$). Age and gender were covariates for the multivariable model base. All odds ratios (OR) present in this paper were adjusted odds ratios from the multivariable models. Statistical analyses were performed using IBM SPSS 24 (International Business Machines Corporation, Armonk, NY, USA) [21] and statistical significance was set at $\alpha = 0.05$ two-sided.

3. Results

Data were collected from 17 September 2018 to 2 October 2018. The final sample size constituted 521 valid respondents (the response rate was 23.8% among eligible people called). The study population were comparable with the Hong Kong 2016 census data, except the study population were proportionally more middle age (age 45–64), more at the post-secondary education level and had higher income. Please refer to the previous paper [18] for further information and detailed analyses.

3.1. Description of the Study Population

For the descriptive comparison (Table 1), it was found that men were more likely to engage in non-essential RBDT ($p = 0.006$). There were no significant associations between RBDT and marital status, income, and respondents with chronic disease. Of the respondents with occupations which require emergency work while typhoon No. 8 or higher was in force, 72.2% reported staying home during Typhoon Mangkhut when the typhoon was at the height of strength. In addition, respondents who had occupations relating to "Sales and services" and "Elementary occupation" were more likely to leave their homes for emergency or work reasons. Respondents who participated in RBDT for emergency or work reasons were found to be more likely to obtain their weather-related information during this typhoon through television and newspapers and less likely through websites and mobile apps.

Table 1. Descriptive table of the study population.

Characteristics		Go Outdoor for Emergency/Work Reasons ($n = 21$)	Go Outdoor for Non-Essential Reasons ($n = 62$)	Did Not Go Outdoor ($n = 438$)	p-Value
Gender	Male	9 (42.9%)	38 (61.3%)	174 (39.7%)	0.006
	Female	12 (57.1%)	24 (38.7%)	264 (60.3%)	
Age	18–24	2 (9.5%)	14 (22.6%)	47 (10.7%)	0.078
	25–44	9 (42.9%)	18 (29.0%)	127 (29.0%)	
	45–64	9 (42.9%)	24 (38.7%)	191 (43.6%)	
	≥65	1 (4.8%)	6 (9.7%)	73 (16.7%)	
Education attainment	Primary or below	2 (10.0%)	5 (8.1%)	49 (11.3%)	0.407
	Secondary	7 (35.0%)	18 (29.0%)	170 (39.2%)	
	Post-secondary	11 (55.0%)	39 (62.9%)	215 (49.5%)	
Marital status	Single	8 (38.1%)	28 (45.2%)	176 (40.2%)	0.734
	Married	13 (61.9%)	34 (54.8%)	262 (59.8%)	
Income	<2000–9999	0 (0.0%)	5 (8.9%)	40 (9.9%)	0.462
	10,000–19,999	2 (10.5%)	5 (8.9%)	66 (16.3%)	
	20,000–39,999	6 (31.6%)	21 (37.5%)	133 (32.9%)	
	≥40,000	11 (57.9%)	25 (44.6%)	165 (40.8%)	
Occupation	Manager/Professional/Clerk	9 (45.0%)	24 (41.4%)	151 (35.4%)	0.033
	Sales & Services	5 (25.0%)	2 (3.4%)	35 (8.2%)	
	Craft related/ Machinery labour	0 (0.0%)	5 (8.6%)	20 (4.7%)	
	Elementary occupation	3 (15.0%)	3 (5.2%)	23 (5.4%)	
	Housewives/Students	1 (5.0%)	14 (24.1%)	115 (26.9%)	
	Unemployed/Retired	2 (10.0%)	10 (17.2%)	83 (19.4%)	
Chronic disease	Yes	4 (19.0%)	10 (16.7%)	77 (17.7%)	0.965
	No	17 (81.0%)	50 (83.3%)	357 (82.3%)	
Routinely work during typhoon signal no.8	Yes	15 (83.3%)	4 (9.3%)	35 (13.4%)	<0.001
	No	3 (16.7%)	39 (90.7%)	227 (86.6%)	
Occupation involving mainly outdoor work	Yes	3 (17.6%)	10 (23.3%)	43 (16.8%)	0.591
	No	14 (82.4%)	33 (76.7%)	213 (83.2%)	
Channel of obtaining weather information	Television	12 (57.1%)	26 (41.9%)	236 (53.9%)	0.015
	Radio	0 (0.0%)	6 (9.7%)	24 (5.5%)	
	Website/Smartphone platform	6 (28.6%)	28 (45.2%)	168 (38.4%)	
	Newspaper or others	3 (14.3%)	2 (3.2%)	10 (2.3%)	
Disaster preparation immediately prior to the typhoon	No	0 (0.0%)	4 (6.5%)	28 (6.4%)	0.489
	Yes	21 (100.0%)	58 (93.5%)	410 (93.6%)	

3.2. Factors Associated with Non-Essential RBDT

In the multivariable logistic regressions (Table 2), the relationship between various sociodemographic details, the subject's perception and preparedness for the typhoon and non-essential RBDT was examined. As reported in the previous article, being male and younger were found to have higher odds in performing non-essential RBDT than those that did not go outside. All factors investigated in this article such as education, disaster risk perception or household preparedness were not found to have a statistically significant association with non-essential RBDT after adjusting for age and gender. Food and water reserves (both routine and specifically prepared for Typhoon Mangkhut) were also not found to be related.

Table 2. Chi-square comparison and multivariable logistic regressions of the associating factors towards non-essential RBDT.

Factors		χ^2 Test			Logistic Regression	
		Stayed Indoor	Non-essential RBDT	*p*-Value	OR (95% CI)	*p*-Value
Gender [a]	Male	174 (39.7%)	38 (61.3%)	0.001	Ref.	
	Female	264 (60.3%)	24 (38.7%)		0.435 (0.248–0.761)	0.004
Age [a]	18–24	47 (10.7%)	14 (22.6%)	0.041	Ref.	
	25–44	127 (29.0%)	18 (29.0%)		0.573 (0.260–1.263)	0.167
	45–64	191 (43.6%)	24 (38.7%)		0.527 (0.248–1.118)	0.095
	≥65	73 (16.7%)	6 (9.7%)		0.297 (0.106–0.833)	0.021
Education attainment [b]	Primary or below	49 (11.3%)	5 (8.1%)	0.144	Ref.	
	Secondary	170 (39.2%)	18 (29.0%)		0.799 (0.269–2.374)	0.687
	Post-secondary	215 (49.5%)	39 (62.9%)		1.110 (0.363–3.392)	0.854
Income [b]	<2000–9999	40 (9.9%)	5 (8.9%)	0.517	Ref.	
	10,000–19,999	66 (16.3%)	5 (8.9%)		0.465 (0.120–1.796)	0.267
	20,000–39,999	133 (32.9%)	21 (37.5%)		0.897 (0.28–2.784)	0.851
	≥40,000	165 (40.98	25 (44.6%)		0.821 (0.264–2.555)	0.733
Perceived Hong Kong to be susceptible to disasters [b]	No	35 (8.0%)	4 (6.5%)	0.669	Ref.	
	Yes	402 (92.0%)	58 (93.5%)		1.474 (0.494–4.398)	0.486
Perceived impact of Typhoon Mangkhut compared to expectations [b]	Less than expected	118 (27.1%)	16 (25.8%)	0.919	Ref.	
	Same as expected	235 (54.0%)	33 (53.2%)		0.919 (0.477–1.773)	0.802
	Larger than expected	82 (18.9%)	13 (21.0%)		1.032 (0.462–2.303)	0.940
Concerned for the safety of oneself and family members [b]	No	159 (36.3%)	17 (27.4%)	0.171	Ref.	
	Yes	279 (63.7%)	45 (72.6%)		1.585 (0.860–2.922)	0.140
Practiced disaster preparedness immediately prior to the typhoon [b]	No	28 (6.4%)	4 (6.5%)	0.986	Ref.	
	Yes	410 (93.6%)	58 (93.5%)		1.077 (0.355–3.264)	0.896
Preparedness: routine food reserves [b]	No	81 (18.5%)	7 (11.3%)	0.163	Ref.	
	Yes	357 (81.5%)	55 (88.7%)		1.663 (0.717–3.857)	0.236
Preparedness: routine potable water reserves [b]	No	223 (50.9%)	32 (51.6%)	0.918	Ref.	
	Yes	215 (49.1%)	30 (48.4%)		0.842 (0.484–1.463)	0.541
Preparedness: food reserves specifically for Typhoon Mangkhut [b]	No	137 (31.3%)	25 (40.3%)	0.154	Ref.	
	Yes	301 (68.7%)	37 (59.7%)		0.666 (0.378–1.174)	0.160
Preparedness: potable water reserves specifically for Typhoon Mangkhut [b]	No	272 (62.1%)	39 (62.9%)	0.903	Ref.	
	Yes	166 (37.9%)	23 (37.1%)		0.894 (0.506–1.581)	0.700

[a] is the multivariable regression of age and gender; [b] is the logistic regression adjusted with age and gender.

4. Discussion

The current study is an extension of the previous published paper [18], which investigated risk perception, household preparedness, and self-reported short-term impacts of typhoons after Typhoon Mangkhut. This study aims to identify the sociodemographic characteristics of those who performed RBDT and investigate correlations between other sociodemographic characteristics apart from age and gender, risk perception and preparedness, and non-essential RBDT. There were no significant associations between RBDT and marital status, income, and respondents with chronic disease. Respondents who participated in RBDT for emergency or work reasons were more likely to watch television and read newspapers to obtain their weather-related information and less likely through websites and mobile apps. Education, income, risk perception and preparedness were found to be insignificantly associated with non-essential RBDT.

4.1. Comparison between Household Preparedness and Risk-Taking Behaviour

Household preparedness and risk-taking behaviour may be negatively associated, as household preparedness represents active protective behaviour, while non-essential RBDT involves potentially injurious active behaviour. Although this study did not find any significant negative association between higher educational level, higher risk perception and routine emergency preparedness with non-essential RBDT, the previous published paper [18] found a positive association of these factors with individuals who engaged in household preparedness. The results suggest these two behaviours may have different perceived levels of risk and/or involve separate rationale, such as respondents not considering non-essential RBDT as high-risk activity but performing household preparedness to ensure adequate supplies for family members. However, there is a lack of data in this study on the magnitude and severity of risk perceived from the typhoon to support this hypothesis. In addition, this study could not indirectly gauge the relative amount of risk respondents were willing to take for RBDT, which could be independent from perception of general risks of the typhoon and disasters.

4.2. Difference between Typhoon Risk Perception and Risk Perception of Non-Essential RBDT

Although there was no association between perceived impact of Typhoon Mangkhut compared to expectations and non-essential RBDT, 80.9% of all respondents thought the impact of the typhoon was similar or less than expected. This may suggest that fewer people underestimate the risks of typhoons, even after the recent typhoon influence, given that Typhoon Mangkhut was objectively one of the strongest typhoons in Hong Kong to date. The literature on sensation seeking involving demographics [17] has also shown that high sensation seekers have lower risk perception of activities they have not engaged in before and are less likely to perceive the negative consequences of risk-taking behaviour. Therefore, there may be a difference between the perceived risk of typhoons or the resulting impacts and non-essential RBDT which is an active behaviour. High sensation seekers may identify typhoons as events that cause harm but do not perceive the negative consequences of non-essential RBDT. As there is a lack of data directly investigating the reasons people performed non-essential RBDT, this study explores other inferred and documented possible rationale.

4.3. Other Reasons for Non-Essential RBDT

This study found food and potable water reserves, whether prepared regularly or specifically for this typhoon, were not associated with respondents going outside for non-essential reasons at the height of the storm. In addition to being markers of household preparedness, the reserves and the lack thereof may indicate situations of non-essential character, which could motivate individuals to leave their homes under the rationale of necessity. The results suggest that seeking these two necessities were not primary reasons for non-essential RBDT.

News outlets have documented a case of an elderly man in Hong Kong stranded at sea and requiring rescue after swimming during Typhoon Haima while the typhoon signal No. 8 was in force [22], highlighting an instance of RBDT which would have caused significant harm if rescue operations did not take place. As the man's motives were not interviewed and reported, the behaviour could have been due to an underestimation of the risk involved or due to sensation seeking. Despite warnings from the Hong Kong government [23] and Hong Kong Observatory [24] before and during Typhoon Mangkhut, people were reported participating in sensation seeking behaviour, such as 'experiencing the wind' and engaging in disaster photography [25,26]. High-risk behaviour during extreme weather has also been documented in the news, with 300 firefighters mobilised to rescue scores of 'frost chasers' and other hikers from Hong Kong's highest peak during the city's coldest day in six decades [27]. Although the news reports did not interview the individuals and verify their desire to seek novel and intense experiences, it is clear that the risk-taking behaviours reported were performed directly to experience aspects of the disasters.

4.4. Ethical Concerns in Rescue Operations

There is also an ethical argument on the duty of firefighters who bear personal risk and danger to help those engaging in sensation seeking behaviour. A fireman in Hong Kong died in 2017 after sustaining a cliff fall while rescuing a pair of hikers [28], highlighting the risk and peril involved even in normal conditions. While rescuers have a duty to respond to emergencies, in cases involving sensation seeking behaviour, this creates a moral issue posing unnecessary risks to the rescuers in such extreme weather events. Rescue operations may also hinder other emergency responses and invoke issues of justice and equitable resource allocation. In total, 160 firemen were involved in a 24 h operation to rescue a pair of hikers who were stuck on a hiking trail during Tropical Storm Pakhar, which struck Hong Kong only days after Typhoon Hato. The entire operation included a total of ten ambulances and thirty-one fire engines, with an estimated total cost of more than 344,000 HKD in staffing costs alone [29].

4.5. What Is the Gap Found in This Study?

One of the major gaps found in this study is that education, disaster risk perception and disaster preparedness were not found to be associated with whether respondents engaged in unexplained risky behaviour. Common understanding would suggest that those with better understanding of the risks presented and especially those concerned about the safety of themselves and their family members during the typhoon would practice less risk-taking or sensation seeking. This suggests that knowledge-based interventions may not be as effective in deterring individuals from engaging in non-essential RBDT.

4.6. Recommendations

As younger aged males were found to be more likely to engage in non-essential RBDT, health promotion targeting this group may be more effective, possibly through official government websites/apps or well-placed advertisements in social media platforms. Legislation limiting accessibility to areas of higher risk during typhoons, such as waterfronts and beaches, may also have a beneficial effect on warding off risk-taking behaviour. Numerous provinces and cities in the Philippines have imposed liquor bans during typhoons to prevent inebriated individuals from hindering relief operations [30–32], but the effectiveness of such legislation have not been investigated. Furthermore, legal restrictions of outdoor movement in the interests of public health may be more socially acceptable due to the experiences of social distancing amid COVID-19.

As some respondents were found to engage in RBDT for work purposes, the updated "Code of Practice in Times of Typhoons and Rainstorms", published by the Hong Kong Labour Department [33], is a crucial document in mitigating health risks to essential workers. Although the guidelines are not compulsory by law, employers and employees must discuss and clearly outline methods to protect the health of those working during extreme conditions. Interventions targeting this group may be more effective if broadcasted through television or newspapers. Thus, a multi-stakeholder approach should be adopted to promote work-related safety and reduce RBDT. This also has a global implication on preventable injury risk reduction, with international planning and discussions necessary in the near future before stronger natural disaster occur driven by climate change.

4.7. Limitations

The main limitation of the analysis is that the results do not demonstrate a causative effect since this study used descriptive analysis and logistic regression as a cross-sectional study. There may also be reporting bias as respondents may present with higher social desirability response bias due to telephone interviews [34]. In addition, analyses involving risk perception asked two weeks after may not correlate directly with risky actions performed during the disaster. This study is also unable to distinguish whether those who executed non-essential RBDT carried out high-risk behaviour due to perception of low-risk or for sensation seeking purposes. There may also be other reasons forcing individuals to remain outdoors during the typhoon, such as street sleepers unable to reach temporary shelters, unaccounted for due to the study design. Recruiting participants using the last birthday method also limits analysis on household preparedness as the recruited participant may not be the decision-maker for household preparedness [35], and thus, unfamiliar with the measures taken.

4.8. Future Research Directions

Future studies can directly investigate the reasons or rationale behind RBDT and explore the extent of such behaviour in detail. The sensation seeking trait and relevant factors could also be examined to determine its association and relevance to RBDT by using a modified version of the sensation seeking scale. Research into interpersonal perspectives through injunctive safety norms [36] and motivating factors for adaptation behaviour, such as descriptive norms [37], may also offer further insight into risk-taking behaviour during disasters. Future studies regarding disaster risk perception may also consider quantifying risk perception using balanced rating scales, as the degree of risk perceived is likely important when analysing risk-taking behaviour.

5. Conclusions

While age and gender were associated with risk-taking behaviour during natural disasters, other sociodemographic characteristics (such as education) and measures of disaster risk perception or disaster preparedness were not found to be correlated with non-essential RBDT. Despite the lack of literature investigating this phenomenon, media outlets in Hong Kong have reported several cases of sensation seeking behaviour during typhoons. Future studies are necessary to investigate the scope of risk-taking behaviour during disasters and the reasons driving this behaviour. Although there have been limited reports of injuries caused by risk-taking behaviour, relevant policy makers should begin to discuss and implement solutions to prevent any accidents and reduce potential extra burden on the emergency response system.

Author Contributions: Conceptualization, E.Y.Y.C.; methodology, E.Y.Y.C. and E.S.W.S.; validation, E.S.K.L. and Z.H.; formal analysis, E.S.K.L. and Z.H.; investigation, E.S.W.S., E.S.K.L., Z.H., E.Y.Y.C., K.K.C.H.; data curation, E.S.K.L. and Z.H.; writing—original draft preparation, E.S.W.S., E.S.K.L., Z.H.; writing—review and editing, E.S.W.S., E.S.K.L., K.K.C.H., E.Y.Y.C., Z.H.; visualization, E.S.K.L. and Z.H.; supervision, E.Y.Y.C.; funding acquisition, E.Y.Y.C. All authors have read and agreed to the published version of the manuscript.

References

1. Doocy, S.; Dick, A.; Daniels, A.; Kirsch, T.D.; Hopkins, J. The human impact of tropical cyclones: A historical review of events 1980-2009 and systematic literature review. *PLoS Curr. Disasters* **2013**, *1*, 1–25. [CrossRef] [PubMed]
2. Republic of the Philippines National Disaster Risk Reduction and Management Council Situational Report No.57 re Preparedness Measures for TY OMPONG. Available online: http://www.ndrrmc.gov.ph/attachments/article/3437/SitRep_No_57_re_Preparedness_Measures_Effects_for_TY_OMPONG_as_of_0600H_06OCT2018.pdf (accessed on 10 January 2020).
3. A New Emergency Management Mechanism Would be Used to Respond to Typhoon "Mangkhut". Available online: http://www.cneb.gov.cn/2018/09/19/ARTI1537354136937520.shtml (accessed on 14 January 2020).
4. The Hong Kong Observatory Super Typhoon Mangkhut (1822). Available online: https://www.hko.gov.hk/en/informtc/mangkhut18/report.htm (accessed on 10 January 2020).
5. Hong Kong Legislative Council. *The Government's Preparations, Emergency Response and Recovery Efforts Arising from Super Typhoon Mangkhut*; Hong Kong Legislative Council: Hong Kong, China, 2018.

6. Tu, J.; Chou, C.; Chu, P. The abrupt shift of typhoon activity in the vicinity of Taiwan and its association with Western North Pacific–East Asian climate change. *J. Clim.* **2009**, *22*, 3617–3628. [CrossRef]
7. World Health Organization. Disaster Risk Management for Health Fact Sheets: Disaster Risk Management for Health Overview. Available online: http://www.who.int/hac/events/drm_fact_sheet_overview.pdf (accessed on 12 January 2020).
8. Chan, E.Y.Y.; Murray, V. What are the health research needs for the Sendai Framework? *Lancet* **2017**, *390*, e35–e36. [CrossRef]
9. Lam, R.P.K.; Leung, L.P.; Balsari, S.; Hsiao, K.H.; Newnham, E.; Patrick, K.; Pham, P.; Leaning, J. Urban disaster preparedness of Hong Kong residents: A territory-wide survey. *Int. J. Disaster Risk Reduct.* **2017**, *23*, 62–69. [CrossRef] [PubMed]
10. Glickman, T.S. *Glossary of Meteorology*; Leif, E.H., Ed.; American Meteorological Society: Boston, MA, USA, 2000.
11. Robertson, D. Beyond Twister: A Geography of Recreational Storm Chasing on the Southern Plains. *Geogr. Rev.* **1999**, *89*, 533. [CrossRef]
12. Cantillon, H.; Bristow, R.S. Tornado Chasing: An Introduction to Risk Tourism Opportunities. Available online: https://www.srs.fs.usda.gov/pubs/19699 (accessed on 10 January 2020).
13. Xu, S.; Barbieri, C.; Stanis, S.W.; Market, P.S. Sensation-seeking attributes associated with storm-chasing tourists: Implications for future engagement. *Int. J. Tour. Res.* **2011**, *14*, 269–284. [CrossRef]
14. Zuckerman, M. Dimensions of sensation seeking. *J. Consult. Clin. Psychol.* **1971**, *36*, 45–52. [CrossRef]
15. Zuckerman, M.; Kolin, E.A.; Price, L.; Zoob, I. Development of a sensation-seeking scale. *J. Consult. Psychol.* **1964**, *28*, 477–482. [CrossRef] [PubMed]
16. Cross, C.P.; Cyrenne, D.L.M.; Brown, G.R. Sex differences in sensation-seeking: A meta-analysis. *Sci. Rep.* **2013**, *3*, 2486. [CrossRef] [PubMed]
17. Roberti, J.W. A review of behavioral and biological correlates of sensation seeking. *J. Res. Pers.* **2004**, *38*, 256–279. [CrossRef]
18. Chan, E.; Man, A.; Lam, H.; Chan, G.; Hall, B.; Hung, K. Is urban household emergency preparedness associated with short-term impact reduction after a super typhoon in subtropical city? *Int. J. Environ. Res. Public Health* **2019**, *16*, 596. [CrossRef] [PubMed]
19. Binson, D.A.; Canchola, J.A.; Catania, J. Random selection in a national telephone survey: A comparison of the kish, next-birthday, and last-birthday methods. *J. Off. Stat.* **2000**, *16*, 53–59.
20. Keinan, R.; Bereby-Meyer, Y. Perceptions of active versus passive risks, and the effect of personal responsibility. *Pers. Soc. Psychol. Bull.* **2017**, *43*, 999–1007. [CrossRef] [PubMed]
21. Downloading IBM SPSS Statistics 24. Available online: https://www-01.ibm.com/support/docview.wss?uid=swg24041224 (accessed on 27 January 2020).
22. Elderly Man Swims While Typhoon No. 8 Signal is in Force, Gets Stranded at Sea. Available online: https://coconuts.co/hongkong/news/elderly-man-swims-while-typhoon-no-8-signal-force-gets-stranded-sea/ (accessed on 13 January 2020).
23. Lam, J.; Ng, N. Hong Kong Leader Carrie Lam Warns Residents Not to Take Any Chances as Super Typhoon Mangkhut Looms. South China Morning Post. Available online: https://www.scmp.com/news/hong-kong/politics/article/2164231/super-typhoon-mangkhut-dont-be-storm-chasers-carrie-lam (accessed on 13 January 2020).
24. Tropical Cyclone Warning Signals Leaflet. Available online: http://www.hko.gov.hk/publica/gen_pub/tcws.pdf (accessed on 13 January 2020).
25. Collier, H. Hong Kong Typhoon Mangkhut: Daredevils Risk Their Lives to Take Selfies in Deadly Storm. The Evening Standard. Available online: https://www.standard.co.uk/news/world/hong-kong-typhoon-mangkhut-daredevils-risk-their-lives-to-take-selfies-at-victoria-harbour-seafront-a3937121.html (accessed on 13 January 2020).
26. Huang, E. The Videos that will Make You Glad You weren't Outside in Hong Kong When Typhoon Hato Struck. Available online: https://qz.com/1060272/photos-and-videos-typhoon-hato-signal-t10-batters-hong-kong-macau/ (accessed on 13 January 2020).
27. Leung, C. Hong Kong Frost Chasers Ridiculed: Hospitalisations, Arguments with Police, 300 Firemen and 8 Helicopter Flights to Rescue Them. Available online: https://www.scmp.com/news/hong-kong/health-environment/article/1905267/hong-kong-frost-chasers-ridiculed-hospitalisations (accessed on 15 January 2020).

28. Lo, C.; Lau, C. Heroic Hong Kong Fireman Dies in Clifftop Rescue Drama. Available online: https://www.scmp.com/news/hong-kong/law-crime/article/2081110/hong-kong-fireman-coma-after-rescuing-hikers-ma-shan (accessed on 15 January 2020).
29. Hollingsworth, J.; Leung, C. Cost to Rescue Two Stranded Hikers in Hong Kong Runs into Hundreds of Thousands. Available online: https://www.scmp.com/news/hong-kong/health-environment/article/2108670/cost-rescue-two-stranded-hikers-hong-kong-runs (accessed on 15 January 2020).
30. Liquor Ban Policy Before and During Typhoon Disaster Prevention Measure. Available online: https://www.culionpalawan.gov.ph/?p=1028 (accessed on 16 January 2020).
31. Ilocos Norte Bans Liquor Consumption, Sale Amidst 'Ompong' Threats. Available online: https://pia.gov.ph/news/articles/1012683 (accessed on 16 January 2020).
32. Mallari, D.T., Jr. Quezon Town Mayor Imposes Liquor Ban as Typhoon Safety Measure. Available online: https://newsinfo.inquirer.net/1196920/quezon-town-mayor-imposes-liquor-ban-as-typhoon-safety-measure (accessed on 16 January 2020).
33. Code of Practice in Times of Typhoons and Rainstorms. Hong Kong Labour Department. Available online: https://www.labour.gov.hk/eng/public/wcp/Rainstorm.pdf (accessed on 12 January 2020).
34. Holbrook, A.L.; Green, M.C.; Krosnick, J.A. Telephone versus face-to-face interviewing of national probability samples with long questionnaires. *Public Opin. Q.* **2003**, *67*, 79–125. [CrossRef]
35. Hung, L.S. Married couples' decision-making about household natural hazard preparedness: A case study of hurricane hazards in Sarasota County, Florida. *Nat. Hazards* **2017**, *87*, 1057–1081. [CrossRef]
36. Pek, S.; Turner, N.; Tucker, S.; Kelloway, E.K.; Morrish, J. Injunctive safety norms, young worker risk-taking behaviors, and workplace injuries. *Accid. Anal. Prev.* **2017**, *106*, 202–210. [CrossRef] [PubMed]
37. Valkengoed, A.M.V.; Steg, L. Meta-analyses of factors motivating climate change adaptation behaviour. *Nat. Clim. Chang.* **2019**, *9*, 158–163. [CrossRef]

Permissions

All chapters in this book were first published by MDPI; hereby published with permission under the Creative Commons Attribution License or equivalent. Every chapter published in this book has been scrutinized by our experts. Their significance has been extensively debated. The topics covered herein carry significant findings which will fuel the growth of the discipline. They may even be implemented as practical applications or may be referred to as a beginning point for another development.

The contributors of this book come from diverse backgrounds, making this book a truly international effort. This book will bring forth new frontiers with its revolutionizing research information and detailed analysis of the nascent developments around the world.

We would like to thank all the contributing authors for lending their expertise to make the book truly unique. They have played a crucial role in the development of this book. Without their invaluable contributions this book wouldn't have been possible. They have made vital efforts to compile up to date information on the varied aspects of this subject to make this book a valuable addition to the collection of many professionals and students.

This book was conceptualized with the vision of imparting up-to-date information and advanced data in this field. To ensure the same, a matchless editorial board was set up. Every individual on the board went through rigorous rounds of assessment to prove their worth. After which they invested a large part of their time researching and compiling the most relevant data for our readers.

The editorial board has been involved in producing this book since its inception. They have spent rigorous hours researching and exploring the diverse topics which have resulted in the successful publishing of this book. They have passed on their knowledge of decades through this book. To expedite this challenging task, the publisher supported the team at every step. A small team of assistant editors was also appointed to further simplify the editing procedure and attain best results for the readers.

Apart from the editorial board, the designing team has also invested a significant amount of their time in understanding the subject and creating the most relevant covers. They scrutinized every image to scout for the most suitable representation of the subject and create an appropriate cover for the book.

The publishing team has been an ardent support to the editorial, designing and production team. Their endless efforts to recruit the best for this project, has resulted in the accomplishment of this book. They are a veteran in the field of academics and their pool of knowledge is as vast as their experience in printing. Their expertise and guidance has proved useful at every step. Their uncompromising quality standards have made this book an exceptional effort. Their encouragement from time to time has been an inspiration for everyone.

The publisher and the editorial board hope that this book will prove to be a valuable piece of knowledge for researchers, students, practitioners and scholars across the globe.

List of Contributors

Nina Lorenzoni, Verena Stühlinger and Margit Raich
Department for Public Health, Health Services Research and Health Technology Assessment, UMIT TIROL—Private University for Health Sciences, Medical Informatics and Technology, 6060 Hall in Tirol, Austria

Harald Stummer
Department for Public Health, Health Services Research and Health Technology Assessment, UMIT TIROL—Private University for Health Sciences, Medical Informatics and Technology, 6060 Hall in Tirol, Austria
Department of Business, University Seeburg Castle, 5201 Seekirchen am Wallersee, Austria

Holly Ching Yu Lam
National Heart and Lung Institute, Imperial College London, Emmanuel Kaye Building, London SW3 6LR, UK
Collaborating Centre for Oxford University and CUHK for Disaster and Medical Humanitarian Response (CCOUC), Faculty of Medicine, The Chinese University of Hong Kong, Shatin, Hong Kong SAR, China
Jockey Club School of Public Health and Primary Care, Chinese University of Hong Kong, New Territories, Hong Kong, China

William Bernard Goggins
Jockey Club School of Public Health and Primary Care, Chinese University of Hong Kong, New Territories, Hong Kong, China

Elizabeth A. Newnham
School of Psychology, Curtin University, Perth 6845, Australia
François-Xavier Bagnoud Center for Health & Human Rights, Harvard University, Boston, MA 02115, USA

Peta L. Dzidic and Enrique L.P. Mergelsberg
School of Psychology, Curtin University, Perth 6845, Australia

Jennifer Leaning
François-Xavier Bagnoud Center for Health & Human Rights, Harvard University, Boston, MA 02115, USA

Bhushan Guragain
Centre for Victims of Torture, Kathmandu 44600, Nepal

Yoshiharu Kim
National Institute of Mental Health, Tokyo 187-0031, Japan

Michael Wright
School of Occupational Therapy, Social Work and Speech Pathology, Curtin University, Perth 6845, Australia

Lalindra Kaththiriarachchi
Department of Physiology, Faculty of Medicine, General Sir John Kotelawala Defense University, Rathmalana 10390, Sri Lanka

Hiroshi Kato and Tomoko Osawa
Hyogo Institute for Traumatic Stress, Kobe 651-0073, Japan

Lisa Gibbs
Child and CommunityWellbeing Unit, Melbourne School of Population and Global Health, University of Melbourne, Melbourne 3010, Australia

Lisa Bross and Steffen Krause
Research Center RISK, Bundeswehr University Munich, Werner-Heisenberg-Weg 39, 85577 Neubiberg, Germany

Ina Wienand
Federal Office of Civil Protection and Disaster Assistance, Provinzialstrasse 93, 53127 Bonn, Germany

Janice Ying-en Ho and May Pui Shan Yeung
Division of Global Health and Humanitarian Medicine, Jockey Club School of Public Health and Primary Care, The Chinese University of Hong Kong, Hong Kong

Tony Ka Chun Yung
Collaborating Centre for Oxford University and CUHK for Disaster and Medical Humanitarian Response, The Chinese University of Hong Kong, Hong Kong

Jarle Løwe Sørensen, Carina Halvorsen and Jens Petter W. Aas
USN School of Business, University of South-Eastern Norway, 3603 Kongsberg, Norway

Eric Carlström
USN School of Business, University of South-Eastern Norway, 3603 Kongsberg, Norway
Sahlgrenska Academy, University of Gothenburg, 413 90 Göteborg, Sweden
Institute of Healthcare Sciences, Sahlgrenska Academy, Gothenburg University, 40010 Gothenburg, Sweden

Viktor Glantz
Institute of Clinical Sciences, Department of Surgery, Sahlgrenska Academy, Gothenburg University, 40010 Gothenburg, Sweden

Phatthranit Phattharapornjaroen
Institute of Clinical Sciences, Department of Surgery, Sahlgrenska Academy, Gothenburg University, 40010 Gothenburg, Sweden
Department of Emergency Medicine, Ramathibodi Hospital, Mahidol University, Bangkok 10400, Thailand

Amir Khorram-Manesh
Institute of Clinical Sciences, Department of Surgery, Sahlgrenska Academy, Gothenburg University, 40010 Gothenburg, Sweden
Department of Research and Development, The Swedish Armed Forces Center for Defense Medicine, 40010 Gothenburg, Sweden
Department of Research and Development, Swedish Armed Forces Centre for Defence Medicine, 426 76 Göteborg, Sweden

Eugene Siu Kai Lo, Sophine Nok Sze Tsang, Tony Ka Chun Yung and Carol Ka Po Wong
Collaborating Centre for Oxford University and CUHK for Disaster and Medical Humanitarian Response (CCOUC), JC (Jockey Club) School of Public Health and Primary Care, Faculty of Medicine, Chinese University of Hong Kong, Hong Kong, China

Nan Zhang, Pak-To Chan, Te Miao, Peihua Wang and Yuguo Li
Department of Mechanical Engineering, The University of Hong Kong, Pokfulam Road, Hong Kong 999077, China

Boni Su
China Electric Power Planning & Engineering Institute, Beijing 100120, China

Volker Winkler
Institute of Global Health, University of Heidelberg, Im Neuenheimer Feld 324, 69120 Heidelberg, Germany

Miguel Antonio Salazar
Institute of Global Health, University of Heidelberg, Im Neuenheimer Feld 324, 69120 Heidelberg, Germany
Graduate School, Angeles University Foundation, Angeles City, Pampanga 2009, Philippines

Ronald Law
Department of Health, Health Emergency Management Bureau, Sta. Cruz, Manila 1003, Philippines
College of Public Health, University of the Philippines, Manila 1000, Philippines

Jarle Løwe Sørensen
USN School of Business, Campus Vestfold, University of South-Eastern Norway, 3603 Kongsberg, Norway

Mohammed Ali Salem Sultan
Model of Care, Directorate of Health Affairs, Najran 66255, Saudi Arabia
Institute of Health and Care Sciences, Sahlgrenska Academy, Gothenburg University, 413 46 Göteborg, Sweden

Hadi Jaber Al Sulayyim
Department of Infection and Prevention and Control, Directorate of Health Affairs, Najran 66255, Saudi Arabia

Fabian Taube
Department of Research and Development, Swedish Armed Forces Centre for Defence Medicine, 426 76 Göteborg, Sweden
Institute of Medicine, Sahlgrenska Academy, Gothenburg University, 41345 Göteborg, Sweden

David Baxter
Infrastructure Development/PPP Consultant and Steering Committee Member for the World Association of PPP Units & Professionals (WAPPP), Washington, DC 22312, USA

Carter B. Casady
Bartlett School of Construction and Project Management, University College London, London WC1E 7HB, UK

Nan Zhang and Yuguo Li
Department of Mechanical Engineering, The University of Hong Kong, Pokfulam Road, Hong Kong, China

Myo Nyein Aung
Advanced Health Science Institute and Faculty of International Liberal Arts, Juntendo University, Hongo 2-1-1, Bunkyo-ku, Tokyo 113-8421, Japan

Virginia Murray
Head of Global Disaster Risk Reduction, Public Health England, Wellington House, 133-155, Waterloo Road, London SE1 8UG, UK

Evan Su Wei Shang
Collaborating Centre for Oxford University and CUHK for Disaster and Medical Humanitarian Response (CCOUC), The Chinese University of Hong Kong, Hong Kong, China
JC School of Public Health and Primary Care, The Chinese University of Hong Kong, Hong Kong, China

Emily Yang Ying Chan
Collaborating Centre for Oxford University and CUHK for Disaster and Medical Humanitarian Response (CCOUC), JC (Jockey Club) school of Public Health and Primary Care, Faculty of Medicine, Chinese University of Hong Kong, Hong Kong, China
Nuffield Department of Medicine, University of Oxford, Oxford OX3 7BN, UK
François-Xavier Bagnoud Center for Health & Human Rights, Harvard University, Boston, MA 02138, USA

Ryoma Kayano
World Health Organization Centre for Health Development, 1-5-1 Wakinohama-kaigandori, Chuo-ku, Kobe 651-0073, Japan

Qiang Zou
Institute of Mountain Hazards and Environment, Chinese Academy of Science, Chengdu 610041, China

Young-Jae Kim, Jeong-Hyung Cho and E-Sack Kim
Department of Physical Education, Chung-Ang University, Seoul 06974, Korea

Eugene Siu Kai Lo
Collaborating Centre for Oxford University and CUHK for Disaster and Medical Humanitarian Response (CCOUC), The Chinese University of Hong Kong, Hong Kong, China

Zhe Huang
Collaborating Centre for Oxford University and CUHK for Disaster and Medical Humanitarian Response (CCOUC), The Chinese University of Hong Kong, Hong Kong, China
JC School of Public Health and Primary Care, The Chinese University of Hong Kong, Hong Kong, China

Sida Liu and Chunlan Guo
Collaborating Centre for Oxford University and CUHK for Disaster and Medical Humanitarian Response (CCOUC), Faculty of Medicine, The Chinese University of Hong Kong, Shatin, Hong Kong SAR, China
Jockey Club School of Public Health and Primary Care, Chinese University of Hong Kong, New Territories, Hong Kong, China

Emily Ying Yang Chan
JC School of Public Health and Primary Care, The Chinese University of Hong Kong, Hong Kong, China
Accident & Emergency Medicine Academic Unit, The Chinese University of Hong Kong, Prince of Wales Hospital, Hong Kong, China
François-Xavier Bagnoud Center for Health & Human Rights, Harvard University, Boston, MA 02115, USA
François-Xavier Bagnoud Center for Health & Human Rights, Harvard University, Boston, MA 02138, USA
Division of Global Health and Humanitarian Medicine, CUHK, Hong Kong 999077, China
Nuffield Department of Medicine, University of Oxford, Oxford OX3-7LF, UK
Collaborating Centre for Oxford University and CUHK for Disaster and Medical Humanitarian Response (CCOUC), JC (Jockey Club) School of Public Health and Primary Care, Faculty of Medicine, Chinese University of Hong Kong, Hong Kong, China

Kevin Kei Ching Hung
Collaborating Centre for Oxford University and CUHK for Disaster and Medical Humanitarian Response (CCOUC), The Chinese University of Hong Kong, Hong Kong, China
Accident & Emergency Medicine Academic Unit, The Chinese University of Hong Kong, Prince of Wales Hospital, Hong Kong, China

Index